THE ENCYCLOPAEDIA OF FLOWER REMEDIES

Thorsons
An Imprint of HarperCollins*Publishers*
77–85 Fulham Palace Road,
Hammersmith, London W6 8JB
1160 Battery Street,
San Francisco, California 94111–1213

Published by Thorsons 1995
10 9 8 7 6 5 4 3 2 1

A catalogue record for this book
is available from the British Library

ISBN 0 7225 3096 X

Printed in Great Britain by
Scotprint Ltd, Musselburgh, Edinburgh

THE ENCYCLOPAEDIA OF FLOWER REMEDIES

*The healing power of flower essences
from around the world*

CLARE G. HARVEY AND AMANDA COCHRANE

Thorsons
An Imprint of HarperCollins*Publishers*

CONTENTS

This book is dedicated to the spirits of the flowers
for the gift of healing they bring.

ACKNOWLEDGEMENTS

A big 'thank you' to all those in the world of flower essences for their generosity of spirit and support throughout this venture.

We would particularly like to thank the following for their continued support: Steve Johnson (Alaskan), Andras Korte (Amazon, African), Penny Medeiros (Hawaiian), Julian and Martine Barnard (Healing Herbs, Bach), Ian and Kirstin White (Australian Bush), Fred Rubenfeld (Pegasus), Tanmaya (Himalayan Enhancers), Philippe Deroide (Deva), Mary Garbely (New Zealand), Patricia Kaminski and Richard Katz (Flower Essence Society), Machaelle Small Wright (Perelandra), Vasudeva and Kadambii Barnao (Living Essences of Australia), Judy Griffin (Petite Fleur), Sabina Pettitt (Pacific), Drs Rupa and Atul Shah (Himalayan Aditi), Simon Lilly and Sue Griffin (Green Man), Cynthia Athina Kemp and Alana Mari Davis (Desert Alchemy), Arthur Bailey (Bailey), Lila Davi (Master), Marion Stoker (Findhorn), Dr Nadhu and Tulsi (Himalayan Tree), Ellie Webb (Harebell), David and Phyllis Lovall (Flower and Gem Remedy Association).

Thanks also to Harry Oldfield and Erik Pelham for their invaluable input; to Gregory Valmis and Marion Bielby for their insight and input on Bach; to Sally Hamilton for the case-study questionnaire; to Zhi-xing Wang (Qigong Master), Wa-Na-Nee-Che (shaman), Vladimir Riabolov (Russian herbalist) for their words of wisdom; to Jane Graham-Maw, our publisher, and Susan Mears, our agent, for their faith and encouragement.

Special thanks to Dr Richard Gerber and Dr George Lewith for giving their valuable time to write the Foreword and the Preface.

Finally, to Dr Edward Bach, for being the father of the flower remedies, our inspiration and for rekindling awareness of the healing powers of flowers.

Clare Harvey and Amanda Cochrane

To my wonderful son Alex, the Harveys, Bijal, Hetti and Ken Russell for their patience and love. To the late J. Krishnamurti and Dr David Bohm for their friendship and influence in my life. To my Grandmother, who taught me the wonders of the remedies when I was young.

Clare Harvey

To Jeremy, for his love, patience and faith in me, and to little Hamish, whose joyfulness and sense of fun were a source of inspiration to us both whilst writing this book, and to Penny for all her invaluable assistance.

Amanda Cochrane

PREFACE

This book provides the first completely comprehensive text for the flower remedies. It is thorough, well researched and offers an excellent resource for the interested patients or practitioners.

In spite of their long history, flower essences began to be used by homoeopaths in the West in the 1920s. This was largely due to the excellent effective range of flower remedies initially developed by Edward Bach in the early part of this century. His painstaking research, based on a combination of intuition and detailed case observation, has resulted in a now-rapidly expanding body of knowledge which will allow the practitioner to treat both physical and mental problems through the unique approaches offered by flower essences. These remedies provide a whole new dimension for medicine – in particular homoeopathic medicine. They allow for the treatment of both mental and physical problems in a safe and well-judged manner.

The Encyclopaedia represents a compilation of various flower remedies available throughout the world, their indications and the clinical experiences that have been used to define their use and support their prescription.

It is my hope that over the coming years more people will use these powerful treatments and more detailed evaluation will become available. At present our knowledge is largely empirical, based exclusively on the clinical observation of individual patients. I believe that it is possible to translate this body of knowledge into approaches that will allow its evaluation in more exacting scientific terms. From my own clinical experience I believe the flower essences offer a powerful approach to the treatment of illness, particularly mental symptoms. If this could be further established in a more scientific context then we may begin to see a real revolution in medical care.

Dr George Lewith, MA, MR, CR, MRC, GP
The Centre for the Study of Complementary
Medicine
1995

FOREWORD

We are living during a unique period in human history. Over the past 50 years, science has discovered many ways of looking at the world and, in the process, has redefined the very nature of what it means to be human. Revolutionary discoveries in medical science have given us an understanding of the way in which the body works and how intricately linked the body and mind truly are. But a new breed of spiritual scientists has begun to explore the links between the body, the mind and the spiritual nature of human beings. Vibrational medicine is the evolving field of healing research that focuses on these links. Although the principles behind vibrational medicine are quite ancient, the development of modern technologies which can visualize and quantify the energetic nature of the links between body, mind and our spiritual anatomy are very new.

The concept that human beings are multidimensional energy systems is an idea that stems, in part, from the Einsteinian realization that matter and energy are dual expressions of the same universal substrate that makes up all things. Quantum physicists have begun to awaken to the concept that the subatomic particles that make up the entire universe, including people, are actually patterns of frozen energy and light. Many other scientists have begun to see the world in a similar light, having been led there by science instead of pure spirituality and intuition. We are literally beings of light and energy assembled in a way that is fundamentally hidden from our limited physical senses. The vibrational medicine perspective ascribes to this light energy link by viewing humans as multidimensional beings consisting of far more than a physical brain and body. The new field of vibrational medicine is actually a fusion of science and spirituality which has defined the energy networks linking the physical body and its energetic substrates to the more rarefied world of spirit. Vibrational medicine views the world from the perspective of vibration and energy with an eye towards how this understanding of our energetic natures can lead to many new and wonderful forms of diagnosis and healing.

Our physical bodies are controlled by many biochemical cellular systems which are, in turn, finely tuned by subtle energy systems including the acupuncture meridian system and the chakra system. While our physical body is nurtured by physical nutrients and oxygen, it is also fed by subtle environmental energies such as ch'i and prana which we absorb through the meridian and chakra networks. These subtle energetic forms of nutrition, understood by the ancients of China and India, are just as important as food and water to sustaining life. The subtle energy networks also connect the physical body to another type of energy system – the etheric body – which is a holographic energy template that invisibly guides human growth and development. Scientific evidence for the existence of subtle energy systems is growing. Modern technology has begun to validate ancient wisdom in a marriage of science and spirituality the like of which has not been seen on this planet for thousands of years.

It is only through a fuller appreciation of a multidimensional model of human functioning that subtle energy therapies, such as flower essences, can be truly understood. Modern medicine has become rigid and locked into a mechanistic model of the body, and the model does not explain how subtle life energies can affect cellular machinery. It is only when one takes into account the larger picture of human beings from a newly evolving multidimensional perspective that flower essences as a healing modality begin to make sense. Flower essences do not work like drugs in which molecular patterns often bind to specialized receptors throughout the cells of the body. Instead they work by influencing the subtle energy structures that feed life energy into the body/mind. Flower essences modify energy flow through the acupuncture meridians, the chakras and the subtle bodies with the end result of affecting the very energetic patterns that influence consciousness.

The essences of flowers have been used in healing for hundreds (and possibly thousands) of years. Dr Edward Bach was one of the first modern pioneers of healing with flower essences. Bach was a medical practitioner as well as a psychic who experienced disturbing emotional patterns within himself when he was near a particular flower. Bach came to learn that taking an essence of the nearby flower would neutralize his psychically induced emotional disturbance. He discovered that the same flower essence would heal similar emotional patterns in others. Bach was among the first vibrational healers of the 20th century to realize how healing the emotions would contribute to the healing of any physical illness, regardless of the cause. It is in this regard, the energetic healing and repatterning of emotional energies, that flower essences have a wide spectrum of applications.

Since Dr Bach's pioneering work in the first half of the 20th century, flower essence usage has undergone a veritable explosion of interest. Working groups that study the effects of local flower essences have sprung up all over the world, from England and North America to the outbacks of Australia. The merging of healing traditions has also begun to occur as practitioners have learned to apply principles of acupuncture to healing with flower essences by applying them to specific acupoints on the body. The wide variety of flower essence applications in healing has become an entire subspecialty within vibrational medicine.

It is because of this renaissance of interest in flower essences that *The Encyclopaedia of Flower Remedies* is of great importance. Clare Harvey and Amanda Cochrane have performed an invaluable service by compiling the knowledge and wisdom of healing with flowers from around the world. It has been said that the answers to curing all of humanity's ills lie within nature. This book is an important step towards revealing the incredible healing wisdom within nature that we have only begun to discover. After all, modern medicine does not have all the answers to healing the afflictions of our techno-industrialized society. Perhaps the real answers to curing modern ailments exist within an exploration of our ancient past in order to synthesize a healing science of the 21st century.

I encourage you to read this book and experiment with the healing and transforming life energy of flower essences. The study and usage of flower essences and flower remedies will allow us to rediscover new ways of healing and remember our true inner spiritual nature as evolving beings of light. Those who take this journey will be richly rewarded for their efforts.

Richard Gerber, MD
Author of *Vibrational Medicine: New Choices for Healing Ourselves*
February, 1995

INTRODUCTION

Have you ever felt happier for surrounding yourself with fresh flowers, been especially attracted to certain kinds of blooms or found solace strolling among fields or gardens filled with flowering plants? If so, you have already experienced the therapeutic power of flowers.

Symbolizing love and friendship, flowers have always been a source of pleasure and happiness – of healing in its quintessential form. From the sensuous rose to the humble daisy, the delicate blooms adorning gardens, fields, hedgerows, mountainsides, woodlands and jungles throughout the world possess special qualities that can ease emotional distress, boost self-confidence, lift energy levels, increase resilience to all kinds of illness and even enrich our relationships. Most importantly, they offer the perfect antidote to stress in its many different guises.

Since the dawn of time we have instinctively known that flowers can lift our spirits and make us feel well again. Flowers and their remedies feature in the traditional healing practices of many cultures around the world. They play an important role in restoring or evoking a sense of harmony in mind, body and spirit. This concept of wholeness is a recurring theme in many ancient philosophies, and we are now rediscovering its relevance to us. We are at last emerging from a time when good health is interpreted as the absence of disease. True well-being is something that lies beyond this limited concept, encompassing contentment and security, peace of mind and an abundance of vitality that are essential if our lives are to be enjoyable and fulfilling.

Many ancient and native cultures believe that everything in nature is infused with a vital energy, the spark of life. Wise men living several thousands of years ago proposed that when mind, body and spirit are perfectly integrated, this life-force abounds, bringing with it a real sense of health and happiness. The way to attain such inner harmony, they claimed, is to respect nature and her ways.

Our existence is becoming increasingly artificial. Cocooned in towns and cities, it is easy to feel isolated from the natural environment. We no longer rely on the flowering of different plants to tell us what time of year it is as our distant ancestors once did. In severing the bond with nature, we risk losing our sense of wholeness. When this happens we become increasingly vulnerable to stress.

Stress is recognized as a major source of unhappiness and ill-health. Too many people feel completely at its mercy, powerless either to avoid or conquer its disruptive effects.

Orthodox medicine offers little in the way to relieve stress-induced turbulence. Drugs such as tranquillizers may ease the discomfort by dulling our perceptions and reactions, but they do not really help us to stay afloat in this sea of turmoil. This is where flower remedies come to our rescue.

Flower essences are not like other medicines. They do not contain active chemicals or possess pharmaceutical properties. They are best described as a sort of liquid energy, a vibrational medicine that brings about benefits by influencing each person's own life-force. Taking these remedies can be likened to surrounding yourself with exquisite flowers which never fade or die.

The state of the world has altered dramatically in the last 50 years and many new sources of stress have arrived on the scene. Horrific events such as wars, famines, tragic accidents, violent incidents and natural disasters may not be new, but thanks to television, radio and newspapers we are now bombarded with their details on a regular basis. We may try not to think about them, but still they often shake us to the core.

Over-population in many areas creates competition for vital resources and work, leading to widespread greed and insecurity. Meanwhile the breakdown of close-knit communities leaves many people feeling lonely and isolated.

Stress tends to be infectious: If you work in an office full of anxious, frazzled people, it will be difficult to keep calm. Add the pressures of feeling hemmed in due to over-crowding, the constant noise of traffic and the almost stifling levels of pollution in some cities and it is hardly surprising that stress has become the twentieth-century ailment. It not only plays havoc with our nervous systems, but also weakens our immunity, leaving us easy prey to the new so-called 'super bugs' that keep appearing on the scene.

Flower remedies are needed now more than ever. Responding to this cry for help, certain people have set out to research and rediscover the therapeutic properties of indigenous flowers growing in countries all over the world. The new flower essences are made from an extraordinarily diverse variety of flora, ranging from the modest hedgerow and alpine flowers to romantic roses, exotic orchids and the blossoms of fruits like the banana and avocado. Some flowers, especially those from the Australian Bush and Himalayan mountains, have a long tradition of being used in natural healing. The beneficial properties of others are only just being discovered.

While some flower essences free us from negative moods and emotions, others go further, helping us to recognize and let go of behaviour patterns that generate negative feelings.

When we feel confused about a situation or relationship in our lives, flower essences help to us to see things from an entirely different perspective – just as escaping to a place of stunning natural beauty leaves you feeling that your problems and worries back home are less daunting than you had imagined.

Some essences act at the physical level, strengthening and re-balancing various areas of the body such as the immune system. Others offer protection against new sources of environmental stress. Many aspire to more spiritual realms, helping us to find our true direction and purpose in life.

Although I have been a professional flower remedy practitioner for more than 10 years, I actually grew up with this form of healing. As a child I would watch my grandmother working with the Bach Flower Remedies. I have always been amazed by the profound ways in which people respond to this gentle form of treatment. I have witnessed the emergence of the newer flower essences and steadily added them to my own repertoire of remedies. Using specially chosen combinations of essences from around the world, I have helped people suffering from all kinds of illnesses back to health. Typical conditions I have treated include infertility, pre-menstrual tension, hayfever, arthritis and nervous exhaustion. I firmly believe that what sets flower essences apart from other forms of remedies and therapies is their ability to address physical, mental, emotional and spiritual aspects of ourselves simultaneously, to bring about complete healing.

The beauty of flower remedies is that they are relatively inexpensive, easy to use and totally free from any unpleasant side-effects. Furthermore, you can prescribe them for yourself. We all have different needs, and the flowers that may benefit one person will differ from those that can help another. You may notice that you are instinctively attracted or drawn to certain flowers such as roses, just as you may choose to use certain herbs when cooking. These are very often the flowers that you probably need.

As you begin to use the flower essences you will embark on a journey of self-discovery. You will become aware of your strengths and weaknesses as well as any stress patterns you have acquired over the years. These are reactions and responses to situations and people that, if left unchecked, consistently undermine your health and happiness.

The remedies will give you the strength and support you need to cope with change in your life, as well as the more far-reaching upheavals occurring on this earth. There is no doubt that anything that calls for a shift in our lives and thinking will generate stress. The more we resist the challenges and transitions we have to face, the more painful the experience of change tends to be. Flower essences can help us to go with the flow, to be more flexible and enable us to respond appropriately to the increasing demands made upon us.

In these testing times, let flower essences play an increasingly important role in helping you regain control of your life and destiny, to find the vitality you need to pursue your dreams and goals – but, above all, to rediscover the true joy of living.

❋ HOW TO USE THIS BOOK ❋

This book is for anyone who wishes to explore the benefits of using flower remedies.

Part I tells you what flower remedies are and how they work. You will discover how to choose remedies that can help you and others.

Part II is made up of an Encyclopaedia of 23 families of flower essences from around the world, giving a brief description of the properties and benefits of over 1200 remedies.

Part III is an Ailment Chart for easy reference, covering a range of typical physical, emotional/psychological, and spiritual problems and suggesting remedies that can help to relieve them. It also includes recipes you can make up for your own use (such as my Stress Buster and Infection Fighter combinations), a chapter of case histories for which I have used remedies to combat successfully a variety of conditions, and further advice for flower essence practitioners.

PART ONE

ONE

THE HISTORY OF HEALING FLOWERS

The idea that flowers possess healing powers
may seem new and revolutionary. It is, however, a very ancient concept
whose origins can be traced back into the mists of time.

For at least 40,000 years the Aborigines of Australia have been using flowers as part of their natural healing system. In other parts of the world where folk medicine is still alive, the tradition of utilizing flowering plants and their essences to restore well-being to body, mind and spirit has continued down the centuries to the present day.

Many of us instinctively turn to flowers to lift our spirits and make us feel better. It is second nature to bring bouquets to those who are sick or ailing. Without floral decorations, any festive occasion or religious ceremony would seem soulless and incomplete.

The task before us is to uncover and rediscover knowledge about the natural world that has existed for aeons.

❋ TALES OF A GOLDEN AGE ❋

LEMURIA AND ATLANTIS

Legend has it that flower essences were first used for healing some 500,000 years ago in a mythical place called Lemuria or Mu. Located in an area now covered by the Pacific ocean, Lemuria was reputedly a veritable 'garden of Eden'. The land was lush and, thanks to a near-perfect climate, all kinds of exquisite flowering plants flourished. Imagine the inhabitants of this civilization as gentle, sensitive souls who truly appreciated the beauty of their environment and were content to live close to the earth.

They were also aware of the natural empathy that exists between human and plant life. To them, every plant was special and had its

3

own personality.

Some believe these people were ethereal beings who could sense the energy or vibration of all living things. It has been suggested that, to them, all living things including plants appeared as luminous or shimmering objects.

These people realized that the highest concentration of life-force in a plant is found in its flowers. Just by being close to a delicate bloom they became aware of its particular healing qualities. The Lemurians were not, however, troubled by physical disease – indeed it is said they lived for around 2,000 years. Instead they used flower essences to evolve spiritually, to attain enlightenment.

According to the myth, Lemuria gave way to Atlantis. Those who believe or suspect there was a civilization known as Atlantis think it probably existed between 12,000 and 150,000 years ago.

Unlike the Lemurians, the Atlanteans were reputedly not content to live in harmony with nature. They wanted to dominate and manage it to their advantage. As their society became increasingly technologically advanced, stress seeped into their lives bringing with it all kinds of new physical, emotional and mental diseases. At this time, so the legend goes, flower essences were first used as a complete system of medicine.

ANCIENT EGYPT, CRETE AND INDIA

The ancient Egyptians certainly harnessed the healing powers of flowers. They did, after all, perfect the art of aromatherapy. Within magnificent temples high priests built laboratories where they distilled flowers to obtain aromatic essential oils. These were then blended to create medicinal formulations for treating a wide variety of illnesses. It should be stressed that essential oils are *not* the same as flower essences, although the Egyptians recognized the therapeutic benefits of both, for they also collected the dew from flowers and exposed it to sunlight to increase its potency.

The lotus flower, which grew in abundance along the banks of the Nile, was sacred to the Egyptians. In their mythology it was the first living thing to appear on earth. When its petals unfurled the supreme god representing intellectual rulership was revealed to them. Its flower essence was used in rituals, as were those of other indigenous plants such as bamboo and papyrus. It has been suggested that the Egyptians imparted thoughts to certain plants, knowing they would reach and help us today.

The Minoans of Crete were another highly cultured people who recognized the healing potential of flowers. They are said to have held rituals devoted to the quest for spiritual understanding; during these rituals they would place a splendid flowering plant such as a wild rose in the centre of the ceremonial chamber. Flowers or sprigs of plants were also floated in bowls of water placed around this room. During the ceremony participants would sip the water or eat the petals to cleanse themselves of any disturbing thoughts or feelings.

At about this time, many miles away in the remote Himalayan mountains, flowers were playing their part in *Ayurveda* ('science of life'), an ancient system of natural medicine dating back at least 5,000 years. We know of it because the Ayurvedic principles have been handed down from generation to generation and are still alive today. Flowers with spiritual significance such as the lotus continue to be used in Ayurvedic healing ceremonies. The petals are traditionally sprinkled into bowls of water, which is then drunk and used to anoint various parts of the body.

✳ FLOWERS AND FOLK MEDICINE ✳

If we look at the folk medicines practised by native peoples around the world, most make use of the flowers and plants growing in each region.

THE AUSTRALIAN ABORIGINES

The Aborigines have always turned to their exotic flora for help in healing mind, body and spirit. They collect the dew that settles on petals at dawn, believing it to enhance emotional well-being and help them enter into the 'dream time'. In some instances they may also eat the flowers themselves.

The Aboriginal story of how flowers were born and came by their healing powers, handed down from generation to generation, is told us here by Ken Colbung of the Bibulmun people:

The Aborigines living in the southwest of Western Australia are known as the Bibulmun people. Their legends were given to them by the Demmagoomba – the spirits of the old people who lived here previously. According to the Demmagoomba, the creator (also known as the Gujub, God, supreme being or senior spirit) sent the Rainbow Snake, Waugal, down to earth as a life-giving element. It landed at a place in the southwest of Bibulmun country known as Broiungarup.

Rainbow colours of the Rainbow Snake gave the flowers their colour at the time of creation. At Broiungarup you will always see beautiful rainbows. Some of the smallest and rarest flowers are only found in this one area.

The Broiunga is a clan. It is where you get your spirituality and your mortal being. You can be clan to birds, to a tree or to flowers. Your Broiunga is a special being for which you are responsible. If your Broiunga is a flower, then you must maintain this flower. It also has a responsibility to you. It gives you a beautiful feeling of colour, of its essence which is the link to the Rainbow Snake.

The flowers of the earth have different link-ups for different people's needs.

There are a lot of occasions when the body needs to be associated with the different types of flowers. The essences are important for our own spirit, or Djugubra. So we have what is known as Kaba nij nyoong (Kaba is the flower essences, nij is the 'I', and ny-oong is the understanding of the person).

We must be aware that when we first see a flower it will bring us happiness; when we have the essence from that flower it will bring us health and with health and happiness we have wealth – the wealth of the spirit Djugubra.

The flower sauna is a unique feature of traditional Aboriginal healing and is arguably one of the earliest forms of flower essence therapy, dating back around 10,000 years. The ceremony, still performed the same way today, is conducted by the *Maban*, a man or woman who is healer and Keeper of the Law. The sauna is prepared by lining a shallow pit with hot coals which are then covered with a layer of earth. Steam is created by sprinkling water over the hot earth. Clay blended with crushed flowers (specially chosen for the occasion) is then smeared onto the body of the person being healed – this helps the flower essence penetrate the skin.

The Maban takes charge of the afflicted person, who enters the pit and is then covered with an animal skin to seal in the warmth. The person remains there until sunrise the next day, when he or she emerges renewed with the spirit of the flowers.

Another ritual sees people sent to sit among a clump of flowers, so that their souls may be purified and they become 'spiritually reborn'.

NATIVE AMERICANS

In ancient times, the Native peoples of North America were blessed with the ability of being able to draw energy from flowers and plants. When they lost this gift they turned to imbibing the therapeutic properties of flowers in the forms of teas and extractions. Some spiritual medicine people can still utilize this energy, but always request the flower's permission first. The Native Americans match the energy of the flower to the particular part of the body that is out of balance and so needs healing. Indeed, in their version of the creation story, when humans came into being much of their physical body was derived from the plants, rocks and waters of Mother Earth, while their spirit or soul came from the heavens or sky. To them this explains why certain plants have a special affinity for certain areas of the body. This idea is echoed in the legends relating to Lemurian times and in the creation myths of other indigenous peoples.

RUSSIAN MEDICINE MEN

Across the Atlantic in Russia, medicine men or shaman also practise a natural form of healing handed down to them by their forefathers. All knowledge is passed on by word of mouth; nothing is committed to print. The medicine people living in the richest floral area of the Caucasus mountains are called the Koldum. Nearly half the flowers growing here are unique to this area. These indigenous flowers are taken in the form of essences and tinctures. So famous are these remedies that people have been known to travel for miles to this region – even the infamous Genghis Khan, who made his pilgrimage from Mongolia. He reputedly prescribed them to his men to give them strength for battle.

THE MYSTICAL PARACELSUS

Healing with flowers was introduced into Europe during the fifteenth century by the renowned physician and mystic Philippus Aureolus Theophrastus Bombast von Hohenheim, better known as Paracelsus.

While still in his early twenties Paracelsus left his home in Austria to embark on a 10-year adventure which took him to Russia, England and North Africa, where he encountered different kinds of folk medicines.

It is said that he would collect the early morning dew from flowers which he took himself and prescribed to treat emotional disturbance in others. Paracelsus was also responsible for reviving the old 'Doctrine of Signatures', a system of equating certain features of a flower or plant – its shape, colour, scent, taste or natural habitat – to its healing properties.

For example, Eyebright, a blue flower with a yellow centre, looks like an eye and is said to help treat eye problems. Similarly the Skullcap flower, resembling the shape of a human skull, may be used to treat headaches and insomnia, while the bark of Willow, a tree that grows in wet places, eases rheumatism and other conditions that are worse for damp weather. We now know that Willow bark contains an anti-inflammatory substance called salicin which eases the pain of rheumatism as well as headaches. Its synthetic form is taken by millions each day as aspirin.

Paracelsus also believed that plants tend to grow where they are needed most – dock leaves, which can be used to treat nettle rash, always grow near nettles, while plants for easing fevers can often be found close to swamps.

❋ THE LANGUAGE OF FLOWERS ❋

With the birth of modern medicine, belief in the healing power of flowers appeared to die out. But this was not so. It simply became channelled into the popular notion that certain qualities or virtues are associated with flowers. Roses, for example, typically signify love and romance, which is why lovers give each other red roses on St Valentine's Day.

Centuries before the birth of the slogan 'say it with flowers', people knew intuitively the special meanings of different blooms. In ancient Egypt the Iris blossom was seen an emblem of power. It adorned the brow of the Sphinx of Giza and the sceptres of kings. To the Egyptians, flowers also represented certain thoughts and feelings. Just as we might send telegrams or cards to wish someone good health during an illness or to show our affection or love, they would send an appropriate flower.

From the earliest times the Rose has been a symbol of love. Cleopatra placed such faith in its romantic charm that she reputedly carpeted her bedroom with millions of fresh rose petals to help her seduction of Marc Anthony.

Flowers had their own language and meaning to the ancient Greeks and Romans as well. It should come as no surprise that the Rose is associated with Aphrodite/Venus, the goddess of love.

The Rose is by no means the only flower linked to love. Others include the Iris, which is named after the goddess of the rainbow who guided the souls of women to their final resting place.

Carnations also express pure love and constancy, while the Tulip denotes a declaration of love.

Many of the classical gods, goddesses and nymphs such as Hyacinthus, Narcissus and Iris are remembered today because they gave their name to flowers. Narcissus owes its name to the young man who, it was prophesied, would have a long and happy life unless he caught sight of his reflection and fell in love with his own beauty. To his cost he did indeed become enraptured by himself. Thus in most books about the language of flowers the Narcissus represents egotism. In the Middle East, however, it is traditionally linked with love, the beginning of new relationships and the enhancement of existing ones.

Flower symbolism occurs throughout the world. In India flowers are associated with various deities and ceremonies, pujas, prayers and certain festive occasions. A sprig of the magical Mimosa is often suspended above the bed to ward off ill-fortune. Its yellow flowers give a sweet aroma which is also said to evoke psychic dreams. To the Chinese, Jasmine represents feminine sweetness, while in India it is considered sacred. The flower of sensuousness and physical attraction, the Jasmine is believed to enhance self-esteem and is always used in traditional bridal wreaths.

Flowers often have religious significance. The Lotus flower is recognized as a symbol of spirituality all over the world. It was not only sacred to the ancient Egyptians. Throughout Asia and the Far East especially it is associated with Buddhism and the state of enlightenment. The figure of Buddha is often depicted sitting on a Lotus flower.

Good fortune, protection and strength have also traditionally been associated with flowers. For this reason they have often been adopted by kings and leaders. The Sunflower became the symbol of Atahualpa, King God of the Incas, for it was believed to hold great magical properties. Like the sun itself it has a strong life-force, encouraging action and strengthening will-power.

The English Plantagenets derived their name from *planta genista* (Latin for Broom) after Geoffrey Count of Anjou wore it as an emblem on his helmet when he went into battle in 1140. The sweet scent of its fresh flowers is said to purify thoughts and feelings. Inhaling the aroma also instils a sense of peace and tranquillity.

The people of Shakespeare's day were well acquainted with the ancient meanings associated with plants and flowers. 'There's rosemary, that's for remembrance,' cries Ophelia in *Hamlet*. It was not until 300 years later that the language of flowers really took shape, however. In 1817 the first real flower dictionary, *Le Langage des Fleurs* by Madame Charlotte de la Tour, was published in Paris. It proved so popular and sparked off such great interest that other versions followed.

With the help of these flower dictionaries, shy Victorians found ways to express what they would not say in words. They sent each other bouquets in which every blossom, leaf and stem was fraught with significance. The language of flowers flourished, and was even given the special name florigraphy.

At the beginning of this century, 'flower fairies' epitomizing the personality or character of various blossoms and buds also became fashionable. These tiny ethereal beings with gossamer wings reputedly lived among the flowers at the bottom of the garden. They captured the imagination of writers like J. M. Barrie, who conjured up Peter Pan's rather wayward guardian angel, Tinker Bell. Sherlock Holmes' creator, Arthur Conan Doyle, was also fascinated by these nature spirits – as his book *The Coming of the Fairies* reveals. Legend has it that these nature spirits, or devas, first made their appearance in Lemurian times. Each fairy was entrusted with a different flower, and together they were said to be responsible for teaching us how to live in harmony with nature.

Folklore tells us that if we wish to see the fairy kingdom we should make a concoction of Rose-water, Marigold water and wild Thyme. After leaving this lotion in the sunlight for three days, apply it to the eyes and the windows of the fairy world will magically open!

FLOWERS AND SIGNS OF THE ZODIAC

When astrology became fashionable flowers, like gem stones,
were also attributed to the signs of the Zodiac.

ARIES:
Geranium, Honeysuckle

TAURUS:
Rose, Violet

GEMINI:
Forsythia, Morning Glory

CANCER:
Acanthus, Jasmine

LEO:
Marigold, Sunflower

VIRGO:
Anemone, Melissa

LIBRA:
Columbine, Orchid

SCORPIO:
Gentian, Hyacinth

SAGITTARIUS:
Pinks, Dandelion

CAPRICORN:
Pansy, Tulip

AQUARIUS:
Orchid, Primrose

PISCES:
Clematis, Hydrangea

❋ REDISCOVERING THE HEALING POWER ❋ OF FLOWERS

In the 1930s healing with flowers was redis-covered by a remarkable man called Dr Edward Bach. Thanks to his pioneering work flower essences have come to the rescue of millions of people throughout the world.

Bach was born near Birmingham in England in 1886. Even at an early age he was fascinated by nature and loved going for walks in the countryside.

He pursued a career in medicine specializing in pathology and bacteriology. In 1920 he established a successful practice in Harley Street, London.

During the next few years he became increasingly disenchanted with the orthodox medical approach, which he felt focused on relieving the symptoms of disease rather than its true cause. At the same time he felt increasingly drawn towards the homoeopathic principle of treating the whole person.

He then began to carry out his own research. He isolated certain bacteria from the intestinal tract and with these prepared vaccines according to homoeopathic principles. These vaccines proved remarkably helpful to people suffering from chronic diseases, and could be taken orally instead of by injection (a method Bach particularly disliked). Remedies prepared from toxins such as viruses became known as the *Bach nosodes*, and are still used by many homoeopaths today.

During his work Bach noticed that his patients tended to fall into distinct personality types, and that those in a particular group frequently responded to the same treatment. Ahead of his time, he also recognized the link between stress, emotions and illness. Bach believed that the disturbing moods or feelings different people experience were a key cause of ill-health. In *Heal Thyself*, a small booklet he wrote which sums up his philosophy of healing and the problems of orthodox medicine, Bach proposed that:

> *The real primary disease of man are such defects as pride, cruelty, hate, self-love, ignorance, instability and greed. Each of these defects...will produce a conflict which must of necessity be reflected in the physical body, producing its own specific type of malady.*

Correcting emotional factors, he reasoned, would go a long way towards increasing physical and mental vitality, which in turn would help to resolve any physical disease.

At the same time Bach became interested in the idea of replacing vaccines based on bacteria, themselves the instigators of disease, with more wholesome remedies. He discovered these in the flowers growing in the fields and hedgerows. Bach was a sensitive soul who relied on his intuition for guidance. During a visit to Wales, he was drawn to two particular wildflowers, Impatiens and Mimulus. These flowers, he felt, emitted a special kind of energy or vibration which could exert a positive influence on certain negative states of mind.

In 1930 Bach decided to give up his lucrative London practice; he spent the next six years living in several parts of rural England in the quest for a new floral healing system.

Aware that personality affects the way we react to stress, the first remedies Bach looked for related to what he perceived to be the 12 key personality types (*see* Chapter 4). To him flowers had their own little personalities rem-

iniscent of certain characteristics in us. The wistful Clematis reminded him of quiet, dreamy people who are wrapped up in their thoughts and fantasies, and who as a result are prone to drowsiness, indifference, sensitivity to noise, poor concentration and difficulty recuperating from illness. As a remedy Clematis would lend support to people with these characteristics, reducing their susceptibility to such tendencies.

The colour, texture, flowering patterns and growth patterns of flowers told Bach something of their healing qualities. The sturdy Oak, for instance, suggested to him the type of strong, reliable, patient, dependable people who shoulder their burdens without complaining.

The next 26 flower remedies he looked for were intended to bring relief from different kinds of emotional discomfort and distress. Bach felt that they could deal with negative mind states like fear, apathy, loneliness and despair, which he believed were not truly a part of our nature but which we only succumbed to in difficult and trying times.

The flowers, Bach has said, have a particular quality which is an exact equivalent to the human emotion. Wild Rose, a remedy for apathy and resignation, is a positive representation of this state. In other words, it replaces these negative feelings with dynamism and optimism.

For Bach the colours of flowers were also indicative of their remedial qualities. Blue flowers such as Cerato express receptive feelings, the red or yellow flowers are more dynamic, while green flowers such as Scleranthus are associated with balance. Remedies for fear have a dynamic colour reflecting their vibrant strength.

Bach confirmed the effects of the various flowers by observing how each one affected his own emotional state. It is said that he would think himself into feeling a particular way, then search for remedies to help restore a sense of calm and contentment.

With a few exceptions such as Vine, Olive, Honeysuckle and Cerato, Bach's healing flowers can still be found growing wild in the fields and hedgerows of Oxfordshire. Almost half of them come from trees, while others (such as Gorse and Cerato) are from shrubs.

In 1936 Bach passed away, satisfied that his work was complete. His close friend and companion Nora Weeks was largely responsible for safeguarding and keeping his work alive. Until recently the flowers continued to be gathered from the Oxfordshire countryside, and prepared and bottled at Mount Vernon as Bach himself had done.

Each year hundreds of people from all corners of the world make their pilgrimage to Mount Vernon, to witness the place where Bach performed much of his pioneering work.

For many years Bach's Flower Remedies stood alone. Then in the mid-1970s interest in the healing power of flowers was rekindled. Richard Katz was one of a few people in the forefront of this revitalization, establishing the Flower Essence Society in California. His aim was to research new flower essences and gather together those working with the essences so they could exchange ideas and information.

Others, too, have been inspired to research the healing qualities of locally growing flowers. From Alaska to Australia, the Mediterranean to New Zealand and Hawaii to the Himalayas, distinct remedies have been rediscovered in the flowers that are indigenous to each particular country or region. The Orchids of the Amazon, for instance, come from the exotic flowers that grow 100 ft up on the branches and tree-tops of the rainforests of Colombia.

These new essences come at a time when they are most needed, for the world has changed considerably in the last 50 years and is continuing to do so at an alarming rate. Many of the flowers address not only emotional problems but also aspire to more spiritual realms, as well as acting at the fundamental physical level, treating the whole person – mind, body and spirit.

ENERGY FIELDS

What they are and how they work

To understand how flower essences work their wonders, we have to become familiar with the idea that all living things are infused with energy, or life-force. We cannot see or touch this energy, but like the air we breathe, it is essential to life.

Most people living in the West find it hard to believe that there may be more to us than meets the eye. In other regions of the world, especially the Far East and Asia, this view is commonplace.

Over 5,000 years ago Indian holy men spoke of a universal energy. Known as *prana*, this energy is still seen as the basic constituent and source of all life. Prana, the breath of life, moves through all things and brings to them vitality. The same idea forms the basis of Taoism, the ancient Chinese philosophy which also emerged during the 3rd millennium BC. It holds that the universe is a living organism infused and permeated with a rhythmic, vibrational energy called 'chi' or 'qi'.

The concept of an energy pervading all things is not as mystical as it may seem. Modern physics is beginning to lend credence to what the ancient wise men supposed all those years ago. In the last century it has become increasingly clear that it is outmoded to think of things as solid objects, as Newton and his colleagues in the late 17th and early 18th centuries suspected.

With the discovery of the atom, physicists felt they had found the fundamental building blocks of the universe. Yet as they delved deeper, they found that atoms are composed of even tinier particles which seem to be constantly on the move. Furthermore, the behaviour of things on this very tiny scale is very different to what one might expect.

In 1905 Albert Einstein shattered the principles of the old Newtonian world view when he published his Theory of Relativity. With this hypothesis came the idea that matter and energy are interchangeable. All particles can be created from energy, and matter is simply slowed down or 'crystallized' energy.

A few years later another important discovery was made by Max Planck. He found that light and other forms of electromagnetic radiation are emitted in the form of energy packets which he called *quanta*. These light quanta, or energy packets, have been accepted as *bona fide* particles. Oddly, though, they also behave as if they were waves rather than individual particles.

The latest 'super-string' theories which first came to light during the 1960s now propose that these fundamental particles are not really particles at all. They are more like snippets of infinitely thin string. In 'string theories', what were previously thought of as pinpoints of light are now pictured as waves travelling down the string, like waves on a vibrating kite string. This means that at the most basic level everything would appear to be shimmering, or moving in light waves all the time.

What all this suggests is that our world of seemingly solid objects is composed of wave-like patterns and energy fields that constantly interact with one another. Indeed, some scientists now view the universe as rather like a vast web of inseparable energy patterns.

In 1964 the physicist John S. Bell came up with what is now a well-known mathematical formula called Bell's Theorem. This supports the idea that sub-atomic particles are connected in some way, so that everything that happens to one particle affects all the others.

The late David Bohm, Professor of Theoretical Physics at Birkbeck College, London, also came to the conclusion that the universe is an interconnected whole after devoting 40 years of research into physics and philosophy. He would have received a Nobel prize for his work had he not died unexpectedly in 1993.

In his book *Wholeness and the Implicate Order*, Bohm discusses the idea that things are not separate and independent of each other in reality, they only exist this way in our minds. We split things up and file them away in neat compartments to make the world around us more manageable. Seeing everything as being separate is purely an illusion which leads to endless conflict and confusion within ourselves and society as a whole. Not realizing this fragmentation is of our own making, humanity has always been driven by a quest for wholeness. Indeed the word 'health' derives from the word 'hale', originally an Anglo-Saxon word meaning whole.

This lends credibility to ancient philosophies which tell us that we cannot enjoy a sense of total well-being unless all facets of us – mind, body and spirit – are in balance. This in turn will come from living in harmony with nature. Should we slip out of this balanced state, nature possesses the remedies to make us whole again.

❋ THE ESSENCE OF A FLOWER ❋

It is believed that the healing power of flowers lies in their special energetic or vibrational qualities. The energy pattern of every flower is unique and has its own special characteristics.

Native peoples have always considered plants as living beings whose energy or life-force is most concentrated in their flowers.

We may not be able to see or touch these energy fields, but many sensitive people claim they can feel their strength and quality. These people use a method called Devic Analysis to attune themselves to the flowers, thus gleaning knowledge of their energetic quality and healing potency. Erik Pelham is one such person who has used this technique to define and describe the nature of the Hawaiian Tropical Flower Essences (*see* pages 150–54).

Evidence to suggest these energy fields do indeed exist came to light back in the 1940s. While investigating electrical phenomenon, Harold Saxton Burr (Professor of Anatomy at Yale University Medical School) accidentally discovered energy fields around living plants and animals. He called these fields bio-electrical or electrodynamic L-fields – the fields of life. After discovering that the electrical fields around tiny seedlings resemble those of the adult plant, not of the original seed, he suggested that the organization of a living thing, its pattern, is established by its electrodynamic field. Like a fingerprint, this electrical field is characteristic of a particular living thing and has a shaping influence on it, maintaining its established energetic 'status quo', or blueprint.

Today, certain techniques can be used to reveal these fields. The most well-known is Kirlian photography, a form of high-frequency,

high-voltage electro-photography which was developed by the Russian researcher Semyon Kirlian. In very simple terms, Kirlian photography captures the interference pattern which is set up when a high-frequency electrical charge interacts with the energy field of a living object. The pattern usually appears as streaks of light surrounding the outline of the object, be it a leaf or a hand.

Erik Pelham is pioneering the use of Kirlian photography to show that flower essences do indeed possess energy fields. Furthermore, he has discovered that the energetic patterns produced by different flower essences vary, often quite dramatically – lending support to the idea that each flower has its own personality or character. The first photograph Erik takes is of a cleansed quartz crystal. Having obtained his 'control', Erik then places a few drops of flower essence onto the crystal and makes a series of exposures.

The individual energy pattern of the essence emerges, reflecting the unique qualities of that particular flower.

❈ CAPTURING A FLOWER'S ENERGY ❈

Flower essences are best described as a kind of 'liquid energy'. They literally encapsulate the energy pattern or vibration of the flower they come from.

Since early times it has been believed that the early morning dew which settles on petals becomes infused with a flower's energy. However, the art of capturing this energy pattern so that it could be used therapeutically was perfected by Dr Bach (*see* Chapter 1). In the beginning Bach would collect morning dew from flowers, just as the peoples of ancient cultures did. He then noticed that the

droplets taken from flowers that had been exposed to sunlight were more beneficial than those which formed on shaded flowers. Sunlight, he concluded, seemed to bring potency to the remedy.

To his delight, Bach also discovered that by floating flowers in a bowl of pure spring water for several hours in the sunlight he could obtain powerful vibrational tinctures. The method he devised is remarkably simple and is still used by many people making flower essences today.

THE SUN METHOD

Flowers for making essences are ideally picked very soon after they come into bloom. Freshly picked and undamaged flowers are floated in a glass bowl filled with spring water so that they cover the surface. The bowl is then left out in the sunlight on a clear, cloudless day for three to four hours (or less if the petals show signs of fading). Bach believed that during this process a flower's energies were transferred to the water. Sunlight plays a role in charging the water with an energetic imprint of the flower's vibrational signature. The blooms are then lifted out with a twig and discarded. The energized liquid or 'essence' is then poured into bottles with an equal volume of brandy to form the flower stock. The brandy acts as a preservative which stabilizes and anchors the flower's energy.

THE BOILING METHOD

A clean enamel saucepan is three-quarters filled with newly picked flowers and stems. These are covered with spring water and brought to the boil, uncovered. After simmering for 30 minutes the liquid is left to cool; when cold the essence is filtered. Again this liquid is bottled half and half with brandy.

(For those who wish to try making their own remedies, these methods are described in greater detail in *The Healing Herbs of Edward Bach* by Julian and Martine Barnard – *see* Further Reading chapter.)

If possible, flowers destined for healing should be growing wild in places that are not often visited and are free from pollution. If they are taken from cultivated plants it is important they are tended with loving care and without the use of chemical pesticides or fertilizers.

New environmentally-friendly ways of capturing a flower's energy are also coming to light. In India, Drs Atul and Pupa Shah have devised a technique which means they do not have to cut the flowers to make their Aditi Flower Essences (*see* pages 100–4). And Andreas Korte has invented a crystal method which he uses to make his Amazonian Orchid and Rose essences (*see* pages 49–51). Ever conscious that increasing demand for some of the rarer flowers may actually jeopardize their existence, many are turning to these and other alternative forms of extraction.

❋ WATER HOLDS THE MEMORY ❋

Water often plays a vital role in making flower essences, for the energy is believed to imprint itself on this liquid. Do not expect to find any dissolved chemicals from the petals in the essence. All it contains is the flower's energy.

It may seem remarkable that energized water alone can possess healing properties.

Yet evidence to suggest this emerged in 1987 when a French immuno-biologist called Dr Jacques Benveniste, working in laboratories just outside Paris, found that certain highly diluted substances can be as potent as vastly greater quantities of the same substance. Using a constant called Avagadro's number, Benveniste confirmed mathematically that it was impossible for water to retain a single molecule of the active antibody, immunoglobulin E. Despite this, the water set off a powerful reaction in the test tube. Somehow the water *had* retained the 'memory' or 'vibration' of the molecule.

Gem or crystal essences are worth mentioning here, as they work in a similar 'vibrational' way to flower remedies and are prepared in much the same way. Flower and gem essences tend to complement each other and work well in combination.

❋ BODY ENERGY ❋

Like all living entities, we are also infused with energy. It permeates every part of our being and its abundance goes hand in hand with good health and vitality. This energy flows freely in newborn babies, but as we proceed on our journey through life it begins to wane for all kinds of reasons which we will discuss in Chapter 3. The traditional medical systems of the Chinese, Japanese, Tibetans, Native Americans and Australian Aborigines all regard this energy as something tangible.

As science has yet to validate this energy's existence, no one knows for sure what form it takes within us, yet for centuries healers have being working with energy systems described by ancient medical and esoteric teachings. As flower essences are believed to have a restorative effect on this energy, it is a good idea to know a little more about these different systems.

❋ RIVER OF LIFE ❋

THE MERIDIAN SYSTEM

Traditional Chinese medicine views all matter as being infused with a subtle energy known as chi or qi, which manifests itself through vibration, circulation and waves of movement. This chi flows along a network of channels called *meridians*, which spreads like an intricate web through the body. It may be likened to a second nervous system which forms a connection between the physical body and the subtler energy system surrounding it. It may also be perceived as an aura of light that may at times be colourful.

According to the Chinese model, there are 12 pairs of meridians, each pair associated with a different organ system or function.

The first reference to this energy network is found in the *Nei Ching*, or *Yellow Emperor's Classic of Internal Medicine*, written during the reign of the Emperor Huang Ti between 2697 and 2596 BC. The concept of chi continues to be very much alive today, and millions of people believe that good health and peace of mind rely on ensuring that this energy flows smoothly and evenly.

Traditional Chinese medicine offers various ways to promote the movement of energy to preserve well-being and encourage spiritual development. The flowing movements of QiGong (pronounced cheegung) and T'ai Chi, and the techniques of acupuncture and acupressure all use knowledge of the meridians to clear energy blockages and heal illness. All QiGong masters have the ability to diagnose illness at a distance by reading the subtle anatomy. According to QiGong master Zhi-xing Wang, any illness can be explained as an energy blockage in the body. Circulation and movements of the subtle energy can clear this blockage and, therefore, heal the illness.

You may be asking, is there any scientific proof that such energy channels or meridians exist?

Over 20 years ago Dr Hiroshi Motoyama, a researcher in Japan, devised a system of measuring the electrical characteristics of the 12 major meridians. It is known as the AMI (ap-paratus for measuring the functions of the meridians and corresponding internal organs) machine. Twenty-eight electrodes are attached to the 'entry points' on the skin for each of the meridians. With the AMI, Dr Motoyama has studied over 5,000 subjects and found strong correlations between meridians that are electrically out of balance and the presence of underlying disease in the associated organ.

A more recent study was carried out at the UCLA School of Medicine. It looked at the electrical conductivity of the distal lung acupuncture (meridian) point in 30 patients. X-ray examination had already shown that four members of the group had lung cancer, but the tester did not know which of the 30 these were. On the basis of the reading of the distal lung acupuncture point, the four patients were identified correctly.

❋ ENERGY CENTRES ❋

THE CHAKRAS

Common to Eastern medical and mystical traditions is the idea that special centres known as 'chakras' play a vital role in moving energy around the body. There are seven major chakras which are inextricably linked to the meridian system.

The chakras may be regarded as 'transformers', simultaneously receiving, assimilating and transmitting energy. They are capable of gathering and holding various types of energy, and can also alter their vibration so this energy can be used for different purposes – for instance by bringing higher vibrations down to the physical plane.

You could visualize the chakras as many-petaled, vibrantly coloured flowers which are attached by invisible threads to the spine.

These 'petals', known as *nadis*, are woven into the nervous system and distribute the energy of each chakra into the physical body. The chakras are continuously opening to receive information about the state of the subtle bodies (*see* 'Fields of Energy', below) and closing again, rather like a periwinkle which unfurls its petals when the sun shines.

The seven chakra centres govern the major glands of the endocrine system and influence both our physical and psychological health. The chakra associations differ slightly from East to West, which may help to explain why people from one culture can find it difficult to feel totally at ease in another. It should be noted that the definitions given below are based primarily on the Western chakra tradition.

Each chakra has its own 'pulse rate'. Some vibrate very quickly, others are more slow, depending largely on the ways in which we use and regard our bodies. Indeed, it is said they each chakra has its own 'note'. If one chakra is not functioning properly it will affect those above and below it. Ideally the top centres should vibrate faster and more subtly than the lower ones, but this is not always the case and heavy vibrations can appear in all the centres.

First or Root Chakra

Situated at the base of the spine and associated with basic raw energy.

- Colour – red.
- Physical connections – large intestine, legs, feet, skeletal structure. Imbalance is linked to problems like obesity, constipation, haemorrhoids, sciatica, arthritis, knee problems and poor circulation in the legs and extremities.
- Psychological influences – connecting with the earth (grounding), survival, letting go of emotional tension. Imbalance is linked to accident proneness, dependency, identity crisis and weak ego.

Second or Hara Chakra

Situated at the centre of the abdomen, just below the navel, and thought of as the seat of power and vitality.

- Colour – orange.
- Physical connections – ovaries, testicles, uterus, bladder, circulation. Imbalance is linked to low back trouble, infertility, reproductive problems, pre-menstrual syndrome, urinary problems and arthritis.
- Psychological influences – sexuality, creativity. Imbalance is linked to a weak personality, depression, hysteria and an inability to be sexually intimate.

Third or Solar Plexus Chakra

Situated above the navel, this is the seat of the emotions.

- Colour – yellow.
- Physical connections – adrenal glands, solar plexus, spleen, pancreas and stomach. Imbalance is linked to nervous stomach, anorexia, diabetes and blood glucose problems, anaemia, allergies, and obesity as well as liver, adrenal and spleen problems.
- Psychological influences – feeling empowered and being in control. Imbalance is linked to addictive and compulsive behaviour, excessive anger or fear, manic depression, sleep problems and all kinds of psychosomatic conditions.

Fourth or Heart Chakra

Situated in the centre of the chest, this chakra is concerned with self-love and universal goodwill.

- Colour – green.
- Physical connections – heart, thymus gland, immune system, circulatory system, lungs and respiratory system. Imbalance is linked to heart and circulatory as well as lung and respiratory problems, high blood-pressure, upper back troubles and childhood diseases.
- Psychological influences – understanding, compassion, unconditional love. Imbalance is linked to inner conflict, self-destructive tendencies, relationship problems and feelings of alienation and loneliness.

Fifth or Throat Chakra

Situated in the throat, this is the centre of trust.

- Colour – turquoise.
- Physical connections – thyroid, parathyroid, lymphatic system, immune system, neurological system. Imbalance is linked to teeth, ear, neck and

shoulder problems as well as to sore throats, bronchial problems and hearing and speech difficulties.

- Psychological influences – trust, expression, creativity and communication. Imbalance is linked to an inability to express oneself in words, poor memory, stuttering and doubt as to the sincerity of others.

Sixth or Third Eye Chakra

Situated in the centre of the forehead and associated with perception, discernment and clairvoyance.

- Colour – indigo.
- Physical connections – the pituitary gland, left-brain hemisphere, central nervous system. Imbalance is linked to nervous upsets, eye and vision problems, headaches, sinusitis.
- Psychological influences – clarity and insight,

interest in spiritual issues. Imbalance is linked to confusion, poor memory, inability to focus, paranoia, detachment from reality and, in severe cases, schizophrenia.

Seventh or Crown Chakra

Situated at the crown of the head, this is the seat of consciousness.

- Colour – white.
- Physical connections – pineal gland, right-brain hemisphere and the ancient mammalian brain. Imbalance is linked to migraine headaches, pituitary problems, epilepsy.
- Psychological influences – intuition, to be open and have faith; connection to higher energies or realms. Imbalance is linked to being gullible, having nightmares, having multiple personalities, being spiritually closed off.

❊ FIELDS OF ENERGY ❊

For centuries mystics have talked about an ethereal body surrounding the physical one, which they refer to as the *aura*. It was first recorded by the Pythagoreans (*circa* 500 BC) as a luminous body. They believed that its light could produce a variety of effects in human organisms, including the cure of disease.

In the early 12th century two well-known scholars, Boirac and Liebeault, suggested that humans have an energy that can cause an interaction between two individuals even when they are some distance apart.

Count Wilhelm von Reichenbach spent 30 years during the 1800s experimenting with a field he named the 'odic' force, but it was not until 1911 that knowledge of the human energy field started to take shape.

Using coloured screens and filters, Dr William Kilner, a medical doctor, described the aura as a glowing mist around the body which had three distinct zones. He found it differed considerably from person to person depending on age, sex, mental ability and health. Certain diseases showed as irregularities in the aura, which led Kilner to develop a system of diagnosis based on the colour, texture, volume and general appearance of this ethereal body.

At around the same time Dr Wilhelm Reich, a humanist psychologist and pupil of Sigmund Freud, became interested in a universal energy he called 'orgone'. He studied the relationship between disturbances in the orgone flow within the human body and psychological and physical illness. He suggested that when strong feelings like anger, frustration, sadness and even pleasure are not expressed, the energy that should have been released became locked in the body, thus sapping vitality.

During the mid-1900s Dr George De La Warr and Dr Ruth Drown invented new instruments to detect the subtle radiation being emitted from human tissues. Dr De La Warr was also responsible for developing Radionics, a system of detection, diagnosis and healing from a distance utilizing the human biological energy field.

Medical science now recognizes that the body does have a weak electromagnetic field which is generated by the activity of brain waves and nervous impulses.

A group of Soviet scientists from the A. S. Popow's Bioinformation Institute recently reported the finding that living organisms emit energy vibrations at a frequency of 300 to 2,000 nanometers (nms). They called this energy field the bio-field or bioplasma.

No one knows for sure whether the aura, electromagnetic field and other forms of radiation emitted by the body are one and the same thing. It is more than likely that the human energy field is composed of many different vibrations. Based on their observations and other findings, researchers have created theoretical models of the aura and subtle bodies.

THE AURA

This is an invisible yet luminous kind of radiation which looks like a halo surrounding the physical body.

From ancient times artists and mystics have 'seen' auras. Ancient Indian sculptures, aboriginal rock paintings in Australia and Native American totem poles all show figures surrounded by light or with lines emanating from their bodies. Highly sensitive or 'psychic' people who claim they can see auras describe them as softly shimmering lights forming a misty outline around people, animals, plants and other objects.

Despite its mystical connotations, the aura has distinct parallels with the body's electromagnetic force-field.

All life forms possess an aura. In humans it varies widely in size, density and colour. Its vibrancy and hue is said to depend upon the spiritual evolution of that person as well as his or her general health. Personality and emotions can also be glimpsed in the aura. Those whose auras have soft-fringed edges are susceptible to the influence of others, while a hard, distinct outline may indicate a person with a defensive and hostile attitude resulting from deep insecurity.

The aura differs remarkably from the other energy fields known as the subtle bodies (see below) in that it is a general field of energy emanating from the physical body whereas the subtle bodies are fixed bands of energy at set distances from the body. The aura surrounds the body with an overall field of bio-magnetic energy which acts rather like a barometer of the body's physiological processes. Although we are not usually aware of it, the aura determines our first responses to people and situations. That sense of unease we feel when close to certain people may be the result of your aura literally clashing with theirs. It is a quicker and more accurate gauge than our more rational faculties.

The aura affects overall balance in the system and is the direct result of the physical body's activities, whereas the function of the subtle bodies is much more specific.

THE SUBTLE BODIES

The seven subtle bodies are specialized bands of different types of energy at fixed distances from the physical body, rather like the rings of Saturn, creating a multi-halo impression. They are said to relate to the soul and its co-ordination on the physical level.

Each of these specific layers of energy emanating from the physical body via the chakras vibrates at a slightly different frequency and has its own specialized function. The layers differ in density, colour and appearance, and each is connected to a different chakra through which it exerts an influence over various psychological and physiological processes. It is helpful to imagine the 'Russian Doll effect': each body maintaining its own space but together creating a whole; each emanating from and attached to a particular chakra which in its turn acts as a porthole.

It is useful to know a little about them in order to understand how the flower essences work their wonders.

Etheric Body or Etheric Lining

Deriving from the base or root chakra, the etheric body is bluish-grey in colour. This is the first subtle body and lies between the physical and other subtle bodies, sustaining the dynamic equilibrium between them. This is one of its key functions.

The etheric body is the exact double, an energetic replica, of the denser visible physical body and contains a blueprint of all the organs. Whether leaving or entering the body, the life-force always passes through the etheric body.

The etheric forces are formative and creative, endowing matter with life, form and power. These same cosmic organizing energies are susceptible to control by the mind and will.

The notion that a particular vibration makes a form out of disorganized matter is known as *cymatics*. Many experiments have shown that certain sounds can create patterns out of a random sprinkling of sand. The classic example is the word Om, which forms a kind of mandala.

If the etheric body is imbalanced for whatever reason, any problems residing in the subtle anatomy (that is, in the aura and subtle bodies) can filter down and express themselves in the physical body, for the body is the medium through which all electromagnetic radiation and energies play.

The Immunofluidium is an integral part of the etheric body. It is a sort of liquid energy which surrounds and nourishes all the cells in the physical body. It transports energy between the ethereal levels and the physical body, fuelling each cell with life-force, or qi. The Immunofluidium flows freely and evenly through the body, maintaining and sustaining good health.

When this liquid energy functions properly, genetic disease, viral and bacterial attacks may be kept at bay.

Emotional Body

This band of energy is linked to the solar plexus and heart chakra. In appearance it is brighter than the etheric body, resembling multi-coloured clouds in constant motion. It is closely aligned with the etheric body; together they balance the emotions.

A strong sense of emotional security and stability at the psychological level is sustained when the emotional body is in balance. Negative emotions dim the emotional body's brilliance, whereas positive feelings of love and enjoyment enhance its colours and sparkle.

Mental Body

This energy band is a vibrant shade of pale

yellow, which varies in tone according to mental activity and is like the emotional body but brighter than the etheric. This mental energy enables people to think clearly and rationally. It contains the structure of our thoughts and ideas. Agitation in the mental body blocks the organs of elimination, especially the kidneys. Stress here results in the build-up of toxins in the physical body, which is often linked to allergies. Mental stress and tension also tend to become lodged in the muscular structure – many of us will be familiar with 'the tension headache', or with muscular pain (particularly in the neck and shoulders) when we are stressed.

Astral Body

More intense but softly multicoloured like the emotional body, the astral body is connected to the solar plexus and heart chakras. It encapsulates the entire personality. When the astral body is in balance the individual is more likely to have an intuitive understanding of events and the flow of life. He or she may even glean insight into what lies ahead in the future. The astral body works to collate all past-life experiences, keeping this knowledge and information from spilling into our consciousness in a way that would disrupt our present incarnation.

It can be visualized as a transparent shield which sifts and filters out karmic information and disruptive patterns acquired from past lives that reside in our subconscious.

Causal Body

Crystal-clear and intensely blue in appearance, this layer is connected to the throat chakra. The causal body is the seat of our willpower. It facilitates the interaction of the individual with other people and events, allowing us to fulfil our personal destiny. It may be regarded as the gateway to higher consciousness. This body is responsible for organizing past-life information before it is released to the astral body when it is needed or appropriate.

Celestial or Soul Body

Vibrantly luminous and golden, this energy band is connected to the third eye (sixth chakra). It houses our spiritual essence and is, in a sense, the Higher Self which allows the soul to move freely through us. This energy band enters the body through the pineal gland.

Spiritual or Illuminated Body

This energy layer is a shimmering composition of pastel colours which is connected to the heart chakra. It represents a combination and fusion of the whole subtle anatomy with the physical body. Our basic energetic blueprint is housed within this subtle body.

The Etheric envelope forms a sort of protective outer-coating around the subtle bodies, separating the subtle anatomy from the other energies around us.

In addition to the ethereal subtle bodies we possess a thermal body which can be likened to a heat source extending beyond the etheric body. The heat is generated by normal cell division and is influenced by our rate of metabolism. It is literally a by-product of physical activity.

THE SUBTLE ANATOMY

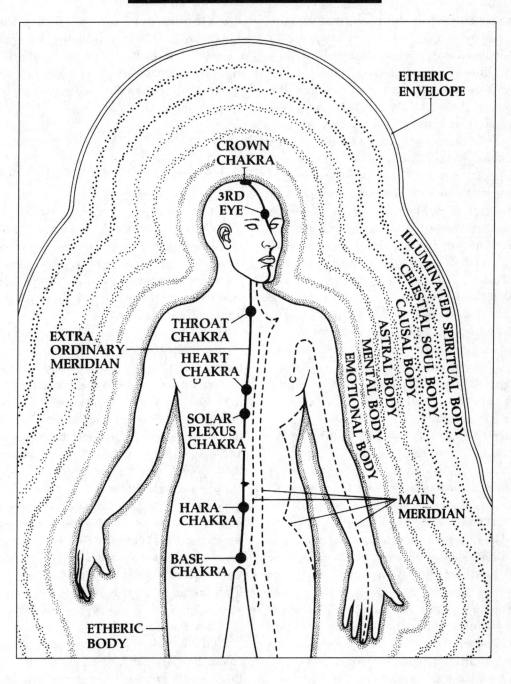

ETHERIC
ENVELOPE

CROWN
CHAKRA

3RD
EYE

ILLUMINATED SPIRITUAL BODY
CELESTIAL SOUL BODY
CAUSAL BODY
ASTRAL BODY
MENTAL BODY
EMOTIONAL BODY

THROAT
CHAKRA

EXTRA
ORDINARY
MERIDIAN

HEART
CHAKRA

SOLAR
PLEXUS
CHAKRA

MAIN
MERIDIAN

HARA
CHAKRA

BASE
CHAKRA

ETHERIC
BODY

❋ HOW THE FIELDS OF ENERGY INTERACT ❋

These energy systems are considered separate entities for simplicity's sake, yet they are all inter-linked and constantly interact with each other, functioning as an energetic whole. The meridians link up and pass through the organs of the body – it may help to picture the meridians as rivers of energy that are constantly on the move, flowing in and out of one another. There are a further eight energy channels (known as the extraordinary meridians) which hover in between the etheric and physical bodies. They act as a sort of energy reservoir, borrowing points from the organ meridians yet forming their own pathways between the nervous and circulatory systems.

These meridians relate strongly to our vitality and emotions/states of mind. Their prime function is to feed the main meridians with energy, qi or life-force. The most important extraordinary meridian travels straight up and down the centre of the body, connecting directly with the major chakras. As we have already seen, these in turn link up with the subtle bodies. All seven subtle bodies enter and leave the body through various chakras, or portholes.

The subtle energy system may be visualized as diaphanous layers held in place with thin membranes which separate yet allow them to diffuse into one another.

The aura has its own unique part to play: It is a reflection of physical vitality. The more balanced and healthy you are, the greater your auric field. This force-field can radiate some three to four feet from the body, its energy infusing the whole subtle body system. In ill-health the aura shrinks back close to the body in an attempt to conserve vital energy.

This entire energy system is in a continuous state of motion. You might want to visualize the different energies as swirling mists of colour and light interacting with and receiving information from each other – a multi-levelled interfusion. These energies are constantly interchanging, redistributing and re-balancing themselves.

ILLUMINATING THE ENERGIES

Scientists have yet to invent a device that confirms categorically the existence of these subtler energies, although many have turned their minds to this. However, some interesting energetic phenomena have been discovered using special techniques akin to Kirlian photography.

Harry Oldfield has dedicated 15 years of his life to illuminating the subtle energies. While working with Kirlian photography he found that sound and radio frequencies as well as light are emitted from an object. This inspired him to invent the electroscanning method (ESM) – a piece of equipment that surrounds an object or person with an electrical reference field which can be measured three-dimensionally around the body. He feels that fluctuations in this field could reflect what is happening on more subtle levels. For his own private research purposes Harry Oldfield has invented a piece of equipment which seems to make visible some interesting energy effects with light using computer technology. This is known as the P.I.P. technique (Poly-contrast-Interface-Photography).

Oldfield feels that the various swirls of colour he sees in and around the body relate in some way to the subtle energies and possibly the chakras.

Over the years Oldfield has photographed the energies of literally hundreds of different people. He now feels he can detect the difference between vibrant energy fields belonging to fit and healthy people and the distorted fields which suggest to him the presence of or potential for illness.

Oldfield uses his various detectors widely as a method of diagnosis to investigate the possibility of weakness, stress or disease in the energy field. On numerous occasions these methods have been verified by doctors using orthodox medical procedures such as X-rays and blood tests. Mr Oldfield insists, however, that his work is still in the research stage and has a long way to go before it can be accepted scientifically.

As we shall see in Chapter 4, flowers and their essences seem to interact with and influence the body's energy field in remarkable ways.

THREE

SHOCK, STRESS AND POLLUTION

Each person's whole energy system –
aura, subtle bodies, chakras and meridians – forms a sort of personal
'blueprint' or 'body map'. We are all born with this energetic blueprint
which, like a thumbprint, is quite unique and different from person to per-
son, however subtly. This energetic pattern holds within it characteristics
that endow us with the potential to be as perfect – physically, mentally,
emotionally and spiritually – as we can possibly be.

When all the elements of your energy system are in balance you experience a deep sense of contentment and well-being. These are the times when life is joyful and everything feels comfortable. Think of those days when you wake up brimming with energy and looking forward to the day ahead. This abundant physical vitality goes hand in hand with a clear, focused mind. You are blessed with a sense of inner calm and cannot be ruffled by other people or the hustle and bustle of life. Deep down you feel safe and secure, as if cocooned from any danger lurking in the outside world, while at the same time totally involved in the here and now. These benefits come from knowing you are following a path or going in a direction that is right for you,

one that will bring real purpose and meaning to your life.

For many of us such sensations are often rare and fleeting. This is because the stresses and strains of living conspire to prevent us from growing to fulfil our potential to be perfect.

We are all, however, capable of feeling this way most of the time because we are blessed with an intelligence or Higher Self that is aware of this energetic blueprint and knows how to keep the entire energy network in order. In other words, we intuitively or instinctively know what is best for us.

Sadly, we do not always hear or heed the wisdom of this inner voice.

In childhood it does not matter too much if our energy systems are thrown off-balance, for there is an abundance of energy or chi which can be used to override any disturbance or misalignment. There comes a point in time when this energy reserve is exhausted, however, and the imbalance begins to become ingrained in the system.

The Higher Self knows when this is happening and sends us warning signals in the form of physical, emotional and psychological symptoms. Typical signs of an energy imbalance are tiredness, feelings of anxiety, irritability and depression, as well as a susceptibility to colds and other infections. If an imbalance is not corrected, it will become firmly entrenched in the energy system and the resulting symptoms will get worse with time. It is my opinion that disease shows itself in the physical body only after disturbances of energy flow have already become crystallized in the subtle structural patterns of the higher-frequency bodies.

I believe that nature holds a cure for every ill, and that the Higher Self will guide us towards certain plants, herbs and flowers that can restore balance in our energetic system. In Chapter 4 you will find out how to follow your intuition and choose a combination of flower essences that will displace the disharmony in your energy system.

Before looking more closely at how flower essences work their wonders, let us first look at ways in which our energy systems can be thrown out of kilter.

❋ SHATTERING THE BALANCE ❋

Shock and stress in their many guises have a devastating effect on the subtle energy system. You can visualize this sudden shock as a pebble being hurled into a tranquil pond, sending ripples or shock waves reverberating through the water or, in this case, the subtle anatomy. This 'pebble', then, can be seen as the root cause of any upset, while the ripples are the physical repercussions of shock. Unlike the pond, however, which becomes still once the pebble has dropped to the bottom, when shock makes an impact on our subtle energy systems the disruptive effects linger unless steps are taken to bring everything back into balance.

As a consequence of shock the subtle bodies are thrown out of alignment and end up becoming either too close or too far apart from one another. When the mental and emotional bodies are not properly aligned to the etheric, for example, we experience feelings of anxiety. When the mental and emotional bodies are too close together we become prone to feelings of frustration and unknown fears, and are unable to make clear-cut decisions. Sometimes the properties of the subtle bodies spill over into each other. This is known as the 'spillage effect'. When the mental body flows into the emotional one, mental lethargy and loss of confidence ensues.

Any misalignment in the subtle bodies ultimately filters down to the physical body, where it triggers a range of symptoms depending on which part of the body is affected.

Shock can be divided into two main categories: traumatic and long, slow shock.

TRAUMATIC SHOCK

We live in an world full of horrific events that are often too distressing even to think about.

Some of these, such as natural disasters, unpredictable violence and the death of a loved one, are age-old. Others, such as car accidents and bomb blasts which can maim and kill, are relatively recent phenomena.

At some time or other we are all likely to experience personally the shock of some traumatic event.

The worst kind are invariably those that are sudden and unexpected because they take us unawares. As they are not part of our ordinary life, we are totally unprepared for them and they shake us to the very core of our being.

The medical profession is only just beginning to appreciate the impact of such shock on our physical and psychological well-being. It has come to realize that such trauma gives rise to a range of symptoms resembling those experienced by shell-shocked war veterans. Such symptoms can last a lifetime unless steps are taken to redress their far-reaching effects.

The so-called Post Traumatic Stress Disorder (PTSD) is now used to describe the aftermath of shock. The repercussions clearly permeate every level of our being.

Physically, those suffering from traumatic shock feel exhausted and drained of energy. In time the tiredness may lift, but it invariably gives way to all kinds of minor ailments such as stomach upsets, stiff necks and so forth. As such symptoms appear some time after the event has taken place, they often seem to have no apparent cause. Little wonder, then, that those suffering from PTSD are often thought of as hypochondriacs.

Shock has a particularly potent influence on the mind. Concentration becomes difficult, thoughts are blurred and decisions about even everyday issues such as when to do the shopping can pose problems. Emotions are volatile and range from anger and irritability to depression and despair. Sufferers often over-react to events that would not normally upset them, and steer themselves away from any kind of pressure. They may even suffer from panic attacks.

Confidence and self-esteem dwindle, making those suffering from shock less inclined to tackle new projects which they would previously have relished as a challenge.

On a spiritual level, many feel compelled to reassess their lives. In the worst cases doubts arise as to whether life is really worth living.

LONG, SLOW SHOCK

This is more insidious than traumatic shock, for we are often unaware of its existence and it becomes an integral part of our lives.

Long, slow shock can start to take its toll even before we are born. Although safe inside the womb, the developing foetus will detect and react to its mother's stresses. Anxieties about her relationship with her partner and her fears and apprehension about motherhood can all be sensed by her unborn child.

In childhood we may experience stress when deprived of the right kind of love, attention and emotional nourishment. Ironically it can be equally stressful to be swamped by too much love (in the form of over-protectiveness or possessiveness). Parents who threaten to withhold their love unless they are obeyed also create a stressful environment for their offspring.

Children whose parents are always quarrelling will also suffer the effects of long, slow shock, as will those whose mother or father has a drinking problem or an incapacitating illness.

As this kind of stress goes unnoticed and is often present for prolonged periods of time, it becomes so familiar that it appears to be normal. We often usually fail even to identify it as shock.

The effects of long, slow shock are cumulative, which means that by the time a person reaches adulthood it has produced the same disruptive effect on the subtle energy system as sudden trauma.

Shock and stress set up an abrasive vibration which is at odds with the natural rhythm of the cells and forces them to 'dance to a different tune'. This ultimately affects the smooth and efficient functioning of all the organs and tissues. If left untreated, such distortion in the energy system ultimately manifests itself as disease of the mind, body and spirit.

The medical profession now agrees that stress can indeed make us more susceptible to illness. This is the reason we often tend to catch cold or fall victim to an infection after a stressful event has taken place or when we feel overly stressed at home or work. Some forward-thinking physicians believe that negative emotions such as anxiety, fear, anger, frustration and irritability play crucial roles in undermining the body's resistance to disease.

Researchers working in the relatively new field of psychoneuroimmunology (or PNI) are attempting to fathom the link between such negative emotions and various disease states. They suggest that psychological and emotional states undermine our resistance in the way that they interact with our nervous, endocrine and immune systems. Seen from an energetic perspective, shock has the effect of throwing the emotional and mental bodies out of alignment. They leak into each other and, in turn, spill into the etheric body.

As a result of shock or stress the etheric body can no longer hold its boundaries and perform its job of defending the physical body from disturbance in the subtle bodies.

The etheric body is also closely affiliated with the nervous system, which in turn is closely bound to the immune system. This then, is how mental and emotional disturbances act as immunosuppressants, weakening the body's natural defences and resistance to illness.

In cases of severe shock or trauma such as a bereavement or being violently attacked or wounded, the astral and etheric bodies are suddenly and dramatically thrown out of alignment. When this happens the aura breaks and holes appear. These gaps are potentially dangerous as the physical body is no longer fully protected and becomes vulnerable.

It is essential to clear the effects of shock out of the system, for if the subtle bodies are misaligned, the chi or life-force that sustains us cannot filter through and replenish our physical body.

Years ahead of his time, Dr Edward Bach (creator of the Bach Flower Remedies), realized that psychological upsets can be a root cause of disease. Bach was also aware that shock and stress provoke emotional or mental distress by heightening imbalances in the personality. Someone who normally has a tendency towards impatience and who prefers to work at his or her own speed, for instance, will become increasingly irritable, impetuous and prone to outbursts of temper and nervous tension as a result of shock or stress.

Bach described and discovered flower remedies for 38 negative states of mind. These remedies aim to bring you back to a state of emotional equilibrium. In keeping with various ancient philosophies, Bach believed that peace of mind and physical well-being go hand in hand.

In his book *Heal Thyself*, Bach wrote:

We must steadfastly practise peace,
imaging our minds as a lake ever to be
kept calm, without waves or even ripples,
to disturb its tranquillity and gradually

develop this state of peace until no event, no circumstance, no other personality is able under any condition to ruffle the surface of that lake or raise within us any feelings of irritability, depression or doubt.

In this book's Encyclopaedia of Flower Remedies and Ailment Chart you will find essences helpful for many almost every permutation of shock and stress, including the urban stress that comes of the loneliness, isolation and loss of identity many of us feel as cozy, tight-knit communities disappear and new technology and pollution insidiously change the very nature of our environment. In Chapter 6 you will also find excellent first-aid combinations to have to hand in case of sudden shocks and emergencies.

❋ CHEMICAL POLLUTANTS ❋

Clean water, fresh air and natural foods are essential for good health, yet slowly and insidiously they are being polluted by synthetic chemicals.

Car emissions contain a noxious mixture of chemicals which irritate the lungs, trigger asthma attacks, exacerbate chest troubles and increase our vulnerability to respiratory infections. Carbon monoxide competes with oxygen in the blood and can, at high levels, suffocate the tissues. Breathlessness, dizziness, nausea, lethargy and faintness are typical symptoms. The situation is exacerbated during the Summer months, for in the presence of strong sunlight the chemicals in exhaust fumes react to form ozone. At ground levels ozone creates a smog that can cause eye irritations, headaches and breathing difficulties. It also damages plants.

Even indoors the air may be far from pure. Sealing buildings hermetically in order to conserve energy also encourages a build-up of irritant substances. While cigarette smoke is often the chief offender, chemicals given off by photocopying machines and carpets add to the load. Toxic gases may even evaporate from the adhesives and preservatives used in construction. Polluted air can cause headaches, difficulty concentrating, stinging eyes, sore throats and skin problems as well as lingering coughs and colds, in part because they create a grey etheric mucus-type substance which clogs up our energy system.

Chemicals in our food and water may come from industrial waste flushed into the seas and rivers, whereby they enter the food chain. Some of these synthetic chemicals, such as chlorinated organics, are extremely persistent. After entering the environment they accumulate in the food chain, sometimes building to high concentrations in certain animals. A typical example are PCBs (polychlorinated biphenyls), which are now banned but are still found in many foods, especially fish.

In addition to these long-lived chemicals, a huge number are also in daily use. Most commercially grown fruits, vegetables and cereals are liberally dowsed with at least one, usually several different chemicals as they grow and are kept in storage. Some crops may be sprayed with up to six different chemicals before they reach the supermarket shelves.

Particularly worrying is the little-known 'cocktail' effect or combined activity of many different chemicals. Emerging evidence suggests that pesticides and PCBs may act as immunosuppressants, contributing to the incidence of allergies and viral infections.

On an energetic level, chemical pollutants cloud the subtle anatomy – preventing realignment and directly affecting the opening and closing of the chakras. If not cleared from the system they can damage these important energy centres.

PROTECTING YOURSELF FROM CHEMICAL POLLUTANTS

- Vitamins A and E help the lungs and air passages to withstand smoke and chemical damage. Together with vitamin C and selenium they work as antioxidants, preventing pollutants from harming the body cells. Vitamin C also helps detoxify pesticide residues, while vitamins A and E protect the liver from chemical abuse and the B-complex vitamins increase efficiency of detoxification systems. The minerals calcium, magnesium and zinc also bolster resistance.
- Ionizers and air purifiers help to remove pollutant particles from the air.
- Plants can help to diffuse office chemicals.
- You should buy organically grown foods whenever possible. Alternatively, wash all fruit and vegetables in a mixture of filtered water and 1 tablespoon of cider vinegar.
- Cold-pressed vegetable oils such as sunflower, olive and safflower reduce the absorption of toxins and speed their elimination.
- Select free-range poultry, eggs and game whenever possible.
- Avoid eating organ meats, as chemicals and hormones can concentrate in an animal's liver and kidneys.
- Opt for bottled spring water and invest in a water filter which will extract pesticide residues as well as nitrates and heavy metals from your tap water.

Flower remedies to combat chemical pollution can be found in the Ailment Chart.

A specific 'cleansing' recipe can be found in Chapter 7.

❊ ELECTROMAGNETIC POLLUTION ❊

The earth has its own electromagnetic field which pulses, like a heart, at 470 beats a minute or 7.83 Hz (beats a second). These pulses are known as the Schumann waves after the German professor who discovered them in 1952.

It is no coincidence that we have in our bodies a pulse that is approximately the same, in the electrical signals – the alpha and beta waves – sent out by our brains. It is thought that this natural electromagnetic pulse may have a role to play in maintaining and sustaining good health. It is well acknowledged that NASA fits its spacecraft with 7.83 Hz oscillators to give its astronauts something to make them feel more comfortable – that is, it helps to regulate their sleeping/waking cycles.

Nowadays, however, the earth's natural pulse is being swamped by other forms of electrically and magnetically generated fields. Electromagnetic radiation from overhead power cables and pylons, televisions, computers, VDUs and radio and satellite transmitters is filling the atmosphere with what is commonly known as electronic smog. It may literally blanket the natural signals needed for good health.

Those which are the greatest cause for concern are the so-called ELFs (extremely low frequencies) because they are so similar to those of our own bodies. Particularly strong electromagnetic fields generated by such frequencies may have the power to influence our brainwaves, resulting in various behavioural and physical problems.

Depression, anxiety, irritability, chronic tiredness, headaches, nausea, sweating and indigestion are among the wide range of symptoms that have been attributed to electromagnetic pollution.

Offices in particular tend to be filled with a wealth of artificial fields, which may contribute to what is known as Sick Building Syndrome.

Electromagnetic radiation can also occur naturally due to geographic faults (also known as 'geopathic stress') or underground streams and rivers. Ley lines are believed to indicate places where the earth's magnetic field is particularly potent. Such forms of radiation impinge on and affect our own electromagnetic force-field. X-rays, microwaves and even ultra-violet rays from the sun can distort the subtle bodies and, if powerful enough, can also alter the structure of DNA, the genetic material of our cells.

The consequences of continual over-exposure to such radiation may not show physically until 20 years after the event.

In his book, *Electromagnetic Fields of Life* the Russian physicist A. S. Presman of the Department of Biophysics at Moscow University explains the detailed experiments he carried out in 1968 which led to his discovery that such radiation was linked to physical problems such as blood disorders, hypertension, heart attacks, sexual dysfunction, lack of energy and nervous exhaustion.

Evidence is emerging that long-term exposure to emissions from VDUs, computers, word processors and television screens can cause chromosomal damage. Studies remain inconclusive and controversial, but some research has linked excessive VDU work with pregnancy problems including miscarriage, still births and birth defects. Embryos are particularly vulnerable to electromagnetic radiation in the first trimester when the cells are rapidly dividing. During this incredible growth spurt, the subtle blueprint has a particularly important role to play in ensuring that everything runs smoothly. It is possible that harmful electromagnetic radiation may damage the blueprint, with far-reaching consequences.

PROTECTING YOURSELF FROM ELECTROMAGNETIC POLLUTION

- Switch off electrical appliances when not in use.
- Prevent static build-up by filling your home or office with bowls of flowers, sprinkling water on all carpets and wearing natural materials like cotton and silk instead of synthetics. Never wear rubber-soled shoes.
- Avoid being in the vicinity of pylons and overhead cables.
- Do not set up home in areas known to be affected by geopathic stress.

Flower remedies to combat electromagnetic pollution can be found in the Ailment Chart.

❋ SOCIAL POISONS ❋

Many of us rely heavily on different kinds of props to boost our energy levels, steady or stupefy our nerves and generally help us to cope with our frantic pace of life. Alcohol, cigarettes and caffeine-laden drinks, however, only provide us with short-lived energy and, once the effects wear off, leave us feeling more depleted than before. These 'social poisons' also have dangerous side-effects.

ALCOHOL

Alcohol damages cells of the brain and nervous system, giving rise to a wide variety of symptoms ranging from lack of concentration, confusion, memory loss, insomnia or lethargy to agitation, irritability and exhaustion.

At an energetic level, alcohol loosens and misaligns the subtle anatomy. It has a particularly disruptive influence on the etheric and astral bodies, making them slip out of sympathy with each other, which is why self-control and will-power are weakened. Alcohol also gives rise to a murky, greenish-brown aura congested with a sticky, mucus-like substance.

CIGARETTES

Cigarette smoke contains a cocktail of noxious chemical substances, many of which are known to be carcinogenic. The health hazards of smoking are well known, but the harm cigarettes cause the energy system is also significant. Smoke clouds and weakens the subtle anatomy, surrounding it with a fog which dulls and discolours the normally bright,

vibrant hues of the aura. It also prevents the aura from cleansing itself. The etheric body is particularly affected by this grey mucus, which undermines the body's first line of defence.

CAFFEINE

Coffee and caffeine-rich foods and drinks stimulate the adrenal glands into producing adrenaline, a hormone normally secreted in times of stress which gives us a sudden rush of energy and mental focus. The effects do not last long, and when caffeine levels fall we invariably end up feeling as tired as before. Increasing caffeine intake acts as an additional stress, which produces feelings of anxiety, irritability and jumpiness. Excessive caffeine intake has also been linked to breast lumps in women.

From an energetic viewpoint, caffeine disturbs the flow of energy in the meridian system. This affects the etheric body, which in turn causes leakage in the emotional and mental bodies. An imbalance in these energies results in emotional instability and disruption to the nervous system. It also upsets the solar plexus chakra, the seat of emotional balance – and the effects then filter down to the stomach.

Importantly, caffeine actually prevents flower remedies from working by misaligning the subtle bodies.

Certain flower essences help to overcome addiction to these social props, while others counter their negative impact on the subtle energy systems (see the Encyclopaedia, Ailment Chart and Recipe sections of this book).

❋ ILLNESS AND MEDICATION ❋

Modern medicines may be essential when it comes to treating physical illness, and they undoubtedly do save lives. On the flip side of the coin, many also have undesirable side-effects.

These vary from drug to drug, but they all have a generally disruptive influence on the energy systems. They tend to cloud the subtle anatomy and cause the subtle bodies to separate from one another. At the same time they also prevent realignment. They also affect the chakras' function of regulating and dispersing energy – especially the throat chakra, which is particularly susceptible to drugs.

Steroids, for example, create congestion in the solar plexus and heart chakras, preventing the nervous and muscular systems from receiving energy or life-force.

Taken in conjunction with orthodox medication, flower essences gently help to buffer these undesirable effects. They can also be taken after a course of medication to realign the subtle bodies and generally re-balance the energy systems.

More importantly perhaps, flower essences actually allay the need for taking orthodox medication, for if taken soon enough they can help prevent disease from occurring in the first place.

Flower remedies may, for example, negate the need for antibiotics by boosting the body's natural immunity. They help by clearing away physical toxins as well as toxic thoughts, emotions and, last but not least, spiritual toxicity which pollutes the energy system. As a consequence the body's natural defence system is strengthened and becomes better able to repel viral and bacterial invasion.

At present there is increasing concern about the repercussions of using drugs like antibiotics too frequently. It is well recognized that bacteria gradually adapt to any antibiotic, so in using these drugs too much they are made less useful for everyone. Yet in the United States sales of antibiotics have doubled since the mid-1980s, and seven out of 10 Americans are prescribed these drugs when they seek treatment for common colds. Is it just coincidence that drug-resistant infections are also soaring?

Resistant germs are hard to treat and can spread through the community. They do not threaten us all equally. A healthy immune system repels most bacterial invaders regardless of their susceptibility to drugs. However, certain people such as the elderly and sick are more vulnerable, and when they contract such bacterial diseases they are harder to treat. While drug companies may see this as the ultimate challenge to invent new wonder antibiotics, surely it is better to strengthen our natural immunity and encourage both doctors and patients to stop abusing the weapons we have.

(For a recipe to help boost the immune system, *see page* 210.)

PHYSICAL INJURY

In cases where disease is already manifest and there is a need for surgery, it is good to know that flower essences can help to reduce the effects of such trauma and aid recuperation.

When tissues are cut and injured during an operation or accident, the subtle energy system receives an almighty jolt. Wherever the physical damage occurs it is accompanied by a rupture in the etheric body print. This must be healed along with the tissues to ensure that the damaged area does not remain weak, vulnerable and prone to recurrent problems. For even when the scars have faded, the subtle bodies may still be misaligned.

Before undergoing any operation it is a good idea to take Bach's Rescue Remedy or Five Flower Remedy, or Australian Bush Emergency Essence to ease the shock and trauma.

As well as the shock of the operation, anaesthetics themselves also throw you into a state of suspension. This results in feelings of disorientation, unworldliness and dragging tiredness. (*See page* 210 for my recipe for clearing the after-effects of anaesthesia.)

✹ INHERITING IMBALANCES IN THE ✹ SUBTLE ENERGY SYSTEM

It is important to clear away any imbalance in the subtle anatomy, otherwise it can become etched in the system and passed on to future generations. These inherited flaws in the energetic bodies are referred to as *miasms*.

The concept of miasms was originally introduced by Dr Samuel Hahnemann, the founder of homoeopathy. He was puzzled to find that some patients failed to respond to treatment, while others who improved relapsed after only a short time. He looked at these 'difficult' cases and found a common 'blocking' factor in their personal or family history – such as the presence of certain diseases which have been passed on from one generation to another. He called these blocks 'miasms'.

We might visualize a miasm as a void or lack of life-force. They are usually stored in the subtle bodies – especially the etheric, emotional, mental and, to a lesser extent, the astral body. Here miasms may lie dormant for long periods of time, only flaring up occasionally and leading to chronic or acute illnesses, trauma, stress and age-related conditions. A bad fall or emotional shock may easily allow them to filter down from the subtle bodies into the physical anatomy, resulting in the development of various symptoms. As we get older, our natural vitality diminishes, making it easier for miasms to emerge. This could help explain why we tend to become more prone to all kinds of disease as we age.

MIASMS

Flower essences help to remove miasms from the system. Once a remedy's life-force filters down to the physical level, an immediate rebalancing and readjustment begins to take place. The essences release the miasm from the cells' genetic material and from the subtle bodies, so that it can be discharged from the system.

It may take some time for these shifts to take place, so do not expect miracles to happen overnight.

Dr Hahnemann described three basic types of 'inherited' miasm (psora, syphilitic and sycosis) which he believed to be the underlying causes of chronic disease. Each predisposes a person to a particular range of health problems. Homoeopaths have since added many more illness-causing miasms to this list, including tuberculosis, radiation and heavy metals.

Psora

Associated with suppressed skin disease, a psora miasm leads to imbalance in the rhythmic bodily functions and causes general mental and physical irritation. Typical symptoms are tiredness, anxiety, sadness or depression as well as skin disorders, congestion in the tissues and bone structure deformities.

Syphilitic

Associated with suppressed syphilis, this miasm has a destructive effect on all the tissues, especially the bones. Cardiac and neurological symptoms are common. Those carrying this miasm are easily upset, sentimental, irritable and suspicious. This miasm may manifest as meningitis.

Sycosis

Associated with suppressed gonorrhoea, this miasm encourages congestion in the skin, the pelvic region, the joints and the digestive, respiratory and urinary tracts. It may cause fearfulness, nervousness and amorality.

Tuberculosis

This miasm may cause susceptibility to respiratory, circulatory, urinary and digestive problems, resulting, for example, in weight loss and poor circulation. Those carrying this miasm typically tend to be escapists who feel unable to make decisions or face life's realities. It may also manifest as mental illness and cancer.

MODERN MIASMS

Most homoeopathic research into miasms was conducted in the 1800s and early 1900s, when infectious diseases such as tuberculosis and syphilis were prevalent. Today we are faced with new threats to our health which derive from modern-day pollutants and are known as 'acquired miasms'.

Petrochemical

Springing from the major increase in petrol and chemical products, the problems this causes are fluid retention, diabetes, infertility, impotence, miscarriage, hair loss/greying hair, muscle degeneration, skin blemishes, or a metabolic imbalance resulting in the storage of fat in tissues. It also blocks assimilation of vitamin K, causing circulatory and endocrine disorders. Those affected find it difficult to resist stress and suffer from various types of psychosis, especially schizophrenia and autism. Leukaemia, skin and lymph cancer can also occur.

Radiation

Associated with the massive increase in background radiation since the Second World War, this miasm primarily affects the skin, connective tissue, circulation and reproductive systems. Symptoms include premature ageing, slower cell division, loss of skin elasticity, rashes, lupus, skin cancer, anaemia, leukaemia, arthritis, allergies, bacterial inflammations (especially in the brain), hair loss, hardening of the arteries, miscarriage, excessive bleeding in women and sterility or a drop in sperm count in men.

Heavy Metals

Resulting from increased levels of toxic metals and chemicals such as lead, mercury, radium, arsenic, aluminium, fluoride and sulphuric acid, the symptoms of this miasm include allergies, fluid retention, an inability to assimilate calcium, viral inflammations and excessive hair loss.

Remedies to combat all these types of miasms can be found in the Ailment Chart.

FOUR

ESSENCES IN ACTION

Learning to use and prescribe flower remedies

No two people are identical. We may share similar physical characteristics, behavioural tendencies and personality traits but deep down each of us is unique. Our individuality determines the ways in which we cope with and react to any kind of stress in our lives.

Two people may exhibit typical symptoms associated with a frazzled nervous system. Each may be anxious, irritable, on edge and suffering from sleeping problems, indigestion and butterflies in the stomach, but each will be this way for entirely different reasons. One may be going through a marriage break-up while the other may be experiencing a conflict at work. Delve deeper and it will become clear that their problems arise from a certain personality trait or a particular behavioural pattern. For this reason it is essential to treat each person as a unique whole, rather than just addressing his or her symptoms or illness. The beauty of flower essences is that they help us to become aware of elements in our nature which are undermining our sense of well-being. They do not work *on* us, but *with* us. They bring our attention to any imbalance that exists within, then lend their energetic support so we can release it gently from our lives. In this way we can begin to take responsibility for our own health and happiness.

❋ KNOW THYSELF ❋

As you begin to use flower remedies, you will be embarking on an exciting adventure of self-discovery which will enable you to understand yourself, why you think and act in certain ways. As the remedies get to work your self-awareness will continue to grow, bringing with it a new freedom to do whatever you wish in life.

In the Encyclopaedia section you will see that there are literally hundreds of flower essences from all over the world to choose from. Each is associated with particular qualities or properties. The real art lies in selecting the essences that are best for you. To do this you need to devote some time to thinking about yourself. This may sound narcissistic, but it is an essential part of self-healing.

Reflecting on your own personality is a good starting point. Although this is as individual as your thumbprint, there are certain personality traits or tendencies which prevail in human nature. These characteristics have a strong influence on how you handle and react to stress.

BACH'S 12 PERSONALITY TYPES AND REMEDIES

Dr Edward Bach identified 12 key personality traits, and the first flowers he searched for related to these:

1. Fear
2. Terror
3. Mental torture or worry
4. Indifference or boredom
5. Doubt or discouragement
6. Indecision
7. Over-enthusiasm
8. Discouragement
9. Weakness
10. Self-distrust
11. Over-concern
12. Pride or aloofness

Take Impatiens, for example. As its name suggests, this flower is for people whose outstanding characteristic is impatience. They tend to rush around and are critical of other people's shortcomings. As a result they are prone to irritability, nervous tension, over-exertion and accidents.

In contrast, Clematis relates to quiet, dreamy, absent-minded people who are wrapped up in their own thoughts and fantasies. Their predominant characteristic is indifference. They tend to lack concentration and are susceptible to clumsiness and sleepiness.

Bach often saw human characteristics reflected in the plants themselves. In each flower family you will find remedies describing many permutations of the basic personality traits. Although some may seem very similar, if you read the descriptions carefully you will see there are subtle differences. You should look for flower essences whose qualities reflect the way in which you see yourself. The remedies will help to emphasize your positive characteristics while tempering negative tendencies which can lead you into trouble.

It is important to remember that such tendencies are not fixed. With the help of flower essences we can alter certain aspects of our personality for the better.

A welcome side-effect of cultivating your better qualities and tempering the less attractive ones is that your relationships with others will be easier and more fulfilling. Many people seem to end up in partnerships that begin beautifully but then, when the magic has faded, become unworkable. When you become truer to yourself, you will automatically draw to you the sort of people who possess qualities you genuinely admire and find attractive. All relationships, be they intimate or purely platonic, will be fun and mutually satisfying.

While personality affects the way we handle other people and life in general, our constitution determines how resilient or susceptible we are to becoming ill. Constitution is best defined as temperament and state of health. It is your genetic inheritance which has been modified by experiences in life and the environment. While a strong constitution can withstand considerable pressure without flagging, a weaker one is more susceptible to illness.

If, for example, all your grandparents died of old age and your parents have been healthy all their lives; if your mother was healthy throughout her pregnancy (she didn't smoke, drink, etc.), if your parents' marriage was happy and your birth uneventful, you should be blessed with a strong constitution.

If, on the other hand, your grandparents died at early ages of cancer or heart disease, one of your parents had tuberculosis as a child and the other suffered from asthma and eczema, then your chances of inheriting a weak constitution are far greater.

Take heart, you can still escape the worst of a poor inheritance if your parents were happily married, they took good care of their health and brought you up with plenty of love and a nourishing diet.

Similarly, you may have inherited a potentially strong constitution but if your parents were always arguing and your emotional needs were neglected, your susceptibility to illness will have increased.

In any case, there is no reason to feel lumbered with a flimsy constitution. Flower essences can improve your resilience to every sort of illness in two ways. First, certain essences help to eliminate, at the vibrational level, the inherited genetic weaknesses known as miasms (see Chapter 3). Secondly, they can clear away the residual effects of any past traumas as well as the long, slow shock of, for instance, an unhappy childhood, which may have weakened your inherent constitution.

TAKING A CASE HISTORY

Making your own case history is a good way of finding out why you are not feeling as well as you could be.

You should list any physical symptoms and psychological problems you would like to treat. These are signs that your mind, body and spirit are out of balance, so it is important to write them all down, no matter how trivial some may seem. They are an expression of need, a call for help from your body.

A thorough case history should take into account your personality, constitution, stress – both past and present – to help you to recognize any underlying patterns.

In addition to noting any symptoms you have at present, it is important to consider your health as a child. Systems that are inherently weak often show up quite early in life. If you frequently caught colds, or suffered from sore throats or ear infections which were treated with antibiotics, your immune system is likely to be a weak area. An allergy to dust mites, pollens or certain foods is another telltale sign. Such immune system weakness does not go away on its own accord although your symptoms may shift to give you that impression.

When a weakness in one system exists, others will compensate for it. Over the years these systems may also begin to exhibit symptoms of upset because they have been overworked or over-loaded. Adding stress of any kind may precipitate or exacerbate such symptoms because stress plays on any inherent weakness. If you are not sure what your symptoms are telling you, refer to Chapter 6 to discover which systems may not be functioning as well as they should.

YOUR OWN CASE HISTORY

Name   Date
Age   Date of birth
Occupation Marital status
Children

MEDICAL HISTORY

Health problems of a) mother b) father
Illnesses running in the family
  Your health as a child
  Your health problems as an adult
Past operations, accidents, injuries
If you are a mother, how did you feel during your pregnancy?
  Birth – was it trouble free or difficult?

PERSONALITY TRAITS

Write down as many different personality traits –
good and bad – you can think of that best describe you
  For example
  – are you impatient or easy going?
  – do you prefer to be alone or crave the
   company of others?
Be as honest and, if possible, ask someone whom
you trust and respect to comment on your character
assessment

LIFESTYLE

Stress levels at home
  – low (not noticeable)
  – moderate (manageable)
  – high (struggling to cope)
  – excessive (not coping)
Stress levels at work
  – low (not noticeable)
  – moderate (manageable)
  – high (struggling to cope)
  – excessive (not coping)
Shock/trauma/loss
  past
  present
Assess your energy levels
  – plentiful
  – sufficient
  – lacking
  – totally drained
Best time of the day
Worst time of the day
Do you smoke?
Do you drink alcohol?
  If so how often and how much?
Are you taking or have you recently taken prescribed meditation?

Addictions
  alcohol sugar/sweet foods
  tobacco chocolate
  coffee   tea
  other

RELATIONSHIPS – DESCRIBE BOTH GOOD AND BAD POINTS

With your mother father
Spouse or partner Children

PRESENT SENSE OF WELL-BEING

Physical – do you suffer from recurring health problems?
  If so list symptoms, for example:
  colds and flu (how often, seasonal or
  consistent throughout the year)
  headaches
  digestive problems
  poor circulation
  poor elimination
  sleeping difficulties
  breathing difficulties
  blood-pressure (high or low?)

For women only – describe your menstrual cycle.
Are your periods regular, do you experience any
pain, pre-menstrual symptoms, mood swings, any
other abnormalities?

Mental – do you have difficulty thinking clearly?
  If so, list problems, for example:
  poor concentration weak memory
  mental fatigue   absent-mindedness
  forgetfulness   learning difficulties
  mental chatter

Emotional – do you feel emotionally calm and content?
If not, list your predominant feelings, for example:
  anger   confusion
  lack of confidence depression
  irritability   mood swings
  tearfulness   night fears

Spiritual – are you happy with and feel in control of your life?
  If not, list reasons why, for example:
  feeling unfulfilled or empty
  not knowing which path to follow
  confusion about beliefs
  disillusionment with life and others

WELL-BEING QUIZ

Give each subject a score of between 0 and 10
0 = no problem 10 = serious problem

Stress	Trauma
Sleep	Health
Fear	Self-esteem
Thoughts	Emotions
Life changes	State of energy
Outside influences	Childhood
Motivation	Sexuality
Fulfilment	Crisis
Relationships	Other

❈ CHOOSING FLOWER ESSENCES ❈

By now you may be wondering how many different flower essences you are going to need to deal with your problems.

Go through your personal case history again and underline those symptoms that stand out clearly and strongly. It is best to leave vague and unclear symptoms alone for the moment – you may refer to them later if you cannot make up your mind about which is the most appropriate remedy for you. If you are new to taking flower essences, begin with your psychological and physical symptoms before attempting to deal with any spiritual issues.

Chapter 7 discusses in some detail the different emotional and spiritual symptoms that can indicate the deeper cause of any imbalance or problem you may be experiencing. The Ailment Chart (Chapter 5), too, will show you at a glance which essences are indicated for a whole variety of physical, psychological and spiritual problems.

If, for instance, you are suffering from insomnia you will see 10 essences listed in the Ailment Chart. Taking each one in turn, refer to the Encyclopaedia section where you will find a fuller description of the essence. You may end up with just one or two that are best suited to your particular type of insomnia.

USING YOUR INTUITION

Read the essence descriptions and determine which ones feel right for you. If you are not entirely sure, follow your intuition. Learn to recognize your instinctive 'yes' to some and 'no' to others. Usually certain essences will tend to catch your eye straight away. They are often flowers you naturally prefer. You may already have chosen them for your garden or they may be the kind you most often buy for your home. These may be the ones you will end up choosing for your combination.

Don't try choosing your essences when you are tired and confused. Come back to it when you are feeling more refreshed and relaxed. Taking a few drops of one of the Emergency or Rescue Remedies beforehand can help you calm down.

BY PENDULUM

If you feel confident about using a pendulum you can dowse for your essences. Most people find they can become reasonably proficient with a little practice.

A pendulum can be anything from a ring to a quartz crystal on a thin chain or string. Its movements provide answers to the questions you choose to ask.

To dowse, hold your pendulum between your thumb and forefinger so that it hangs downwards. Swing it gently back and forth. With practice you will find that when you concentrate or think 'yes' the pendulum will start to move in one direction. When you change this to a 'no' it will start to move in another, probably the opposite direction. It may swing back and forth or in circles – there are no hard and fast rules.

Once you have your positive and negative responses when you ask your pendulum certain questions (such as 'Is this an appropriate essence for me at this time?') it should give you either a yes or no. If it is indecisive, there may be no clear-cut answer.

❋ CREATING YOUR PERSONAL PRESCRIPTION ❋

Ideally you should select no more than seven flower essences for your personal prescription. These should be the ones you feel will be most helpful at this particular time.

When purchasing a flower essence from any supplier you will be getting what is known as the Stock Essence. This is a concentrated form which will need to be diluted to the proper dosage level to make your personal prescription. (Full directions for making up your personal prescription are given in Chapter 6.)

❋ THE SELF-HEALING PROCESS ❋

Self-healing is invariably a slow and gradual process, so it is important to be patient.

It may have taken many years for negative behavioural patterns or deeply ingrained emotional states to have become a part of your life, so you cannot expect them to vanish overnight. Similarly, physical problems do not appear without warning. Tiredness and mood changes are early warning signs that our internal balance is disturbed, and other symptoms will follow if we do not take stock of our current situation.

Flower essences are not magic bullets – they are subtle remedies which act as catalysts for change. Don't be concerned if you become more aware of your physical or emotional symptoms when you start the course of treatment. This is natural and shows that the remedies have begun their conversation with the blueprint. My clients often report that a part of them (the Higher Self) is watching the whole process, making them more aware of what their symptoms are telling them.

Often a physical condition or emotional state will clear, only for a deeper emotion to surface. This particular emotion may be associated with an earlier stressful experience or trauma in your life. It is often important to retrace your steps, as if going back in time in order to release that emotion, before you can move forward. This is nothing to be alarmed about. You will not have to relive the emotional intensity or pain of the experience. It is more like being a passive observer who remains detached from what is happening.

Those using the flower essences for physical and psychological problems may find that as time goes on they are drawn to the more spiritually-orientated remedies. It is rather like peeling back the petals of a rosebud until you finally get to the real source of your problems.

❋ TIPS ON CHOOSING REMEDIES FOR OTHERS ❋

Flower essences are wonderful remedies for babies, young children, animals and even plants because they are so gentle and free from harmful side-effects. They are incredibly effective – and you do not necessarily have to believe in them to reap their benefits!

As babies and animals cannot say how they are feeling, you will have to use your intuition and read the signs to select the most appropriate flower essences. This is not difficult. After all, mothers instinctively know when their children are anxious, irritable, insecure, frustrated or angry.

For babies and young children you will find symptoms such as teething, restlessness, disturbed sleep, night terrors, temper tantrums and colic listed in the Ailment Chart (Chapter 5). Flower essences for these conditions are often best used individually. If you are making a combination, it is best to keep it simple – a mix of two or three flower essences is plenty. It is helpful, too, to have an all-purpose Emergency or Rescue Remedy (*see page* 80) on hand for minor accidents or traumas which end in tears, such as falling over or being given routine inoculations.

Pets and other animals can also benefit from being given flower essences, especially those that are deemed to be neurotic or aggressive. It is worth bearing in mind that most animals are very sensitive to the emotional states of their owners, so if you are giving remedies to your cat, dog or horse, it may be a good idea to take some yourself as well.

In the Himalayan Aditi Flower family (*see pages* 100-104) you will find specific remedies for plants, to aid their growth, reduce infection and minimize the shock of transplanting, pruning or any harm brought on by poor weather or accident.

❋ TAKING FLOWER REMEDIES ❋

It is important to get into the habit of taking a remedy regularly to reap its full benefits.

Take two to three drops in the morning (on rising) and in the evening (on retiring). At these times your mind is usually most relaxed and receptive to the essences. It may be a good idea to keep your chosen remedy beside your bed so you remember to take it as you wake up and before you go to sleep.

Some people find it helpful to focus on the positive qualities of the essence and visualize their symptoms lifting as they take their remedy.

For severe cases you may need to take the remedy more frequently. In addition to your morning and evening dose, take another one at midday. If the symptoms become more intense or get worse – particularly those of a physical nature such as headaches or skin problems – double the number of drops you would normally take until they clear.

Towards the end of the two-month treatment course you may find you need to take the essence less frequently. You may even forget to take it altogether, signifying that you no longer need that particular essence or combination of essences.

❀ WAYS TO USE THE ESSENCES ❀

These flower essences are vibrational remedies, so the best way to experience their effects is to surround ourselves with them, both inside and out.

BY MOUTH

The traditional way of taking flower essences (diluted to the dosage level) is to drop them under the tongue. Placing them under the tongue seems to enhance their absorption. This method also hearkens back nicely to the way ancient healers would sip the dewdrops of flowers to cull their precious benefits.

- **Try to avoid letting the dropper touch your mouth, as this tends to create bacterial growth in the essence.**
- **The drops can also be added to drinks such as herbal teas, spring water and juices, but on no account to coffee or tea.**
- **You may dilute the remedies quite a bit. Rather like homoeopathic remedies, flower essences are equally effective, if not more so, when they are very dilute.**

ON THE SKIN

Flower essences can also be beneficial when gently rubbed onto the skin. Good places to apply them are your forehead, lips, wrists, soles of the feet and palms of the hands.

This method is useful if someone is unable to take the essences by mouth. He or she may, for instance, be unconscious, in which case it may be helpful to give an emergency, first-aid essence to ease the state of shock (*see page* 211).

Another way to apply the flower essences is to add them, usually at Stock concentration, to compresses, body packs, creams, lotions, ointments and oils.

To enhance the effectiveness of a relaxing massage, add a few drops of one or two of the soothing flower essences to your body oil.

Good ones to try are Chamomile (Cal), Dandelion, Lavender (Fes), or Yellow Ginger (Haii).

Another idea is to add a few drops to your favourite moisturizer or skin cream, one you use every day. Some flower essences are particularly helpful for revitalizing and rejuvenating tired, ageing skin (*see page* 178).

BATH THERAPY

You can create a remedy bath by adding a few drops of flower essence to your bath and soaking for up to 30 minutes. In these relaxing conditions the energy of the remedy is readily absorbed into the system.

Choose one that is most appropriate to

your needs at that particular time. After a fraught day at work you may benefit from an essence to clear your mind and promote relaxation (such as White Chestnut , Chamomile [Cal], or Five Flower Rescue [Bach]). If in need of a morning pick-me-up, it is best to choose an essence that helps counter lethargy (such as Morning Glory [Cal; Haii]). A good way to enhance the benefits of the essences is to add a few handfuls of pure sea salt to the bath as it is running.

For a curative night-time treatment, add five drops of your personal prescription to the bath. Stay in the water for 30 minutes.

BODY SPLASH

Splashing or spraying your body with flower essences (diluted with pure spring water) is an effective way of treating sensitive skin conditions such as eczema, cold sores, blisters, blemishes and surface grazes.

Add seven drops of essence to a bowl of spring water and, if possible, leave out in the sun for a day. Splash the potentized flower water onto the part of your body needing treatment and allow it to dry naturally. Alternatively you could use an atomizer to spray the diluted essences onto your skin.

For burns, insect stings, animal bites or cuts where there is an element of shock or trauma combine a few drops of an emergency/first-aid combination with an appropriate flower essence (*see pages* 211). Spray night and morning, or more frequently for shock.

Another way to benefit from the essences is to spray your clothes and pillow cases before ironing them. For those who have sleeping problems such as insomnia or nightmares, it may be a good idea to place a few drops of an essence on your pillow before going to bed. This can be particularly helpful for babies and children who have a tendency to wake during the night because of nightmares.

ROOM SPRAY

Spraying flower essences into the air is an excellent way to improve the atmosphere of any room. Add 4–5 drops to a 250-ml plant spray filled with still spring water and spray the mixture around the room every couple of hours.

Cleansing and protecting essences are beneficial for city environments as well as offices filled with cigarette smoke and chemicals given off by photocopiers and so forth (*see page* 180 of the Ailment Chart).

This method of using the flower essences is also recommended if you have a cold or influenza, as well as for breathing difficulties brought on by asthma or hayfever. An essence for boosting the immune system can help to protect you from infection if a bacterial or viral epidemic has broken out in your place of work. Some essences are particularly helpful for improving the general atmosphere. (*See pages* 209-10)

❋ STORING THE ESSENCES ❋

It is important to remember that these remedies are *pure* energy. They are activated and will start to work on your energy system the moment the combination is made up and the spring water is added.

Being 'vibrationally alive', they are highly susceptible to negative influences in the environment. Always store the essences in tinted glass dropper bottles to protect them from sunlight. Keep them away from any electrical- or radiation-emitting appliance such as a television, radio or computer.

Don't leave them on your dressing table or in your medicine cabinet next to prescribed medication, essential oils, perfume or herbs. If stored in these conditions the liquid may go cloudy, or a mucus-type substance or tiny specks of impurities may form. If this happens, throw it away.

The best place to keep your personal prescription is beside your bed, provided again it is not sharing a space with a clock-radio or other appliance!

PART TWO

ENCYCLOPAEDIA
OF
FLOWER ESSENCES

*This encyclopaedia is a compilation of flower essences from all around
the world. Each floral family offers a wide variety of different essences,
many of which are made from flowers that grow locally or
are indigenous to a particular country.*

You will notice that the properties of one type of flower, for instance Chamomile, may vary slightly according to the family to which it belongs. Just as wines from different regions have their own distinct characteristics, so have flowers. The same rose growing wild in the hedgerows of Britain may have slightly different qualities to that found several thousands of miles away in New Zealand, due to differences in habitat, climate and so forth. The description of each flower essence also depends on the interpretations of the person who discovered and originally prepared it.

The essences listed address a broad spectrum of physical, emotional, mental as well as spiritual issues. You may wonder why it is important to have so many different essences at hand. Once you begin to use the remedies this will become clear. As your awareness expands, there will be times when you find that you need remedies of an increasingly refined or higher vibration.

AFRICA AND THE AMAZON

Andreas Korte Essences (AK)

AUSTRALIA AND NEW ZEALAND

Australia:
Bush Flower Essences (Aus B)
Living Essences of Australia (Aus L)

New Zealand:
New Perception Flower Essences (NZ)

EUROPE

Britain:
Bach Flower Remedies/Healing Herbs
Company (B)
Bailey Essences (Ba)
Findhorn Flower Essences (F)
Green Man Tree Essences (GM)
Harebell Remedies (Hb)

France:
Deva Flower Elixirs (Dv)

INDIA

Himalayan Aditi Flower Essences (Him A)
Himalayan Flower Enhancers (Him E)
Himalayan Indian Tree and
Flower Essences (Him I)

USA AND CANADA

USA

Alaska:
Alaskan Flower and Environmental Essences
(Ask)

Arizona:
Desert Alchemy Flower Essences (DAl)

California:
F.E.S. and Californian Research
Essences (Cal)
Flower Essence Society (Fes)
Master's Flower Essences (Ma)

Colorado:
Pegasus Essences (Peg)
Hawaiian Tropical Flower Essences (Haii)

Texas:
Petite Fleur Essences (PF)
Virginia: Perelandra Virginian Rose and
Garden Essences (PVi)

CANADA
Pacific Essences (Pac)

Gem Essences:
Flower and Gem Remedy Association (Gem)

AFRICA AND THE AMAZON

*The Amazon is home to
a vast number of different species of flowering plants. In Colombia over
4,000 species of orchid can be found, many of which live 25–35 m (80–115 ft)
up in the trees. Here, at the top of the tropical rainforests, they obtain
sufficient light to support their existence. Their roots have adapted to
anchor them to the branches so they have no direct contact with the earth.
The continent of Africa has
many regions of total wilderness and is also home to many unusual
flowering plants, as well as many that have yet to be discovered.
It was the promise of such
untapped potential that attracted Andreas Korte to these subtropical
regions in his quest for new and unique flower essences. The names of some
of the flowers from which he prepares his essences are protected because
they are so rare – to these he gives only code letters/numbers.*

❋ ANDREAS KORTE ESSENCES ❋

Andreas Korte is a researcher and specialist in the field of essences. Brought up in a small village by a forest near Lake Constance in Germany, he has always believed in the flower devas. He regards Orchids as queens of the plant kingdom, feeling that they have an exceptionally high vibrational rate and are responsible for creating a link between the cosmos, ourselves and the earth. The orchids often take the form or shape of angels and appear to have human features.

Andreas has invented a gentle, ecological method of preparing essences so that the flowers are not harmed in any way. This involves cleaning and preparing one half of a quartz geode (a naturally occurring stone containing crystals split into two semi-spherical halves) and filling it with natural spring water. He then carefully places the geode into the energetic field of the blossoms and leaves it in the sun for a length of time (which differs from flower to flower). The special crystal formation of the geode acts to focus and capture the energy of the flowers.

Co-author of *Orchids, Gemstones and their Healing Energies*, he is currently involved in research projects in Europe, Africa and South America.

ORCHIDS OF THE AMAZON

AGGRESSION (*Asinetas superba*) For blockages in lower chakras. Releases basic energy, sexuality, impulsiveness and aggression.

AMAZON RIVER For loosening energetic blockages, especially in the back. Brings free-flowing energy, understanding and comprehension of the planet.

ANGEL (*Epidendron secundum*) For opening up to higher states of consciousness. Brings lightness, stepping up the vibrational rate in order to open us to the higher levels of consciousness and allow communication with our spirit guide (guardian angel).

ANGEL OF PROTECTION (*Miltonea phalenopsis*) For fragile, sensitive people who need shelter from hostility and harsh environments. Provides a protective shield for sensibilities and vulnerabilities. Improves communication with our spirit guides.

CHANNELLING (*Oncidium incurvum*) For increasing direct contact and communication with your spirit guide and universal being. Allows channelling – the receiving and passing on of messages.

CHOCOLATE (*Stanhopea wadrii*) For those who take spirituality too seriously. Allows you to walk the path of joy.

COLOUR (*Oncidium landeanum*) For those who have a tendency to be sad, thinking life is grey and hopeless. Helps you to recognize that your thoughts guide your life experiences.

CO-ORDINATION (*Cymbidium lowianum*) For those with co-ordination difficulties. Promotes cell growth and stimulates self-healing.

DEVA (*Epidendrum prismatocarpum*) For opening up to communication with devas or the spirits of flowers and trees. Brings integration with the natural environment and an opening up to healing from nature.

FUN (*Vandas tricolor*) For laughter, harmony and love of life. Increases humour and zest for life. Allows you to see life's problems from a different and wider perspective.

HEART (*Laeliocattleya hybr*) For raising self-centredness to the heart level. Transforms ego-centred love to pure spiritual love.

HIGHER SELF (*Laeliocattleya anceps clara*) For communication and self-knowledge. Connects you to your Higher Self and increases your capacity to act as a messenger.

HORN OF PLENTY (*Cattleya warcsewiczii*) For experiencing infinite, 'universal' love. Brings the ability to give and receive this love freely.

INSPIRATION (*Carrleya trianae*) For inner inspiration. Helps you get in touch with higher spiritual levels, bringing inspiration that can be used creatively.

LOVE (*Oncidium abortivum*) For opening the heart chakra. Allows energy and love to flow freely. Opens the heart, allowing this love to be utilized for healing and compassion.

PAST LIFE (*Paphiopedilum hairysianum*) For enhancing self-knowledge, understanding and inspiration. Facilitates access to past-life stream of consciousness to retrieve lost skills, meanings and stored knowledge.

PSYCHE OR SOUL (*Paphiopedilum insigne*) For knowledge of life. Allows access to the subconscious in order to discover the reason for our existence.

SUN (*Cymbidium*) For balance and harmony. Connects us directly with the energy of the sun by opening and harmonizing the solar plexus and re-balancing the ego.

VENUS (*Anguloa cliftonii*) For understanding, tenderness, love and listening skills. Stimulates the female receptive energy, promoting these qualities.

VICTORIA REGIA (*Victoria amazonica*) For explosive energy and transformation. Brings a powerful release of natural energy, or kundalini. Supports the transformation process of dying and death itself.

ROSE ESSENCES

APPLE/ROSE HYBRID ('Sarah of Fleet'/'White Rose') For opening the heart centre to the deeper experience of life. Allows love to flow and teaches us to give this love without expectation.

APPLE/ROSE HYBRID ('Souvenir de Philemon Cochet') To achieve unity of mind, body and soul. Allows love to flow through the entire system, reconnecting head to heart and recreating a single unit. Helps the energy of love to run through our entire being, infusing the crown, upper chakras and beyond.

CINNAMON ROSE Restores hope at times when there seems to be no way out. Sustains the principle of hope when there is darkness in our souls.

JAPANESE ROSE For humble, modest people needing to learn the principles of hope and love of life. Brings the knowledge that hope is the original source, and love the elixir of life.

SPRING GOLD Links the solar plexus to the heart chakra. Helps you to accept yourself as you are, enabling you to love and express this love through the solar plexus.

TIBETAN WHITE ROSE Integration process, connected with love energy – for those who need help in learning to love themselves.

WILD ROSE HYBRID Helps to integrate into one's being the incoming higher energies and outgoing love. Allows an all-encompassing love to flow back to the earth.

ESSENCES OF WILD PLANTS

ALMOND TREE For those who are afraid of the accelerated ageing process. Eases this fear.

ALOE VERA For restoring inner balance. Helps in states of exhaustion, replenishing life energies.

ARNICA For re-establishing the connection to the Higher Self, especially after anaesthetics, drug addiction or shock.

ARUM LILY For conflicts concerning sexual identity. Helps you to learn to accept the male and female aspects of yourself.

BASIL For times when sexuality gives rise to conflict or fear. Integrates sexuality as a natural part of life.

BLACKBERRY For those who have problems initiating protects. Helps us realize our creative power to execute projects and follow them through.

BLEEDING HEART For all affairs of the heart; admitting love. Offers support to those who have lost someone dear, or when a relationship ends.

BLUE FLAG IRIS For accessing creative potential. Helps you to receive impulses for creative work.

BORAGE For feelings of darkness, depression and discouragement. Rekindles cheerful courage and joy.

BUTTERCUP For those feeling weak and inferior. Increases self-esteem and boosts self-confidence.

CHAMOMILE Especially for those who are easily worked up and have difficulty calming down again. Soothes and calms.

CORN Ideal for town-dwellers searching for contact with the earth. Promotes connection with the earth.

DAISY For integrating many different thoughts. Ideal for children during the learning process. Helps make it easier to take in and analyse new information.

DANDELION For reducing tension. Loosens emotional tensions, especially those manifesting in the muscles.

DILL Ideal for children of which too much is expected; for going on journeys. Enables us to digest and process seemingly overwhelming impressions and experiences.

FIRE LILY For achieving the correct attitude towards sexuality. Brings self-understanding and helps to direct sexual energy towards the heart.

FORGET-ME-NOT Stimulates the subconscious and dreaming. Helps us remember friends who are no longer here.

FRENCH LAVENDER For digesting spiritual experiences. Calms in cases of overstrain. Helps us to open ourselves for spirituality and to integrate it into our daily lives.

KNOTGRASS For those who have a tendency to be in several places at one time in their thoughts. Helps put you entirely in the present moment.

LOTUS The universal flower which kindles harmony in all areas. Opens the crown chakra to higher energies.

MISTLETOE For help with going through a radical process of change. Aids transformation on both the physical and psychological levels.

MORNING GLORY Supports withdrawal and rehabilitation. Helps us become conscious of our negative living habits and addictions.

MULLEIN For helping us listen to our inner voice and conscience. Aids in the ability to be true to ourselves, even in teamwork, and to develop ourselves.

PASSION FLOWER For raising energy so that we can open ourselves to spirituality. Helps us to integrate spirituality as a reality in our lives.

PINK YARROW For those who are too easily influenced by the emotions of others. Improves protection of the heart and emotions.

PUMPKIN For integrating femininity. Brings harmony during pregnancy, promoting bonding between mother and child.

RED CLOVER For panic and fear. Helps us stay calm and centred in the face of dread.

ROSE BOY WILLOW HERB For comprehending shock and traumatic situations, for example after an accident. Brings resolution.

ROSEMARY For forgetfulness. Helps us to be more aware and conscious of what is happening in our lives.

ROSE OF SHARON For childish fears and nightmares. Increases ability to experience inner light as the guide of consciousness and to trust in the protection of a divine guide.

SAGE 'Purifying'. Promotes dawning of consciousness to help us integrate our life experiences.

SELF-HEAL Stimulates self-healing powers, especially on the cellular level. Brings courage to be healthy.

SUNFLOWER Helps in conflict situations with the father figure, both natural and archetypal.

VALERIAN For cases of severe stress leading to insomnia. 'Soothing.'

VIOLET For people who feel lonely in a group. Brings increased openness so you can interact with others better. Develops warmth and faith.

WHITE LILY Promotes Christ-consciousness. Opens the crown (seventh) chakra and fills the body with white light.

WHITE YARROW For sensitive people exposed to negative environmental influences. Strengthens the light of aura protecting us from negative environmental influences. Increases our protective shield.

WILD CARROT For when the same thoughts persistently invade the mind, swirling round and round in your head. Soothes and eases worries and anxieties.

WILD GARLIC For fear. Doubly active essence for strengthening our psychological defence mechanisms against all forms of fear in a soothing and calming way.

ZINNIA Stimulates childlike humour. Helps us relax and loosen up emotionally, so we re-learn how to laugh and see things less tragically.

AFRICAN RESEARCH ESSENCES

BANANA Stimulates the male sexual energies.

BIRD OF PARADISE For those who view themselves as unsightly or ugly. Helps in finding one's inner beauty.

CANARY ISLAND BELLFLOWER For the conscious integration of female sexuality.

CANARY ISLAND WORMWOOD To help those who have been ill for a long time to re-adopt the life force or energy.

CERATO 'Liberating'. Helps those who are not able to set themselves free from something.

COCONUT PALM For sensitive people. Helps you to learn to develop a hard outer shell.

EUCALYPTUS For helping to accept life as it is. A freeing influence.

GERANIUM For those lacking joy and happiness. Helps you to see and bring more colour into life.

HOOP PETTICOAT DAFFODIL For despair. Brings light in moments when we are not able to see the light.

MILK THISTLE For emotional tension. Relaxes and loosens the emotions. Excellent when added to massage oils.

K9 (the name of this flower is protected) For the immune system. Strengthens the body's natural defence system on all levels. Antiviral effect. Still being researched.

K14/VIPER'S BUGLOSS For humourless people. Helps those who need to feel free to be themselves.

K18 (*Echium wildpretii*) For those who have had to face strong resistance and who give up too easily. 'Breakthrough.'

ROCK ROSE For low self-confidence. Promotes integration in a group, helping to strengthen and encourage the ability to say yes to yourself.

PIMPERNEL For learning to integrate in a group situation. Promotes the integration of spirituality.

POINSETTIA For those who are unable to express their emotions. Links the heart and throat chakras.

RED HIBISCUS For integrating and being at ease with female sexuality.

SWISS CHEESE PLANT Strengthens the male sexual energies and re-balances everything.

TREE HEATHER For people who are over-emotional and only able to fulfil themselves through others.

YELLOW MIMOSA For those who feel unable to dedicate themselves to opening up and realizing their own inner richness.

SPECIAL ESSENCES

T1 CHERNOBYL RESEARCH ESSENCE Soaks up radiation like a sponge. Brings regeneration after exposure to radioactivity, electromagnetic fields, earth radiation.

Made by Andreas at the Chernobyl plant itself seven years after the nuclear explosion occurred, when tested after leaving the site these essences showed no trace of radioactivity.

DELPH [DOLPHIN] ESSENCE A re-energizer and cleanser that activates all the chakras and subtle bodies. Made in the Caribbean where seven wild dolphins were playing. It is said dolphins are the guardians of the ancient wisdom and secrets. The essence has a special role to play in cleansing the seas, rivers, lakes and waters of the earth.

Recommended for childbirth to ease the trauma of coming into the world. Helps babies to be peaceful and serene.

ESSENCE SKIN CREAMS

Andreas Korte makes a range of Essence Skin Creams which (with the exception of Amazon and Emergency, can be personalized by adding a few drops of your own prescription mix (*see page* 42) or other specially selected flower essences.

Amazon Skin Cream is recommended for massaging into areas of the body when the energy flow is stifled or blocked.

Emergency Cream, containing seven different flower essences, is for shock or injury to the skin such as bruising. It also energizes and stimulates.

Venus Orchid Skin Cream is a deeply relaxing preparation for the face and body which enhances feminine softness of the skin.

Lotus Skin Cream restores energetic harmony and balance to the skin through its relaxing properties.

Self-heal Skin Cream stimulates self-healing for irritated or chaffed skin. Ideal for using as an after-shave balm.

AUSTRALIA

Australia was once part of the
southern landmass known as Gondwanalan. The land has a powerful and
vibrant energy that has not been weakened by civilization, war or pollution.
Native Aborigines have long acknowledged
the power of the flower kingdom and have been using flowers to heal
emotional imbalance and physical injuries for over 10,000 years.

❋ BUSH FLOWER ESSENCES ❋

Some of the oldest flowering plants in the world can be found growing in the wilderness of the Australian Bush. They draw upon and reflect the power, strength and vitality of this extraordinary region.

The collection of Australian Bush Flower Essences described below were created by Ian White, a fifth-generation herbalist who spent much of his childhood in the Bush learning from his grandmother about the healing properties of Australian plants and flowers. He spent many years travelling and researching the properties of flowers growing in areas as diverse as the Northern Territory wetlands, the Olgas, the Kimberleys, the South Australian deserts, the Victorian heathlands and Sydney's sandstone region before he, together with Kirstin White, developed the Australian Bush Flower Essences in the early 1980s.

The main focus of these remedies is to bring out and cultivate the positive qualities present in everyone. The Waratah flower, chosen to represent this collection of essences, is unique to Australia. It comes from one of the oldest plant groups in the world whose origins date back 60 million years to Antarctica. Known by its Aboriginal name, meaning beautiful, the Waratah has a magnificent red bloom comprising many individual flowers which are tightly packed together. The Waratah is a survival remedy. It embodies the Australian Bush-dweller's qualities of adaptability and the ability to cope with all sorts of emergencies. Ian believes that in the years to come there will be major economic, social, physical and spiritual upheavals which will take us by surprise. The Waratah will help by aiding people to find the courage and strength they need to deal with such change.

ALPINE MINT BUSH For mental and emotional exhaustion, lack of joy, feeling the weight of responsibility. Brings revitalization, joy and renewal.

ANGELSWORD For those who are spiritually possessed. Helps in attaining spiritual truth/protection and access to gifts from past lifetimes. Repairs the whole energy field.

BANKSIA ROBUR For people who are normally dynamic but are suffering a temporary loss of drive and enthusiasm due to burn-out, frustration or illness. Restores energy and the enjoyment of and interest in life.

BAUHINIA For resistance to change and rigidity. Encourages the embracing of new concepts and ideas, bringing acceptance and open-mindedness.

BILLY GOAT PLUM For sexual revulsion, physical loathing or self-disgust. Brings sexual pleasure and enjoyment, acceptance of one's physical body. Good for skin conditions such as eczema, psoriasis, herpes and thrush.

BLACK-EYED SUSAN A remedy for stress. For those always on the go, rushing, constantly striving and impatient. Slows you down, enabling you to turn inward, be still and enjoy inner peace.

BLUEBELL For those cut off from their feelings, fearful of emptiness and vulnerable to greed. Opens the heart, encourages sharing and belief in abundance, gives a sense of joy and universal trust.

BOAB For those who adopt family thought-patterns, repeating negative experiences of the past. Releases negative thought-patterns and actions within families. Good for abuse and prejudice.

BORONIA For obsessive thoughts, grieving over recently ended relationships, feeling broken-hearted. Brings mental calmness, serenity, clarity of mind and thought.

BOTTLEBRUSH For those going through and overwhelmed by major life changes such as puberty or pregnancy. Holding on to the past and old habits when approaching the end of a phase in life. Restores ability to cope with serenity and to be calm by letting go. Good for pregnant women and new mothers who feel inadequate. Assists bonding between mother and child.

BUSH FUCHSIA For poor ability to learn, dyslexia, stuttering, ignoring 'gut feelings'. Unsurpassed for resolving learning problems, balancing and integrating the left and right hemispheres of the brain. Brings clarity to expression and speech. Develops intuition.

BUSH GARDENIA For those caught up in their own world and affairs, taking for granted and being oblivious of those close to them. For stale or failing relationships. Brings passion, renewed interest in a partner; improves communication.

BUSH IRIS For fear of death, of materialism, of atheism, addiction to sex and drugs. Brings spiritual awakening and insights, understanding of things beyond the physical. Assists in making transitions in life.

CROWEA For individuals who continually worry; feeling out of balance. Brings peace, calm, vitality and a sense of being centred and balanced.

DAGGER HAKEA For resentment, bitterness

towards close family, friends and old lovers. Brings forgiveness and enables feelings to be expressed.

DOG ROSE For fearful, shy, insecure people who are apprehensive of others. For niggling fears. Promotes confidence, courage, belief in oneself and a love of life.

DOG ROSE OF THE WILD FORCES For those who fear losing control, for physical pain with no apparent cause. Brings emotional balance, ability to overcome fear.

FIVE CORNERS For low self-esteem and self-dislike. For those who repress or 'hold in' their personality. An important remedy for bringing love, acceptance of oneself and a celebration of one's inherent beauty.

FLANNEL FLOWER For those who dislike being touched, lack of sensitivity, especially in males, an aversion to physical activity and agoraphobia. Encourages emotional trust, sensuality and gentle, sensitive touching. Makes physical activity joyful.

FRINGED VIOLET For shock and trauma, damage to the aura and lack of psychic protection allowing energy and vitality drained by other people and environmental factors like radiation. Poor recuperation. Removes the effects of recent and old trauma, realigns the subtle bodies after shock and gives psychic and energy protection.

GREEN SPIDER ORCHID For nightmares, phobias. Those needing acceptance. Brings release from terror and the ability to guard information.

GREY SPIDER FLOWER For terror, panic and fear of psychic attack. Nightmares. Gives faith, calmness and courage.

GYMEA LILY For proud, dominating and controlling personalities. Brings humility and the ability to let go of control.

HIBBERTIA For fanaticism, excessive self-discipline, addiction to acquiring knowledge for self-improvement. Allows you to accept yourself, your own knowledge and experiences. Dispels the desire to be superior to others.

ILLAWARRA FLAME TREE For those suffering from a sense of rejection and feeling left out, especially for children undergoing temporary setbacks at school. Fear of responsibility. Brings self-approval and reliance, confidence and inner strength.

ISOPOGON For poor memory, senility, an inability to learn from past experience. For a stubborn, controlling personality. Brings learning from past experiences, retrieval of forgotten skills and memories. Allows you to relate to others without manipulation and control.

JACARANDA For those who are changeable, dithering, aimless, scattered, always rushing around and accident prone. Brings decisiveness, quick thinking and a clear mind.

KANGAROO PAW For socially immature, clumsy or gauche individuals who are insensitive to the needs of others. Encourages relaxation, sensitivity, *savoir faire* and enjoyment of company.

KAPOK BUSH For people who are easily discouraged and give up easily, resigned and apathetic. Brings persistence, common sense, practicality and a willingness to apply yourself to any task.

LITTLE FLANNEL FLOWER For denial of the child within, over-serious adults, precocious children who grow up too quickly. Restores sense of playfulness and joy. For having fun.

MACROCARPA For those who are tired, exhausted, burnt out and, as a result, have poor immune resistance. A tonic, quick pick-me-up which regenerates the adrenal glands, restoring energy, strength and vitality.

MINT BUSH For spiritual trial and tribulation, despair, feeling overwhelmed. Brings calmness, the ability to move on, readiness for new beginnings.

MOUNTAIN DEVIL For hatred, anger, jealousy, holding grudges and suspiciousness. Brings unconditional love, forgiveness and happiness.

MULLA MULLA For trauma associated with fire, heat or even sunburn. Fear of flames, fire and hot objects. Brings a feeling at ease with fire. Releases stored radiation and aids rejuvenation.

OLD MAN BANKSIA An Aboriginal symbol of female spirituality. For lethargy, low energy levels, sluggish thyroid activity, obesity. Restores energy, enthusiasm, the enjoyment of and interest in life.

PAW PAW For those overwhelmed and burdened by decision who are unable to resolve problems. Malabsorption of food. For assimilating and integrating new ideas and information. Improves access to the Higher Self for help in problem-solving. Aids the absorption of nutrients.

PEACH-FLOWERED TEA-TREE For mood swings, lack of commitment to completing projects due to boredom. For hypochondriacs. Brings emotional balance, completion of goals and projects. Encourages trust and taking responsibility for health without becoming preoccupied by it. Balances the pancreas.

PHILOTHECA For an inability to accept acknowledgement, excessive generosity. Brings an ability to accept praise and receive love and acknowledgement.

PINK MULLA MULLA For deep hurt, isolation, being guarded and feeling blocked. Helps in overcoming obstacles, opening up and finding forgiveness.

RED GREVILLIA For feeling stuck, knowing the goal but not how to attain it. For those who are easily affected by criticism and unpleasantness, too reliant on others. Gives strength to leave unpleasant situations. Encourages boldness.

RED HELMET For rebellious, hot-headed, selfish people who resent authority due to a poor relationship with their father. Helps men bond to children; develops sensitivity and respect.

RED LILY The sacred lotus embodying Aboriginal spirituality. For daydreamers who are vacant and accident prone. Balances spiritual and earthly aspects, enabling you to be grounded and practical while evolving spiritually. Good for autism and countering the effects of drugs.

RED SUVA FRANGIPANI For turmoil, emotional upheaval, sadness. Brings feelings of acceptance, equanimity and nurturing.

ROUGH BLUEBELL For those who lack concern for others' feelings, who are openly malicious. Brings openness, compassion and unconditional love.

SHE OAK For infertility, especially when there is no physical reason; hormonal imbalance in females, especially PMT. Restores fertility and hormonal balance; aids conception. Helps with fluid retention.

SILVER PRINCESS For lack of direction in life, aimlessness and despondency. Gives life, purpose and direction, motivation.

SLENDER RICE FLOWER For racism, narrow-mindedness, and comparing yourself to others. Encourages co-operation, humility, pride, interconnectedness and the ability to see goodness in others.

SOUTHERN CROSS For victim mentality; those who think life has been hard on them and feel hard done by; complaining, feeling impoverished. Brings personal power; taking responsibility for situations and being able to effect a positive change.

SPINIFEX For herpes, chlamydia and surface cuts or grazes. Heals physically by helping you realize the emotional issues involved. Heals skin conditions when applied topically.

STURT DESERT PEA For deep hurt, sadness and emotional pain. A powerful essence that diffuses and allows you to let go of sad memories. Motivates and re-energizes.

STURT DESERT ROSE For guilt and lack of self-esteem stemming from past actions. For those who are easily led. Helps you to follow your own inner convictions and morality.

SUNDEW For those under the age of 28 who are vague, indecisive, dissociated, lacking focus and prone to procrastination. Encourages grounding, focus, inspiration, attention to detail, enabling you to live in the present with interest. Speeds recovery from fainting and anaesthetics.

SUNSHINE WATTLE For struggle, feeling trapped in the past and expecting the worst for the future. Brings optimism and an acceptance of the beauty and joy in the present.

TALL MULLA MULLA For feeling scared and unsafe, lack of integration with others. Brings the ability to interact socially and feel secure with people.

TALL YELLOW TOP For alienation, loneliness and isolation. Brings a sense of belonging and knowing that you are 'home'.

TURKEY BUSH For creative block and disbelief in your abilities. Inspires creativity, self-expression and renewed artistic confidence.

WARATAH For black despair, suicidal thoughts, feelings of hopelessness and an inability to respond to crisis. Brings courage, tenacity and adaptability. Strengthens faith and survival skills.

WEDDING BUSH For difficulty in committing to relationships, whether business, social or intimate. Encourages commitment in and to relationships. Restores dedication to life purpose.

WILD POTATO BUSH For a sense of being physically encumbered and weighed down; for a body that is slow to respond to will. Brings freedom and vitality to move on in life.

WISTERIA Specifically for women who are tense about and unable to enjoy sex for fear of intimacy, frigidity. Also for the macho male. Brings sexual enjoyment and gentleness.

YELLOW COWSLIP ORCHID For critical, judgmental, bureaucratic attitudes. Fosters humanitarian concern, impartiality and constructiveness. Enables you to step back from emotions and develop a sense of arbitration. Balances the pituitary gland.

COMBINATIONS

EMERGENCY ESSENCE *Fringed Violet, Grey Spider Flower, Sundew and Waratah*

Calms and stabilizes, rapidly alleviating fear, panic, severe mental stress and tension. Excellent and beneficial for all psychological and physical stress.

PERSONAL POWER ESSENCE *Dog Rose, Five Corners, Southern Cross and Sturt Desert Rose*

Rekindles self-esteem and confidence, allowing us to take full responsibility for situations and events in life. Helps us to realize that we have the power to change and create our own destiny.

RADIATION ESSENCE *Bush Fuchsia, Crowea, Fringed Violet, Mulla Mulla, Paw Paw and Waratah*

Negates or reduces all forms of radiation including natural earth radiation, electrical force-fields, solar rays and radiation therapy for cancer. Also good against nuclear radiation. Prevents accumulation in the body and helps to emit already-stored radiation to keep the body's energies intact and the neurological systems functioning normally.

SUPER LEARNING ESSENCE *Bush Fuchsia, Isopogon, Paw Paw and Sundew*

A powerful combination of essences which brings about mental clarity and focus, enhancing all learning skills and abilities.

VITALITY ESSENCE *Banksia, Crowea, Macrocarpa and Old Man Banksia*

Encourages abundant energy, vitality, enthusiasm and joy for life. Balances the major glands, the thyroid and adrenals, and the muscles associated with generating and utilizing energy.

❊ LIVING ESSENCES OF AUSTRALIA ❊

The Living Essences of Australia have been researched and developed by Drs Vasudeva and Kadambii Barnao, PhD. They are mostly made from flowers that grow in the southwestern region of Australia, called the Wildflower State, an area known for its prolific and unique flora.

After moving to Australia from New Zealand, Vasudeva began his pioneering research into the native flowers of Australia in 1977.

In 1982 Vasudeva and his wife Kadambii

started working together, setting up the Australasian Flower Essence Academy and the Living Essences Clinic in Perth, Western Australia. Together they have made and researched over 200 flower essences and developed the Microvita range of creams and lotions for the relief of pain, arthritis, hypertension, stress and lethargy which are now used in hospitals and by orthodox practitioners (*see page* 249). This has led to the Baraos being invited in 1994 to create the first university flower essence course in Perth, WA.

Kadambii's work from 1985 with an Aboriginal community brought her into contact with an elder who had been entrusted with the secrets of native folk-healing. He still used the traditional flower sauna, one of the oldest-known forms of flower essence therapy dating back at least 10,000 years.

They also initiated research into the benefits of combining flower essences with the ancient Chinese art of acupuncture/acupressure to strengthen the potency of both modes of healing. Their findings led to the creation of some of the world's first Floral Acu-maps, which pinpoint specific flowers for specific acupuncture points. This therapy is proving highly effective in the treatment of pain and stress.

They have pioneered many new flower essence diagnostic techniques such as Baihui diagnosis, Field of Flowers technique and Flower Photography Diagnosis, all of which are taught internationally through their academy's video correspondence course.

At the 1990 World Congress of the Open University of Complementary Medicine and Medicina Alternativa, Drs Vasudeva and Kadambii Barnao were awarded the Gold Star of Excellence for their pioneering research work.

ANTISEPTIC BUSH For cleansing oneself from negative influences in the environment which may have built up over some time. Maintains inner sanctity when living among negative or harmful aspects or people.

BALGA BLACKBOY For those who are unaware that their personal desires and goals can create emotional or environmental catastrophes. Brings an awareness of the impact your desires may have on others, so that you understand and do not resent any natural obstacles placed in your path. For the naturation of the masculine principle.

BLACK KANGAROO PAW For those unable to forgive parents for controlling them in the past. Replaces hate and resentment with love and forgiveness.

BLUE LESCHENAULTIA For those who can be emotional and physical 'Scrooges', self-sufficient, unmoved by the needs of others. Breaks down the walls of selfish isolation, allowing you to see the needs of others and learn to share with them.

BROWN BORONIA For an overactive mind, working excessively without rest in an attempt to solve pressing problems yet being unable to find adequate solutions. Brings patience and acceptance so you do not worry unnecessarily about things you cannot change, as well as the realization that the journey of life will deliver solutions.

BRACHYCOME For lack of empathy, intellectual arrogance, over-criticism and contempt of others. Encourages appreciation of people for who they are, not how intelligent they seem.

CAPE BLUEBELL For those who have a chip on their shoulder and can be negative, displaying hatred and malice. Confers the ability to let go of the past and be loving and empathetic.

CAT'S PAW For depression, sadness and anger caused by the insincerity and selfishness of others. For families and close-knit groups with undefined problems. Helps you to drop expectations of fairness while refusing to let others take advantage, so that they too can learn fairness. Promotes mutual consideration.

CHRISTMAS TREE (KANYA) For those times when duties and everyday pressures cause you to become distant and avoid your share of the load, causing resentment among others. Helps you to meet your responsibilities and reap the rewards of consistency and shared goals. Brings inner contentment which enhances your enjoyment of your family or group.

CORREA For those who are too hard on themselves. Teaches acceptance of our limitations and shortcomings without regret. Enables us to see how we make mistakes unintentionally, and helps us to do better next time.

COWKICKS For the unsuspecting optimist who is devastated by an unexpected crisis and trauma, making him or her the depleted, hopeless victim of circumstance. Helps you to rebuild and pull the pieces back together after a shattering experience to create a wiser perspective.

DAMPIERA For those who are fearful and unable to relax, blowing all situations out of proportion. Allows you to let go and be open, to let things happen in different ways and allow people their own style.

FRINGED LILY TWINER For those who blame others for their misery when thwarted. Also for spoiled children and manipulative parents who can be vengeful and brooding. Allows you to see that selfishness lies at the root of misery. Teaches you to turn your focus away from yourself, and stimulates love.

FUCHSIA GREVILLEA For those who tend to be two-faced. Brings the realization that hidden negativity is destructive, as well as a release from smugness, anger and a dislike of being exposed.

FUCHSIA GUM For claustrophobia, both physical and emotional. Prevents feelings of panic in confined spaces.

GERALDTON WAX For those who feel trapped and resentful, who feel they are under someone else's thumb (for example a parent who always tries to appease a demanding child). Helps you to become strong enough not to be pressured against your will or influenced by the desires of others.

GODDESS GRASSTREE For maturation of the female principle (in both men and women). Brings inner strength, nurturing, sensitivity and loving wisdom that is not emotionally dependent. Releases the female aspect into society.

GOLDEN GLORY GREVILLEA For those whose trusting, open, relaxed nature has been abused, creating within them an uneasy feeling about the motives of others. Rekindles a sense of trust and confidence to allow other people into your life, not to expect or worry about being judged.

GOLDEN WAITSIA For those who worry about details as well as those needing to accept their present imperfect state of health and well-being while convalescing from illness or trauma. Re-ignites spontaneity and carefree feelings, healing all aspects of the anxiety that is caused by perfectionism.

GREEN ROSE For people intolerant of advice when needing to break through a problem, becoming agitated when challenged by new ideas – and stagnating in their isolation. Maintains progressiveness, helping you to embrace new thoughts and ideas, not to stagnate, become negative or blame others for your situation.

HAPPY WANDERER For those who doubt their abilities and need others for security and support, either emotionally, mentally or physically.

Helps you stand on your own feet, knowing you are strong enough to do things by yourself. Clears insecurity.

HOP'S BUSH For those who cannot sleep or relax due to frenetic energy. Earths excessive, scattered energy, re-establishing a natural and healthy flow which feeds your need for activity without over-stimulating you. Brings inner mental and physical peace, restoring your control over life and balanced states of rest and activity.

ILLYARRIE For those who have been badly hurt and suppress the memory. Allows you to realize that you have the strength to face and deal with any pain, that it is never as bad as you fear and it will not overwhelm you. Useful in past-life therapy to uncover forgotten experiences affecting the present.

MACROZAMIA For balancing basic flows of Yin and Yang. Balances sexual energy to free blockages brought about by bad experiences such as rape or incest. Heals and restores all aspects of the male/female – releases blockages, corrects under-development and adjusts hormonal fluctuations.

MANY-HEADED DRYANDRA For those seen as irresponsible or 'fly-by-night', displaying erratic behaviour and panic. Brings composure and strength. Helps you to confront and deal with life's problems rather than running away from them.

MAUVE MELALEUCA For the emotional idealist who has been hurt and is sad. Also for the unloved spouse, parent or child. Eases despondence about an uncaring world. Allows you to find fulfilment within and tap into the source of eternal love.

MENZIES BANKSIA For clearing the fear that history will repeat itself, in the form of past experiences of hurt and rejection. Also for psychic paralysis. Allows you to let go of past pain, move on through present pain with courage, and have no fear of new experiences.

ONE-SIDED BOTTLEBRUSH For those who are over-burdened and depressed, caught up in themselves, complaining about their workload. Brings the realization that others also have burdens to bear and keeps you from getting caught up in the 'poor me' syndrome.

ORANGE LESCHENAULTIA For true survivors, tough-skinned people who have become insensitive and lacking compassion. Encourages benevolence and caring and puts you in touch with the softer qualities of life.

ORANGE SPIKED PEA FLOWER For those who feel undermined by what others say, feeling angered to the point of violence. Helps you to let words spoken by others pass over you and not destroy your poise. Promotes self expression.

PALE SUNDEW For unscrupulous people who use people and situations for their own benefit, such as the business shark or ambitious politician. Brings the realization that being manipulative and predatory is senseless and destructive. Increases repulsion to wrong-doing. The essence is conscience.

PARAKEELYA For quiet, passive people who become the unappreciated work-horse in the family, business or community; for deep-seated loneliness and pain that comes of feeling used and uncared for. Helps you to stand up and be respected so you become the inspired worker who can enjoy belonging to the group. For self-esteem and assertiveness.

PIN CUSHION HAKEA For those whose feel their beliefs may be threatened or their logic undermined by new ideas, such as scientists and religious people. Allow you to be open to new ideas, not to fear the views of others, to relax and be more accepting without compromising your own ethics.

PINK EVERLASTING STRAW FLOWER For those who perceive others' feelings but cannot respond to them emotionally due to feeling 'dry' and depleted. Renews springs of love and joy. Helpful for teachers and care-givers.

PINK FOUNTAIN TRIGGERPLANT For those losing their inner vital force which keeps us alive, either by a slow draining on the physical level or a rupture in the subtle bodies. Re-ignites the vital flame and restores its dynamism.

PINK IMPATIENS For the idealist, the moralist who compromises through struggling to maintain his or her standards. Helps you to retain ideals and standards no matter the obstacles, to have determination and creativity to carry on without compromising.

PINK TRUMPET FLOWER For those who find it difficult to maintain their sense of purpose, who get lost during a thought-process or activity. Brings clarity and focus. Harnesses inner strength of purpose and directs it towards important goals. Encourages achievement through new mental directness.

PIXIE MOP For sensitive, emotionally needy people who have become hard because they feel let down. Brings the realization that forgiving those who let you down frees your heart, so that you can help others as you would hope to be helped yourself.

PURPLE EREMOPHILA Very helpful during relationship upsets. Helps you to gain and maintain serene objectivity amidst very personal issues of the heart, without compromising your richness of feeling and sensitivity towards loved ones.

PURPLE FLAG FLOWER For those who push themselves to their stress threshold, making them feel extremely anxious and unable to relax. Brings healing relaxation of mind and body. Helps you to unwind, releasing built-up pressure and tension.

PURPLE NYMPH WATERLILY Helps those wishing to share their treasures with others but finding themselves holding back. Brings selfless service, while making sure you are not caught in emotional traps in your dealings with others.

PURPLE AND RED KANGAROO PAW For clearing negativity and non-constructive criticism, such as blaming others all the time. Encourages you to do something positive and constructive.

QUEENSLAND BOTTLEBRUSH For clearing a conflict of desires and unsettled behaviour. Allows us the freedom to be ourselves, to know that people and experiences come and go; we do not have to be isolated from them to stay safe.

RED FEATHER FLOWER For the laziness and dishonesty that can arise in those who feel life owes them a living. Teaches that it is better to give than to receive; that we should not exploit the goodness of others or feel resentful when they feel they have given enough; to rely on our own energy and resources; to be there for others.

RED AND GREEN KANGAROO PAW For being in touch with the here and now, and realizing that those close to you are a priority. Encourages sensitivity and patience; brings joy.

RED LESCHENAULTIA For those who feel contemptuous of weaker people, are harsh, lacking in sensitivity. Turns harshness and lack of empathy into sensitivity. Helps you to become caring and considerate towards those weaker than you.

RIBBON PEA For those who feel a sense of nameless dread, but don't understand why. Helps you to rise above the fear and foreboding that prevents you from having a positive attitude and real direction for a fulfilling life. Heals the panicky fear of annihilation.

ROSE CONE FLOWER For those who feel frazzled and touchy, have difficulty coping, are easily disturbed, want to be alone, need space and peace (such as the parents of babies or young children). Helps you to discover peace amidst the storm, releasing tension so you can enjoy being around others.

SILVER PRINCESS GUM For those who lose interest or give up easily, displaying rebellious and frustrated behaviour. Teaches you to persevere when things are not working out, to keep caring and not rebel – thereby overcoming obstacles and achieving your goals.

SNAKE BUSH For those who give but are motivated by the need to be loved. For people emotionally unsettled and frustrated in love. Helps you to learn to be self-contained and to care for others without seeking anything in return, so easing disillusionment and anxiety.

SNAKE VINE For victims of destructive gossip or character assassination. Also helpful during relationship break-ups, when bitter feelings can undermine your self-confidence. Replenishes confidence and appreciation for your own achievements when others are sowing the seeds of negativity and doubt.

SOUTHERN CROSS For those with comfortable lifestyles who feel bewildered when life deals them a sudden blow and have to struggle for survival. Brings a realization of how life is for others and how, one day, it could be for you.

STAR OF BETHLEHEM (AUSTRALASIAN) For resignation, frustration and lack of initiative due to a feeling that there is no hope of improvement. Brings the realization that there is always hope; helping you to see all the solutions life can offer, and to know that you can find happiness by breaking through problems with creativity.

URCHIN DRYANDRA For those who feel downtrodden, the underdog in unequal relationships. Encourages you to rise above the feelings of inferiority stemming from ill-treatment by others.

URSINIA For idealists who are cynical, critical and frustrated with being part of a group or organization. Allows the bright-eyed enthusiastic to see the reality of group dynamics and still retain his or her idealism. Fosters co-operation and productiveness to ensure healthy progress and growth despite problems with selfish members of the group.

VERONICA For isolation and alienation stemming from the feeling that you go unnoticed and are misunderstood. Teaches you to relate to others differently, not to dwell on loneliness and the belief that no one understands you.

VIOLET BUTTERFLY For those feeling emotionally shattered during and after relationship traumas such as break-ups. Calms flaring sensitivities and emotional pain, speeds emotional recovery, heals the damage and allows you to get on with the rest of your life.

WESTERN AUSTRALIAN SMOKE BUSH For those feeling pressurized to achieve when they have no desire to, resulting in loss of mental control, nervousness, anxiety, fearfulness and severe stress. In extreme cases, fear of going mad. Promotes mental stability; reconnects mind and body and re-integrating the subtle with the physical aspects. Helpful for concentration, faintness after anaesthesia – promotes quick recovery.

WHITE EREMOPHILA For developing a broad perspective when messy situations threaten to drag you down. Brings clarity to complexities and difficulties. Helps maintain your equipoise, consistency and direction in life.

WHITE NYMPH WATERLILY For uncovering your deepest spiritual core. Brings tranquillity for reaching into the soul and use your Higher Self to integrate and respond to life from a universal rather than personal perspective. Helpful for spiritual practices such as meditation.

WILD VIOLET For pessimists and worriers who are apprehensive, depressed, complaining and single-minded. Balances caution with the willingness to be carefree and optimistic, to take a chance on happiness.

WOOLLY BANKSIA For those who are losing heart when the struggle seems too much. Rekindles the desire to go ahead with ideals and goals, to face new aspirations without fear of inevitable failure. Helpful during long, tiring, seemingly pointless phases in the journey to reach your higher ambition.

WOOLLY SMOKEBUSH Helpful for maintaining forward progress without getting distracted. Offers perspective and humility. Helps you avoid the traps of glamour and self-importance, so that you look at life objectively.

YELLOW BORONIA For an overactive mind, scattered thinking, those who are easily distracted. Helps you to remain calm and centred so the mind can be focused and follow thoughts through.

YELLOW CONE FLOWER For a sense of inferiority and lack of self-esteem. Brings acceptance of inner worth and freedom from the need to seek recognition from others. Prevents situations arising in which you are used.

YELLOW FLAG FLOWER For those stressed by daily chores, who feel unable to cope with the trying events in life. Brings calmness and brightness during times of stress, to help you to find the fortitude to handle all situations without making life one long, difficult grind.

YELLOW AND GREEN KANGAROO PAW For the perfectionist, hard task master, uncompromising parent or boss who is super-critical and intolerant. Teaches tolerance, the value of mistakes and the importance of being non-judgmental and patient with imperfections.

YELLOW LESCHENAULTIA For those who always know better – teachers, parents, teenagers who dismiss out of hand the views of others. Helps you to become open to others, to listen, be patient and tolerant.

AUSTRALIAN ORCHIDS

BLUE CHINA ORCHID For addictions of one sort or another, the inability to control yourself, feeling overwhelmed or unfulfilled, lack of will-power. Breaks the spell of addiction, strengthens the will, helps you to take back control of yourself. Brings the realization that you no longer need a crutch.

COWSLIP ORCHID For those with a superiority complex, who crave recognition and over-rate their own importance, use arrogant, pompous behaviour and are negative and contemptuous to those who do not acknowledge them. Helps to deflate egos and to reveal the value of interacting with and enjoying people from all walks of life.

FRINGED MANTIS ORCHID For the destructive, psychic predator, or the busybody with an unhealthy curiosity and no conscience. Brings conscience into one's activities; curbs unhealthy curiosity about the affairs of others. Confers the realization that you should only use information for benevolent reasons

HYBRID PINK FAIRY (COWSLIP) ORCHID For those who take others' attitudes too personally, feeling unfairly persecuted or threatened; for over-sensitivity, paranoia, tearfulness over-small matters. Enables one to get on with life concerned with others' reactions. Generates contentment, inner tranquillity and self-contained positivity. Also helpful for PMS and the sensitivity of pregnancy.

LEAFLESS ORCHID For those who feel bogged down – such as the uninspired therapist who is drained, tired and lacking vitality. Promotes attention to central not peripheral needs in yourself and others. Allows you to find the energy deep within to keep positive and active in your work for others without becoming depleted and tired, mentally and physically.

PINK FAIRY ORCHID For those who feel panicky due to circumstances, creating mental instability and the feeling of being overwhelmed by the environment. Filters the stress of environmental situations which can cause feelings of panic and being overwhelmed. Calms the inner core and helps to lessen over-sensitivity to the environment.

PURPLE ENAMEL ORCHID For those who begin a task feeling unmotivated and useless, then behave like workaholics to prove themselves. Maintains a consistent and healthily balanced energy input – not too much, not too little and not all at once – to gain a healthy equilibrium between rest and work.

RABBIT ORCHID For those who tend to be superficial and insincere – socialites. Bestows sincerity and straightforwardness, not shallowness and emptiness. Provides the ability to see the rewards of meaningful, honest relationships. Helps you to find your true self.

RED BEAK ORCHID – BURNOUT ORCHID For the frustrated housewife or husband, lethargic employee, lazy student or truant. Resolves the clash between desire and responsibility that often causes a sense of burden and mental paralysis. Counters lethargy, rebelliousness, boredom and depression.

SHY BLUE ORCHID For to those dedicated to the path of light. Gives a sense of protection and dynamism where powerlessness had prevailed. Focuses spiritual energies that dispel negative forces in the environment.

WALLFLOWER DONKEY ORCHID For those who feel they are the victim of circumstances, becoming vengeful, cynical, empty and disillusioned. Allows 'letting go' rather than feeling the sickness of revenge. Allows you to take responsibility for making life positive so that you do not live with a chip on your shoulder.

WHITE SPIDER ORCHID For spiritual, humanitarian people such as volunteer workers with a tendency to introversion, sadness, hypersensitivity, and anguish deep in their souls. Brings love and caring without devastation at the insensitivity and suffering of others. Allows you to empathize while not being brought down by the world.

RUSSIAN ESSENCES

With the political and social turmoil in Russia, these remedies reflect the problems that beset the Russian people, and are relevant to all those facing suppression, oppression and the subsequent reactions to these forces.

Made by Vasudeva Barnao, who was invited to the then Soviet Union in 1989 to begin research on essences collected from flowers in the Bush about 125 miles (200 km) from Moscow. Their contribution to the essence repertoire is unique and invaluable.

BLUE-TOPPED COW WEED For the escapist or joker who avoids life's deeper issues – the superficial good-timer who avoids responsibility, lacking empathy, depth of character. Brings a more responsible attitude. Engenders the strength to deal with problems rather than avoid them.

KOLOKOLTCHIK For conquering adversity after a long history of struggle when the will to fight has faded. Restores the desire to fight on and not succumb.

RUSSIAN CENTAUREA For brave people who stand up and oppose injustice, regardless of the consequences; for risk-takers who feel opposed or trapped. Teaches that there are times when you cannot act because of negative forces stronger than yourself, when you must keep your flame hidden so as not to attract undue attention from those seeking to destroy you.

RUSSIAN FORGET-ME-NOT For the follower, looking to others for leadership, underestimating his or her own abilities and strengths. Helps you to find hidden strength.

MICROVITA CREAMS

The Microvita creams in the Living Essences of Australia range contain specially selected flower essences in combination, cold-pressed and essential oils in an aqueous cream base. These creams and lotions are designed to relieve states of mind associated with physical discomfort, to bring long-term benefits.

Massage Lotion 1
For stressed-out adults, fretting babies, overactive children. For anxiety, depression, sleeplessness, devitalized skin.

Massage Lotion 2
For general muscle pain, energy loss, cramping, sun burn, stiffness, menstrual discomfort, bruising, sports preparation and invigoration.

Skin Rejuvenation Moisturizer
For wrinkled, devitalized skin and stress-related lines. Brings back the vital energy to your face, which is where stress first shows.

Arthritis Cream
Designed to alleviate arthritic pain. Relief should occur within four to eight weeks.

Pain Cream
Concentrate for pain, bruising, cramping. Also used for menstrual or birth cramps. Has invigorating effect.

NEW ZEALAND

*New Zealand is an unspoiled land which boasts
spectacular scenery and vast open spaces. Since c. AD 500 the North Island
has been inhabited by the Maori people, who recognize and respect the
spirituality of nature.
Despite being a traditionally warrior-like people,
they show great appreciation for every fish or bird they catch, every seed
they pick, every tree they use for building their houses – realizing that these
things are provided by their god, Tane. They communicate with the spirit
in nature and have no wish to exploit the gifts it has to offer.
Their respect and love of nature has contributed
to the energy of New Zealand. Many early European settlers were drawn by
the philosophy that everything is alive, a philosophy shared by Celtic and
Oceanic people as well as the Maori, and brought with them their desire for
freedom which has added to the positive feeling of this land.
The flowers growing here
are imbued with this combination of energies.*

❋ NEW PERCEPTION FLOWER ESSENCES ❋

The New Perception essences are made from indigenous and imported flowers that grow wild or in gardens and parks throughout New Zealand.

They are made by New Zealand New Perception Flower Essences, run by Mary Garbely and her husband Dolf under the aus-

pices of the New Zealand Flower Essences Co-operative Charitable Trust. Mary's interest in flower remedies was kindled by her own miraculous healing experience. At the age of 41 she was crippled with rheumatoid arthritis. Specialists told her she would probably have to live on drugs and be confined to a wheelchair for the rest of her life. She came across an article about Dr Bach and the relationship of fear to illness, then began to use the remedies. While using meditation and the Bach Flower Remedies alone, she slowly began to regain movement in her spine; later X-rays proved that much of the calcification had dissolved.

In the winter of 1979, auspiciously at the solstice, Mary met with two women both with Maori maternal grandmothers who had cured themselves of serious illnesses with flower remedies. By the following Spring they had formed a charitable trust to explore and develop essences from flowers growing in New Zealand. The first essences were developed for lay people and naturopaths to use. Then Mary herself created more spiritually-orientated essences.

Mary suspects that the North Island was once part of ancient Lemuria, which to her accounts for the strong sense of spiritual awareness here. She feels that the essences have a special role to play in fulfilling the potential for shifting consciousness which exists at this time.

Developing the essences has been an exciting journey of self-discovery which has taken place simultaneously to her own spiritual growth and healing. Mary feels that the flower that best symbolizes the mood of New Zealand is Koromiko, which is for peace – a dynamic state that is never static but holds within it the potential for progress and movement.

1. ABELIA For those whose 'take apart' thinking is too analytical, rational, assertive, or authoritarian – or too imaginative, with the imagination feeding fears, airy-fairy and impractical. Balances left and right hemispheres of the brain, co-ordinating their use.

62. ACORN For those who feel unable to cope

with their life, struggling on, constantly tired, unaware of solutions for self, world, planet.

2. AGAPANTHUS For hereditary problems, racial or collective unconscious fears, fears formed at conception, *in utero*, at birth or in early childhood.

41. AUTUMN CROCUS For those who want to change direction, be flexible yet retain their spiritual soul purpose. Helps you to take responsibility for your own reality, for knowing and applying this.

3. BASIL To help those needing to put aside what was useful before, but now hinders the life purpose. A basis for humanitarianism movement.

4. BELLADONNA For periods of confusion, mental, emotional and spiritual instability, mental breakdown. For adults who are intolerant, inappropriately strict and constantly angry.

60. BLESSINGS MIX – ACIANTHUS

61. BLESSINGS MIX – KAURI (Totara Leaves, Acianthus Kauri, Kowhai and Puriri) For those who believe that life is all struggle, pain and sorrow. Gives the ability to see that gratitude and appreciation for the Creator and all Creation brings blessings back to us.

55. CABBAGE TREE For loss of success or abundance, and the feeling that because you didn't succeed in the past you cannot succeed in the future. Fosters the need to have soul-directed individuality.

6. CHOKO For deep subconscious fears about one's present situation, leading to an inability to move or think with clarity, especially in cases of old age, acute loneliness or childhood terror.

63. CLEMATIS Brings the ability to 'stay with' a task or idea, not to fantasize. To be idealistic *and* practical, to have freedom but accept responsibility.

8. DAISY For recurring problems concerning health, friends, relationships or money. Gives clarity to know what it was and why it came about. Allows you to move on.

9. DANDELION For strictly conformist people, rigid-thinking, 'delay, refer, consider' attitudes; for those seeing no good in their present situation. Also for muscular tension, especially in the neck, shoulders and back.

10. DILL Need for change and growth, when there are issues, problems and illnesses festering away within; needing to come to a head and burst so regrowth can happen.

64. ERIGERON DAISY AND 65. WHAU For confidence, faith and certainty, so that the body can be healed by the mind and spirit.

11. EUCALYPTUS For fearing to be alone; for children feeling unwanted and in the way, who leave but who are afraid of being alone. For those adults who claim not to need anyone.

12. EUPHORBIA To cleanse and purify for when we reject ourselves, deny ourselves true life by feeling and wishing we were different or had not lived that way.

13. EVENING PRIMROSE For those smothered by love, who feel stifled, suppressed, feeling unsafe, so unable to be independent.

43. EVERLASTING PEA To give consistency, self-discipline and flexibility in applying your talents so that you do not limit your talents nor paint yourself into a corner.

14. FIVE FINGER For enclosing situations which are heavily negative and emotional; for those who feel boxed in, claustrophobic – and for those afraid of jumping insects. Often stemming from an 'addiction prone' family.

5. FLAX For fear of the future because its situations have not been experienced before. Fear of unknown social, economic, health aspects. Group fears of nuclear Armageddon.

15. FORGET-ME-NOT For the needy child, feeling a loser in life, never a winner. To rid oneself of self-pity. For those who choose games in life that fail and feel left out by others.

16. GINGER BLOSSOM For anger, irritability, hate, frustration, futility – for relationships that are too intense. Especially useful for single parents. Swinging from love to hate, hate to love.

7. HANGEHANGE To facilitate learning at any stage of life for those who believe they are slow learners or unable to remember. To change old thought-patterns that prevent learning. Builds success.

17. HEATHER For those who feel the need to isolate or withdraw, making barriers between themselves and others because they have been hurt and 'choose' to work alone.

18. HIMALAYAN BLUE CLOVER For those swayed by the opinions of others, or those easily caught up in a mass hysteria or pessimism. Confers steadfast hope and optimism.

44. IMPATIENS (BALSAM SHRUB) For deep emotionalism concerning family, nation and race. For upsets when the link is broken. Bestows the need for humility and an increasing capacity for compassion.

45. IRIS Gives you the ability to just be guided from your inner resources. For loss of surety and security, leading to continual obsessive planning for your safety, progress or happiness.

46. JASMINE For loss of your soul's purpose, or a misunderstanding of it and lack of ambition towards it. For the realization that the future is healed now.

19. JONQUIL For those who feel 'it will never be the same again' due to trauma, stress and death fears.

47. KOHEKOHE For those who are one of the silent majority, not doing or acting on environmen-tal issues, social, economic or global issues. Helps you to accept stewardship.

66. KOHIA For the fear that negative thoughts will take over your mind; the feeling of continual darkness – almost mental breakdown, with sudden destructive impulses.

20. KOROMIKO For indecisiveness, stagnation, conflict; having a desire for peace but being unwilling to 'rock the boat', to be open to alternative solutions or to co-operate.

67. KOWHAI When a spiritual understanding is needed to assist the desire for nature energy with which to transform and work for global and national communal issues, not for achieving mere possessions and physical desires.

68. LASIANDRA For handling worry, concern and anxiety that are constantly present, preventing inner peace and increasing negative feelings towards yourself and others. On the sympathy level, not the compassion level.

48. LEMON BALM For loss of natural good health and spiritual growth; for finding your spiritual progress blocked by poor health. Also for those who have trouble saying 'no' to requests for assistance.

49. LOBELIA For those who have no patience with themselves or no kind feelings towards themselves. Gives you the courage to accept yourself as you are, imperfections and all.

50. LONDON PRIDE For loss of tolerance, perceiving the negative in others, belief in bad/evil influences.

21. LOQUAT For fear of change, thereby creating what is feared; for self-centredness and a need to 'walk alongside' new ideas.

69. MANUKA To strengthen the will so that the intention is to find and remove all blocks in one's self, to be open to the awareness of love and interdependence.

23. MARIGOLD (French) For those who are not really in touch with what others say, for nervousness, those who do not listen to their body's messages, or their own intuition. For nervousness, for those who jump at noises.

24. MEXICAN SUNFLOWER For those who feel held back by thoughts of loss, who use the past to guide them. For those for whom material possessions are important and who are unable to give them up in order to gain. A mistaken security.

25. MINGIMINGI For emotional stress in home situations: broken homes, quarrelling children; problems of adoption, step-parenting problems. When love, service and co-operation are needed.

26. MONTBRETIA For those feeling like victims and thinking, 'I am unable to handle my life.' Helps the body to ward off illness.

51. MORNING GLORY For loss of belief in your spiritual being, loss of spiritual faith and certainty that you were created in the Creator's likeness.

52. NEW ZEALAND ORCHID For those who feel life has betrayed them, that life has never given or provided them with anything. For those lacking enjoyment in life or excitement about participating fully in life.

27. OAK For doubting your will to accomplish your destiny. For those who need help with balance, strength and vision, and constructiveness. Balances the body/soul fusion.

28. PAPAYA (Mountain Pawpaw) For those who do not wish to claim responsibility for their own health when they 'burn out' from working for others' health, welfare and safety. For those who are overly concerned for others.

22. PASPALUM GRASS For those who demand care and attention, controlling others by manipulating their feelings or using fear or their own health to direct others – sufferers may be elderly or teenagers.

29. PEACH A catalyst essence for speeding up all healing processes, including grief.

30. PENNYROYAL To correct the inability to speak out about your own values, opinions and faith. For sore throats, tonsillitis, the inability to sing in public – for energy blockage in the throat chakra.

53. POHUTUKAWA For fearing your own power or loss of your power. For the perpetual seekers for the need for power with wisdom, that is spiritually-based.

54. POLYANTHUS To eliminate the self-blame and guilt that prevents you from loving yourself. Feeling that you could have done something to prevent an event from happening, or you haven't done something you feel you should have.

70. PURIRI To express, recognize and use wisdom. To help control arrogance and dominance, and use power with true humility.

31. RAGWORT To combat the fear of commitment that leaves you unable to put down roots, make friends or have loving relationships.

71. RATA BERRIES, WHITE To counteract resignation and apathy, lift above present plateaus and be involved in co-creating your own reality. Also boosts the immune system.

72. RAUPO To handle a dislike of self, physically, and handle shocks at the solar plexus level that panic you into feeling 'I'm not good enough. I don't know enough.'

42. RED RATA VINE For loss of function and balance of body/mind/soul; low energy and vitality. Helps the ego and soul to co-operate for when a melding is needed.

57. RHODODENDRON (SIR ROBERT PEEL) For those who always attack the negative in themselves. For those wanting to be the warrior that fights it to death instead of the adventurer who uses the negative emotion for understanding.

32. RHODODENDRON FRAGRANTISSIMA For those taking on overwhelming responsibility, pushing themselves too hard, waking early but feeling tired and unrefreshed, for closing down the heart chakra because 'loving hurts'.

33. ROSE PEACE For those at a crossroads in life. To re-channel energy in a new direction. Brings the need of awareness of choices and decision making in the spirit of harmony and tranquillity and understanding.

38. SALVIA For those who do not like themselves, so become 'rebels'. For selfishness, intellectual hostility, defiance, criticism of others and life, irresponsibility.

34. SUNFLOWER To overcome the superiority that hurts others' feelings, the 'better than' attitudes and righteousness 'for the good of the children/community' and so forth.

58. TOTARA SEED Loss at a physical level; believing you are 'body' only. Assists you in seeing the whole body/mind/soul being.

35. VALERIAN For exhaustion, disturbed sleep, tension, stress. Helpful in times of convalescence.

36. VERBASCUM For small fears built into mountains. Bestows the ability to laugh at yourself and your fears.

37. VERONICA For laziness; for those who make bargains or pay-offs to gain advantages for themselves; for a weakness in their individuality. Loving because you need, dominating for gain.

59. VIOLA WHITE For those who have lost the sense of their own value, continually questioning it; for those who feel 'I am a burden. Should I be here?' Brings on a feeling of being completely worthy.

39. WATERMELON For those with an inferiority complex, weak convictions, resentment, 'so mad you can't speak' and for a fear of speaking up/speaking out or of authority.

40. WILD FENNEL For those who are unable to resist the influences that lower their vibrations; for those needing survival help. Combatting negativity in their own aura.

EUROPE

*Throughout Europe there exist ancient traditions
of healing with plants and flowers. In many countries such as Britain,
France and Switzerland, folk remedies handed down from generation to
generation are still alive today. Not surprisingly, many of the most
renowned herbalists – from Nicholas Culpeper to Paracelsus – came from
this part of the world. Dr Edward Bach himself was a native of Britain and
prepared many of his remedies from flowers growing in the fields and
hedgerows of Oxfordshire. Throughout Europe many others are
following in his footsteps.*

❃ BACH FLOWER REMEDIES ❃

In the 1930s Dr Edward Bach rediscovered the art of healing with flowers and created 38 remedies from flowers growing in the British countryside. After his death his close companion Nora Weeks kept his work alive; she in turn entrusted the Bach Centre to Nickie Murray for many years. Since then it has changed hands again: John Ramsell and Judy Howard now run the Bach Centre and are responsible for preparing the Bach Flower Remedies. To meet increasing demands the company Nelsons, makers of homoeopathic preparations, are now involved in their production.

Julian Barnard and his wife Martine also prepare a range of remedies according to the dictates of Dr Bach at their home on the edge of the largest area of national park in Britain (Hertfordshire). They were invited to work at the Bach Centre by Nickie Murray in 1984 and were involved in establishing the Bach Educational Programme before setting up their own Healing Herbs company in 1990.

Julian, a medical herbalist, feels it is important to follow Dr Bach's instructions to the word, so he and his wife adhere scrupulously to his original methods. They go to some of the wildest and most inaccessible places to seek flowers, and use only pure, fresh mountain water to make the essences. They are the only company, as far as is known, who make the remedies with full-strength brandy as did Dr Bach himself. The remedies are endorsed by Nickie Murray, who has said, 'The Healing Herbs are genuine flower essences prepared according to original methods with great care, love and integrity...I wholeheartedly give them my recommendation and support.' The Remedies have earned a reputation for integrity and quality and the Barnards now run a flourishing education programme, and lecture throughout the world.

AGRIMONY For those who appear cheerful, jovial and uncomplaining, hiding mental torture and anxieties behind this mask – they may be restless and seek excitement to overcome their worry, or may use alcohol/drugs to dull and forget their pain. Helps us acknowledge and transcend such feelings so real peace and humour can be found.

ASPEN For irrational, vague, inexplicable fears of unknown origin; sudden apprehension, fear of unseen power or force, of sleeping and dreams; headaches, sweating, trembling, sudden faintness, sleep walking/talking, fatigue and anxiety. Brings a sense of security and an ability to trust that we are safe and protected.

BEECH For those who are critical, dissatisfied, intolerant, unsympathetic, irritable, always finding fault, seeing only the negative things; for tension affecting the upper-chest area, jaw and hands. Brings compassion and tolerance, relaxing strict attitudes.

CENTUARY For timid, quiet, kind, gentle, conventional people who are anxious to please. They may have a tendency to lose their identity and direction, be submissive and be exploited. Physical symptoms affect the shoulders

and back. Encourages self-determination and an ability to trust and follow our good judgement, to act decisively.

CERATO For those who doubt their own abilities, lacking faith in their own intuition and judgment, always asking others' advice – they tend to be mercurial and are easily led astray.

CHERRY PLUM For desperation, fear of being unable to control negative thoughts, feelings and impulses of losing control, suicidal feelings, obsessive fear, delusions, nervous breakdown. Enables us to feel strong and safe enough to deal sanely with issues that scare us.

CHESTNUT BUD For those who do not learn by experience, repeating the same mistakes over again, always looking ahead and failing to see what is happening. They can be careless, clumsy, slow to learn and inattentive. Enables us to observe, remember and make logical connections which help us make sense of life and formulate wise responses and choices.

CHICORY For those feeling empty inside who become manipulative and possessive to get the attention they crave, who dislike being alone, needing their loved ones near to control and direct their activity. For 'the mothering type' as well as children who demand attention. Helps those who are self-pitying, fussy, bossy, critical, smothering, tearful and thwarted. Nourishes by instilling feelings of love and security.

CLEMATIS For dreamers who are absent-minded, lacking concentration and vitality; for quiet people preferring dreams and fantasy to reality, who are romantic and imaginative but unrealistic, prone to drowsiness, excessive sleep, sensitivity to noise and faintness. Helps transform ideas and visions into actuality, developing talents and creating a life that is interesting and fulfilling.

CRAB APPLE A cleansing remedy for those who feel unclean and polluted, leading to despondency and self-disgust. For those obsessed with and repelled by what is seen as bad in themselves and the environment. Enables us to process impurities and negativity, and create sensible priorities.

ELM For capable people who shoulder responsibility and occasionally take on tasks that are unreasonably demanding, making them feel exhausted, overwhelmed and temporarily inadequate. Enables you to let others handle the excess responsibility, so you are free to enjoy what you are doing.

GENTIAN For those easily discouraged by difficulties, who doubt and lack faith in their ability to succeed. For the negativity that breeds feelings of failure, disappointment, scepticism, gloom and sadness. Encourages perseverance and the realization that we cannot fail when our goal is to learn more about ourselves and the nature of life.

GORSE For times when life seems a misery, bringing hopelessness and despair. For those resigned to feeling nothing can be done to help and that any attempt will be futile. These feelings can result in conditions that apparently cannot be cured, or repeated failure or disappointment. Heals the inner will to see light in the darkness and embrace suffering as a positive aid to self-realization.

HEATHER For whose who feel needy of and greedy for attention of others. They may be obsessed with their own affairs, constantly chattering, unable to bear being alone, seeking sympathy and living off the energy of others. For those who are self-centred, over-concerned with themselves, lacking interest in others, or prone to hypochondria. Enables you to stand alone and find a wider, less self-centred view of life.

HOLLY For when we are enveloped in negative and aggressive emotions such as anger, jealousy, bitterness, envy, rage, suspicion, revenge, hatred, bad temper, contempt, selfishness, frustration. Encourages the ability to show goodwill and love to others, in the awareness that what enhances us, enhances all.

HONEYSUCKLE For nostalgia, getting stuck in the grief, regrets and memories of the past, longing for happier days gone by, romanticizing the past. Also for homesickness. Helps us to live in the moment, using past experiences as a guide and solid foundation, rekindling interest in life.

HORNBEAM For temporary feelings of being overwhelmed, mental/physical weariness, lack of energy, boredom, the feeling that everything seems too much, an inability to get up in the morning and face the day. Also for convalescents. Encourages creation of a balanced lifestyle which is sufficiently stimulating and varied to allow inspiration to flow.

IMPATIENS For impatient, impulsive people who dislike restraint and are driven by urgency and hastiness, who like working at their own speed, act quickly and are critical of others. For those prone to nervous tension, overexertion and accidents, temper outbursts, irritability, sudden pains and cramps, indigestion. Releases pent-up tension and encourages the patience to enjoy being as well as doing. Brings sensitivity to situations and relationships.

LARCH For lack of confidence, feeling trapped in self-doubt and inferiority, expecting failure so not bothering to try, hesitating and procrastinating. Also for the despondency and general depression often associated with impotency. Develops our sense of realism about our talents, builds confidence and self-assurance, clears old patterns of limitation.

MIMULUS For fear of specific or known origin, often undisclosed due to shyness; fear of illness, death, others and being alone. Symptoms may include stuttering, blushing, shallow breathing and over-sensitivity to noise, crowds and confrontations. Allows us to value our sensitive disposition and have the strength, courage and safety to enjoy life.

MUSTARD For overwhelming black clouds of depression of unknown origin, causing deep sadness and melancholy that lifts as unexpectedly as it descends. Brings the realization that every day is an opportunity to get more deeply in touch with ourselves, to grieve for what is amiss so healing can occur in preparation for new growth.

OAK For strong, reliable, responsible and patient people who shoulder their burdens without complaining, though have a tendency to take on more than they can manage. Their perseverance can lead to exhaustion, though they find ill-health frustrating because it imposes limitations.

OLIVE For total mental/physical exhaustion. Useful after prolonged illness or during convalescence, for combating the effects of overwork and over-worry, and to help you get through crises such as divorce or conflict.

PINE For those taking the blame for others' mistakes or situations not of their making. For the guilt and self-reproach that has become part of their lives. Also for those who are self-critical, over-conscientious and constantly striving, leading to tiredness and depression. Allows forgiveness of shortcomings, releases responsibility, brings true understanding and acceptance of the human condition.

RED CHESTNUT For those who are fearful and anxious for the welfare of loved ones, anticipating trouble, imagining the worst, being over-concerned about world problems and projecting their anxiety onto others. Develops trust and calm confidence in the ability of others to look after themselves.

ROCK ROSE For fear, panic, feeling paralysed by terror, and the hysteria due to emergencies, sudden illness or accidents. Symptoms include coldness, trembling and loss of control; nightmares. Brings calm so you can respond adequately and appropriately to problems.

ROCK WATER For rigidity and self-repression, being ruled by logic and hard on oneself and others. Also for fantasists and idealists prone to obsession, punishing self-discipline and spiritual pride. Facilitates open flexibility and a sense of balance in your approach to life.

SCLERANTHUS For indecision, mood-swings, lack of concentration and balance, restlessness, changeable outlook, problems making oneself understood. Also for those prone to travel sickness. Helps us to discover inner balance so we can become clear and decisive.

STAR OF BETHLEHEM For all forms of shock: sudden and traumatic, long and slow over a period of time, delayed from the past, the shock of birth. Clears shock from the system bringing a sense of being centred, soothed and comforted. Restores the body's self-healing mechanisms.

SWEET CHESTNUT For anguish and despair,

desolation, feeling at the limits of our endurance, that nothing is left but destruction and oblivion – the dark night of the soul. Reveals the light at the end of the tunnel, restoring hope and an awareness that all transforming processes have a purpose. Brings the understanding that we must experience darkness to appreciate the light.

VERVAIN For those who are over-zealous and forceful in their beliefs, enthusiastically trying to convert others by imposing their own will and ideas. For those who are highly strung, argumentative, strong willed and prone to over-exertion, thus setting up a stress pattern for physical tension, muscle strain, headaches, migraines, eyestrain and exhaustion. Releases the stress pattern and built-up tension, enabling us to relax and let others lead their own lives.

VINE For self-assured, proud, dominating, bossy people who use authority to gain power; leaders who are of great value in emergencies but who can be ruthless in pursuing their goals; tyrants and dictators; those prone to back problems and high blood-pressure. Brings flexibility, allowing us to put our skills and abilities to the general good while letting others develop their potential.

WALNUT For protection from outside influences and from major life changes (puberty, a new career, etc.) which have unsettled our foundations. Helps us to break with the old and those influences that impose on our free will. Enables us to establish new patterns, to break free and be ourselves.

WATER VIOLET For loners who retreat and isolate themselves, appearing aloof and quiet. They are self-reliant and contained, knowing their own minds, seemingly condescending because they believe they are different and special, never interfering with others and intolerant of interference; prone to physical tension, stiffness and rigidity. Brings the ability to ask for help when needed; allows us to appreciate and enjoy others.

WHITE CHESTNUT For persistent unwanted thoughts, restless mental chatter, congestion, preoccupation, insomnia, confusion, depression, nervous worry and headaches. Quietens and calms mental processes, allowing the mind to function clearly and efficiently.

WILD OAT For feeling uncertain of one's direction in life; dissatisfied, undefined or unfulfilled ambitions; despondency, frustration and boredom. Gives definite knowledge of and clarity to one's purpose in life.

WILD ROSE For resignation and apathy; feeling unable to cultivate interest or make an effort; being fatalistic, lacking vitality; prone to dullness and fatigue. Restores motivation, creativity and energy; rekindles enthusiasm.

WILLOW For resentment and bitterness, blaming others, feeling hard done by, being self-centred and self-pitying, bearing grudges, feeling wronged. Often linked with arthritic problems. Brings the ability to take full responsibility for life in order to make a fresh start. Cultivates optimism and a sunnier disposition.

SPECIAL COMBINATIONS

RESCUE REMEDY AND FIVE FLOWER REMEDY A blend of Cherry Plum for loss of control, Clematis for unconsciousness, Impatiens for stress, Rock Rose for panic/terror, and Star of Bethlehem for shock.

❋ BAILEY ESSENCES ❋

These flower remedies have been developed over a period of 20 years by Dr A. R. Bailey at his practice in the north of England.

As a child, Arthur Bailey was drawn to flowers and loved going for long walks in the woods and fells near Grange-over-Sands, England, with his 'Uncle George' (his grandmother's housekeeper's husband), who taught him the names of wildflowers growing locally.

Bailey first discovered flower remedies when he was suffering from post-viral syndrome. He consulted Dr Aubrey Westlake, a homoeopathic doctor whose wife assisted in the selection of appropriate homoeopathic and Bach Flower Remedies by dowsing. Bailey made a speedy recovery and subsequently found he could heal others by laying on of hands and working with the Bach Flower Remedies. At times none of the remedies seemed suitable, although Bailey instinctively felt flowers could help. He began his own investigations, preparing flowers from his own garden. To his surprise, he found them effective. The range steadily expanded. Some plants, like Firethorn, gave good results when their fruits were used. Bailey finally realized that the flowers were specifically for attitudes of mind – how people see and relate to the world around them. Only when old conditionings and beliefs go can we truly 'come into the present moment'.

The Bailey essences, then, are mainly prepared from flowers found in the Yorkshire Dales and Ilkley Moor, though many come from all corners of England. The remedies are primarily concerned with personal growth and transformation. The original six essences have steadily expanded since they were first developed nearly 30 years ago. There are now 48 essences, three of which – Grief, Tranquillity and Obsession – are composites made from the essences of several flowers (not included here, though they can be purchased from Bailey Essences – see Useful Addresses). All are hand-made by members of his family using pure spring water and vodka as a base.

BISTORT For protecting those who tend to self-destruct during a period of great change.

BLACKTHORN For the depths of despair – 'the valley of the shadow of death'.

BLUEBELL For after a depression, when we feel as if we are falling apart inside.

BOG ASPHODEL For the 'willing slave', always wanting to help others yet ignoring his or her own needs.

BRACKEN (Alcoholic Extract) For those who habitually play the role of child in life.

BRACKEN (Aqueous Extract) For psychic sensitivity that has been blocked since childhood, with the resulting fear of addressing one's psychic senses.

BUTTERBUR For blocked off self-love and low self-esteem. Helps you to realize your own inherent 'goodness'.

BUTTERCUP For those with a jaundiced view of life who refuse to let the sunshine in.

CHARLOCK For those suffering from the 'Peter Pan' syndrome, clinging to childhood states. For those who want to be liked and who therefore often become habitual victims.

DOUBLE SNOWDROP For those with a frozen attitude and approach to life. Brings openness and a lighter touch.

EARLY PURPLE ORCHID For unblocking the energy centres in the body and protecting any vulnerable spaces so created.

FIRETHORN Balances the fire energy within – imbalance can arise from long-suppressed emotions.

FLOWERING CURRANT For those who have lost heart but still keep going, often feeling they are facing inevitable defeat.

FOXGLOVE For those who feel confused in life and suffer from woolly thinking. Brings the needed stillness of mind.

HAIRY SEDGE For poor memory caused by mental attitudes where there is a chronic lack of attention to the present moment.

HONESTY For help with bringing openness and receptivity where there were previously subversive negative characteristics.

LEOPARDSBANE For those who are at the point of major change but feel as though they are living on a knife-edge.

LESSER STITCHWORT For possession – that is, those whose behaviour is dominated by strongly held ideas or by other beings.

LILY OF THE VALLEY For yearning, for those who have become blocked by desiring the unattainable.

LILAC For those whose personal development has been stunted, often by a dominating parent.

MARIGOLD For those with a rigid, materialistic approach to life, often with a total denial of their psychic and spiritual dimensions.

MARSH THISTLE For those locked in the past, who cling to old, outmoded patterns of thought and behaviour.

MILK THISTLE For those who do not love themselves, often trying to make up for this by struggling always to please others.

MONK'S HOOD For long-standing difficulties that have their roots in the distant past. Helps bring us to the present.

MOSS Helps those who fear freedom and lightness in their lives, often fearing the dark spaces within their being.

NASTURTIUM For those who know they need to make changes in their lives but seem unable to make the first move.

OXALIS For things that 'have you by the throat' and seem to be so overpowering that there appears no way out.

PINE CONES For those who are trapped by the authoritarian powers of others and feel unable to escape from them.

PINK PURSLANE For the self-opinionated; for those who go about with blinkers on.

RED CLOVER For those who are blocked off by fear of their own emotional nature.

RHODODENDRON For those who lack flexibility and keep trying to push through blind alleyways.

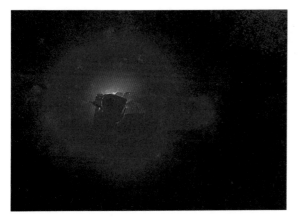
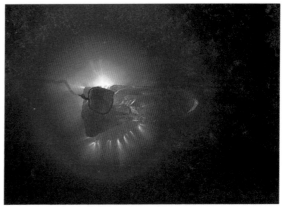

Kirlian photograph of Australian Bush Fringed Violet essence,
control (left) and showing effect of flower essence (right)

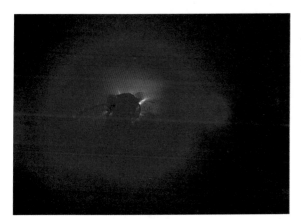
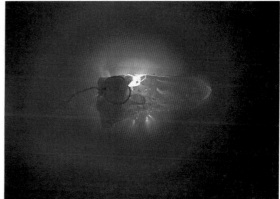

Kirlian photograph of Amazonian Fun Orchid essence, control (left)
and showing effect of flower essence (right)

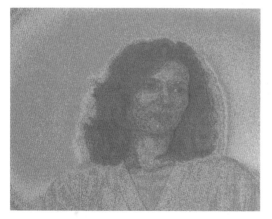 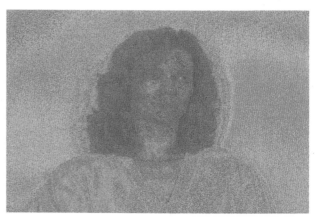

These aura photographs show changes in the body's energy field when holding a flower essence using Harry Oldfield's electro-scanning machine – his method of diagnosing imbalance in the body.

The first aura photograph is the 'control'. Harry has interpreted it for us:

The red/pink area in the throat region shows congestion in the throat chakra. Clare had in fact a slight sore throat at the time.

Red/pink in the right shoulder area shows a build-up of muscular tension here – Clare had just driven for two hours up the motorway.

The overall colours in Clare's aura are turquoise with yellow – turquoise is a colour indicating a healer with a strong connection with nature. Yellow in the aura indicates a lot of mental vitality. These colours in combination indicate a person who heals through changing consciousness. This Clare agrees with.

The second photograph shows the colour change in the energy field when Clare held Pansy flower essence – an antiviral remedy. Notice the red/pink areas lessening and clearing the throat and discharging negative energy out through the right side.

Essence of Pansy is also useful for drawing out toxins, such as for driving viral infections out of the system. This also shows Pansy's ability to bring or draw violet-coloured energy or life-force into the auric field from above, in order to heal imbalances.

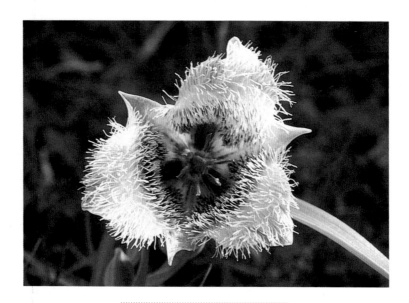

Star Tulip
FLOWER ESSENCE SOCIETY

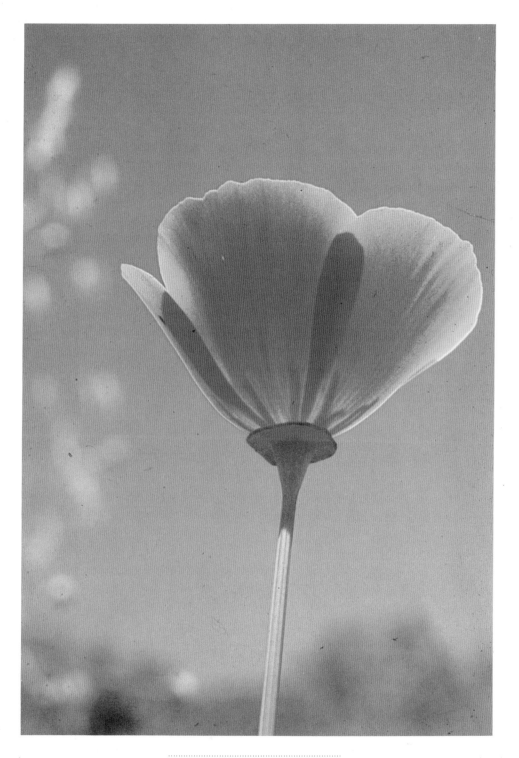

California Poppy
FLOWER ESSENCE SOCIETY

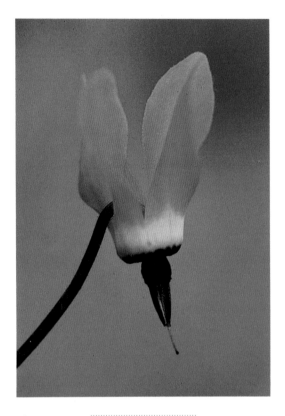

Shooting Star
FLOWER ESSENCE SOCIETY

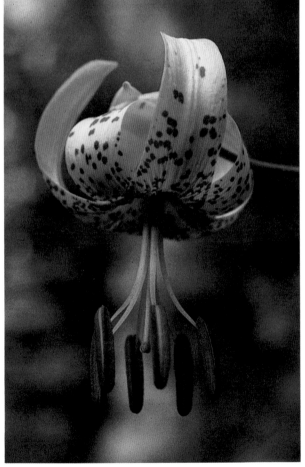

Tiger Lily
FLOWER ESSENCE SOCIETY

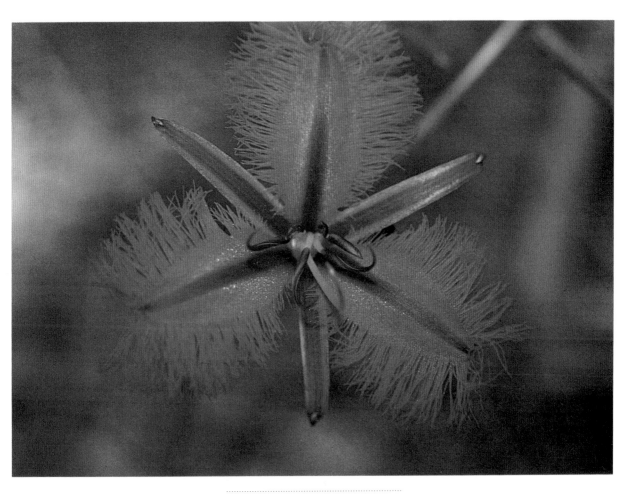

Fringed Violet
AUSTRALIAN BUSH FLOWER ESSENCES

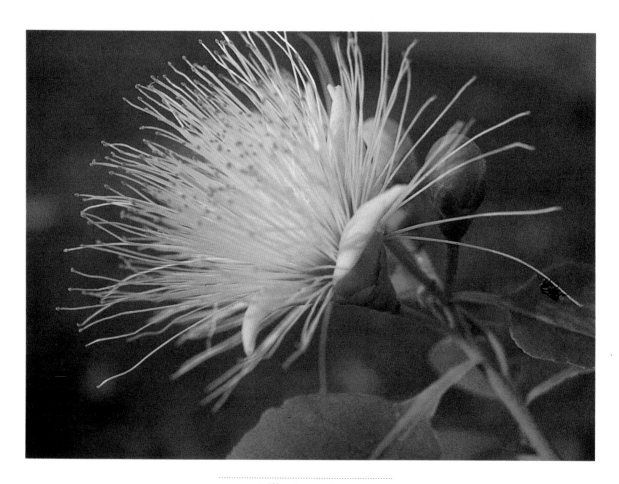

Billy Goat Plum
AUSTRALIAN BUSH FLOWER ESSENCES

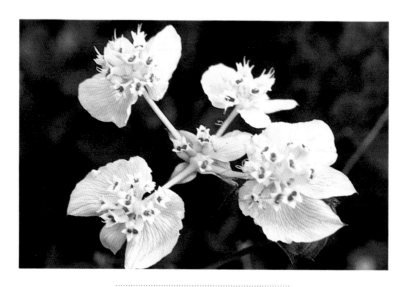

Southern Cross
AUSTRALIAN BUSH FLOWER ESSENCES

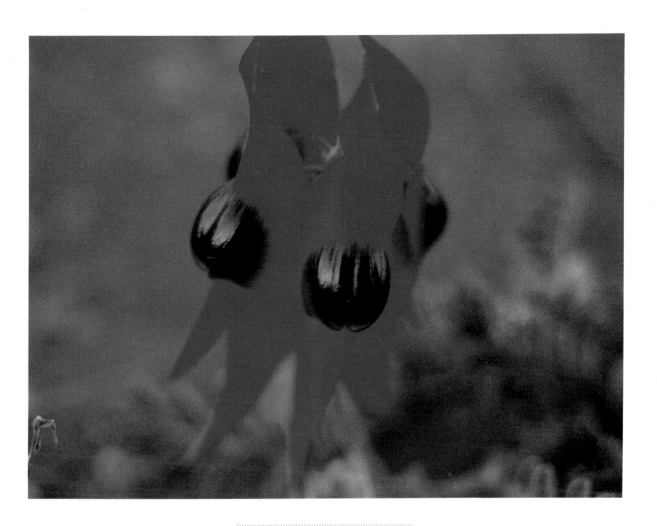

Sturt Desert Pea
AUSTRALIAN BUSH FLOWER ESSENCES

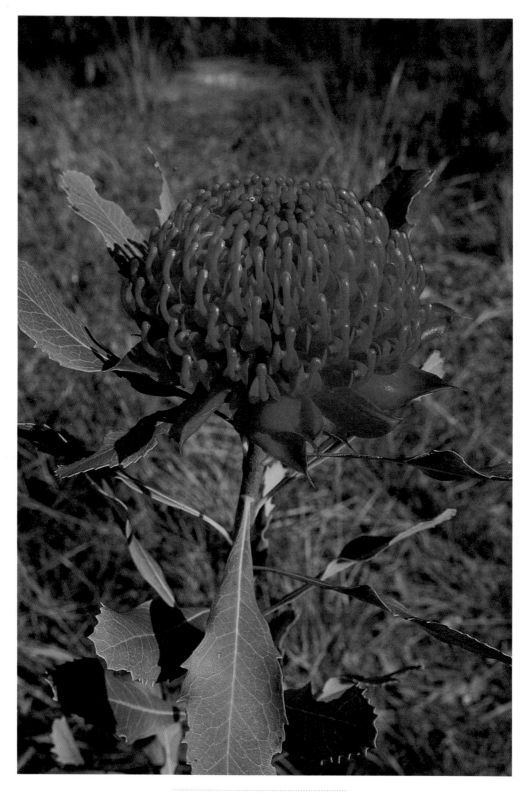

Waratah

ERIK PELHAM

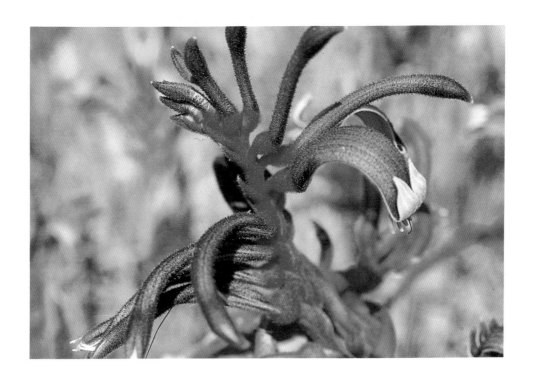

Red and Green Kangaroo Paw
LIVING ESSENCES

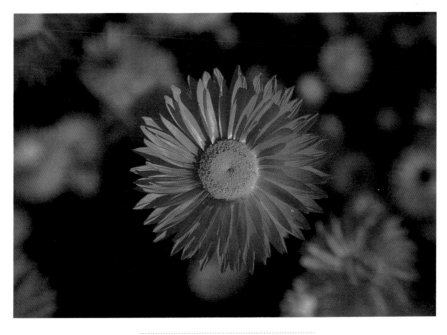

Pink Everlasting Straw Flower
LIVING ESSENCES

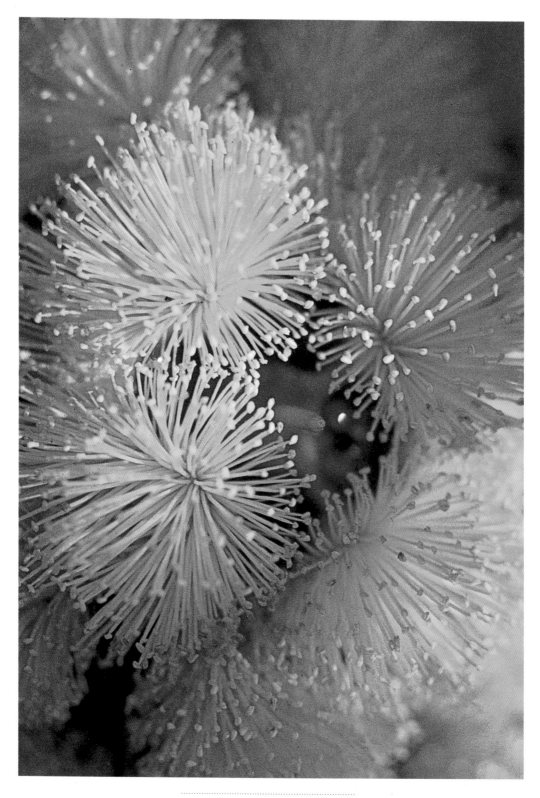

Illyairie
LIVING ESSENCES

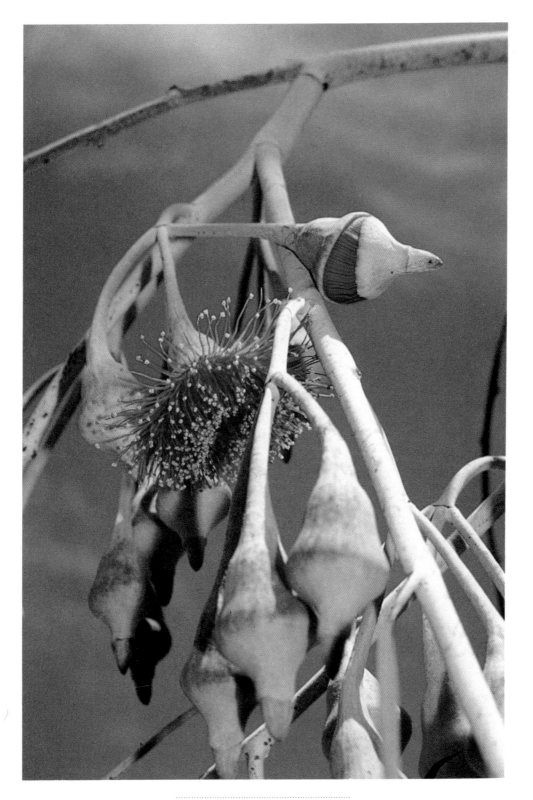

Silver Princess Gum
LIVING ESSENCES

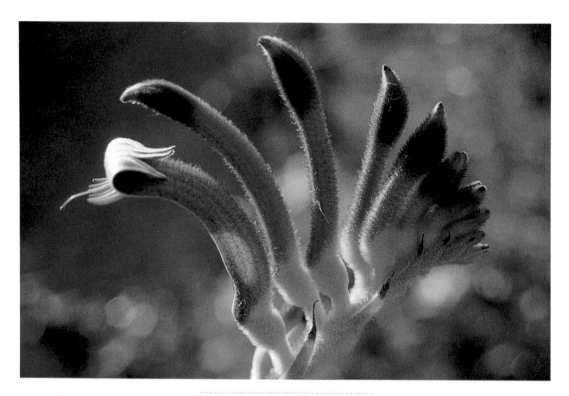

Formosa Orange
LIVING ESSENCES

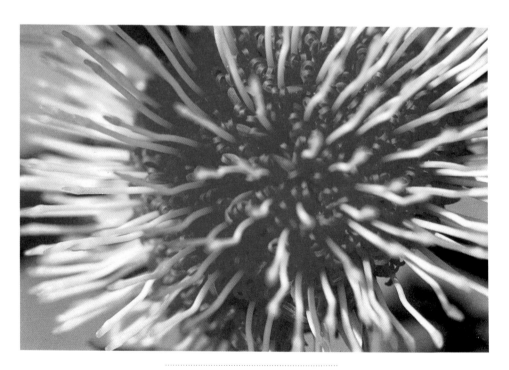

Pin Cushion Hakea
LIVING ESSENCES

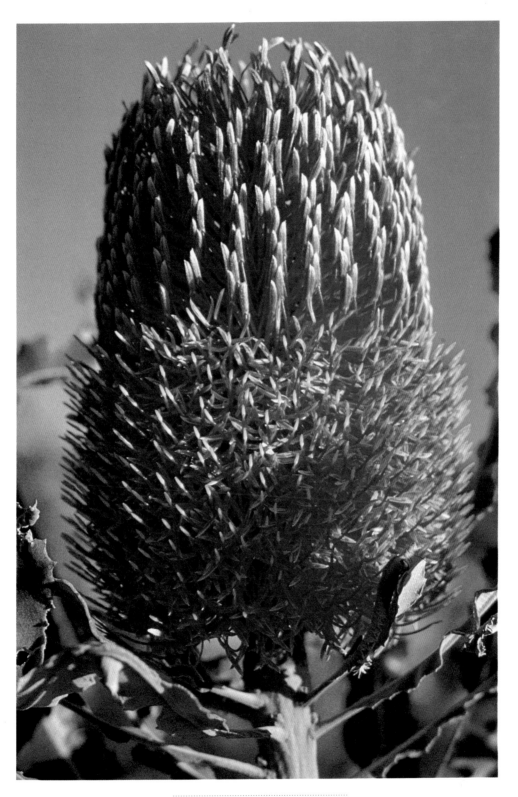

Menzies Banksia
LIVING ESSENCES

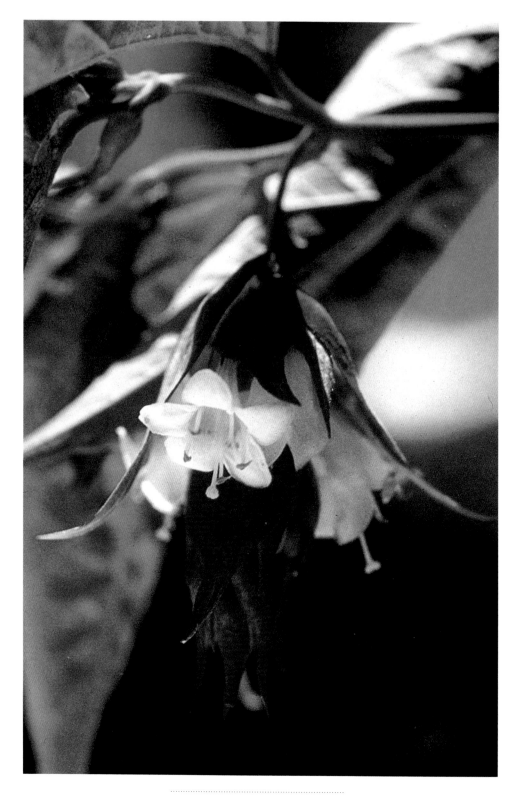

Down to Earth, Leycestra Formosa
HIMALAYAN

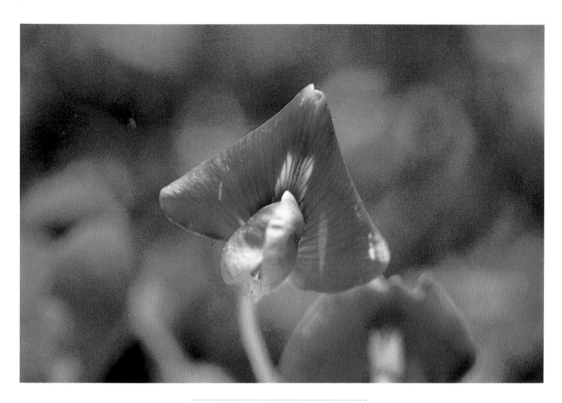

Clarity, Parochetus Communis
HIMALAYAN

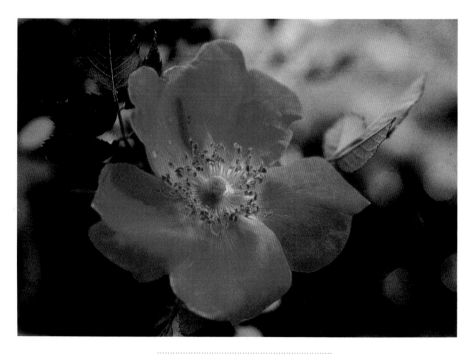

Ecstasy, Rosa Webbiana
HIMALAYAN

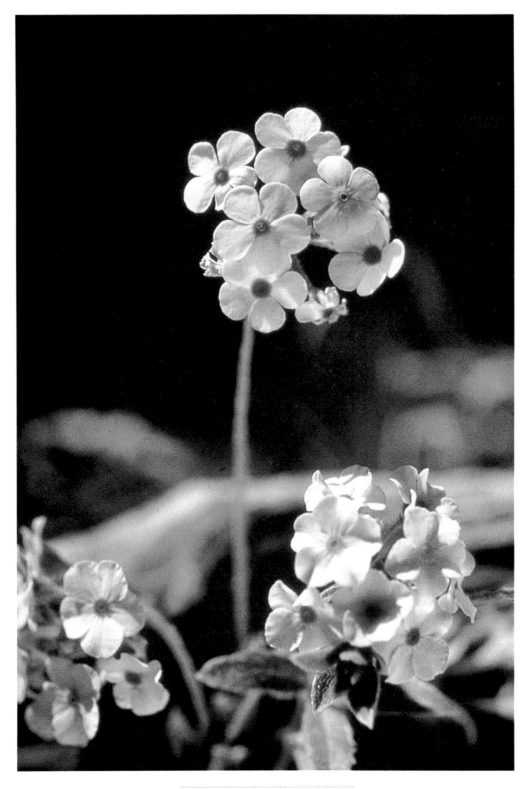

Children's Flower
HIMALAYAN

SCARLET PIMPERNEL For those who are emotionally trapped or psychically dependent on others.

SIBERIAN SPRUCE For those whose 'male' energy is lacking, producing frustration and a lack of clarity.

SINGLE SNOWDROP For those experiencing difficulty breaking through to new levels of awareness and consciousness.

SOAPWORT For those who feel a sense of bewilderment and lack of vision. For the feeling of 'What am I doing here?'

SOLOMON'S SEAL For the busy mind. Helps to bring quietness and detachment.

SPRING SQUILL For points of major change in a life when one is prepared to open up to a new view of reality.

SUMACH For those who ignore their potential due to fear of losing their old identities.

THRIFT For helping to open up the psychic sensitivity while remaining firmly grounded at the same time.

TUFTED VETCH For sexual difficulties caused by an incorrect sexual self-image, usually due to childhood conditioning.

VALERIAN For those who have not had their need for love fulfilled in childhood.

WELSH POPPY For those who have lost their fire and inspiration and have become daydreamers.

WITCH HAZEL For those who sacrifice themselves trying to live up to the expectations of others.

WOOD ANEMONE For those with ancient difficulties – genetic or karmic.

YEW For resilience where previously one had been too brittle. For strength to avoid bowing to the inevitable.

❀ FINDHORN FLOWER ESSENCES ❀

The Findhorn Flower Essences are subtle infusions of Scottish wildflowers which, when used for healing, can enhance spiritual awareness and growth by restoring equilibrium throughout the different levels of being. They are made by Marion Stoker, who first joined the Findhorn Foundation in 1976, then temporarily returned to her native Australia to become a qualified homoeopath. Through her study of homoeopathy and work with the Australian Bush Flower Essences she came to appreciate the extraordinary healing proper-

ties of flower essences. On returning to Findhorn she found the whole region carpeted with gorse in full bloom, and was drawn to preparing an essence from this flower. She decided to use water collected from an ancient secluded ancient local well with known healing properties.

Marion feels the flowers tend to find her when the time is appropriate. One exception was the rare Scottish primrose, a plant found only in certain areas on the north coast of Scotland and in Orkney. Marion actively went in search for this flower after receiving a message that its essence had remarkable powers for promoting feelings of inner peace and stillness in times of struggle, strife and conflict.

KIT 1

BELL HEATHER Stability. For loss of faith in oneself, lack of confidence, loss of direction or purpose, mood swings or feeling fragile, easily swayed or victimized by circumstance. Helps to access inner strength and resolve in order to stand firmly grounded after stress, trauma or conflict: self-confidence.

BROOM Clarity. For memory loss, dullness, feeble-mindedness, bewilderment, confusion or lack of integration, co-ordination or communication. Stimulates mental clarity and concentration, facilitating ease of communication and creative thought when in a state of bewilderment: illumination.

DAISY Innocence. For distraction, confusion, inconsistency, fickleness, indifference, over-sensitivity, feelings of being overwhelmed, fearing the loss of control, being easily swayed. Allows us to remain calm and centred amid turbulent surroundings or overwhelming situations, creating a safe space in which to be vulnerable: grace.

GORSE Joy. For apathy, burn-out, low immunity, listlessness, lack of motivation or joy. A light-bringer, stimulating vitality, enthusiasm and motivation, bringing light-heartedness and enjoyment of life: passion for and celebration of life.

HAREBELL (SCOTTISH) Prosperity. For fear of

want, possessiveness, lack of faith, attachment, being out of alignment with oneself and one's environment. Helps us become realigned to the spirit of abundance and release material concerns following fear of want: faith.

RAGGED ROBIN Purity. For congestion, toxicity, obstruction, blockages, unclean living, hindrance of spirit. Aids in releasing congestion, obstruction and toxicity on all levels. Facilitates the free flow of life-force and energies: inner purification.

SCOTTISH PRIMROSE Peace. For fear, constriction, panic, shock, paralysis, hysteria, anxiety, inner struggle, conflict in relationships, disheartenment. Brings inner peace and stillness to the heart in times of crisis: unconditional love.

SILVERWEED Simplicity. For over-indulgence, fussiness, narrow-mindedness, self-centredness, greed, pretentiousness, disconnection from the spirit. Helps foster detachment from material concerns and over-indulgence by promoting moderation and self-awareness: self-realization.

SPOTTED ORCHID Perfection. For cynicism, self-centredness, pessimism, an inability to see beyond ourselves and our personal circumstances, nostalgia. Enables us to go beyond pessimism and self-interest to see the best in everyone and everything: creative expression.

STONECROP Transition. For resistance to change, those who are stuck in the past; for loneliness, isolation, inertia, stagnation, stubbornness. Helps us to maintain inner stillness while we are in the process of breaking through inertia and resistance to change in the face of imminent transformation: transcendence.

THISTLE Courage. For fear, dread, the fight-or-flight syndrome, powerlessness. Helps us to find true courage in times of adversity and to respond with positive action: self-empowerment.

WILLOWHERB Power. For those who are self-important, judgmental, authoritarian, oppressive, angry, hot-tempered. Helps to balance the personality expressing self-seeking, authoritarian or over-bearing behaviour, bringing about the responsible integration of will and power issues: self-mastery.

KIT 2

APPLE Higher purpose. Helps us to integrate our desires and our will-power to realize our goals and visions. By aligning with the higher or divine purpose we channel these powerful energies into the right action: will-to-do-good.

BIRCH Perception. Helps us to broaden our perceptions and transcend limitations of mind. By expanding our consciousness and seeing our cosmic connections we gain understanding and peace of mind: vision.

ELDER Beauty. Stimulates the body's natural powers of recuperation and renewal. Helps us to contact and radiate the beauty and joy of our inner eternal youth.

HOLY-THORN Rebirth. Opens our hearts to love and the acceptance of ourselves and others, allowing intimacy and the expression of our truth and creativity: creation.

LAUREL Resourcefulness. Represents the abundance of the universe. Enables those wise in heart to empower themselves to find the resources to bring their ideas and ideals into form: manifestation.

LIME Oneness. Helps us open our hearts to the light and love of our universal being. From this awareness we experience our interelatedness on earth and create harmonious relationships in our lives: universality.

ROWAN Forgiveness. Helps us to let go of resentments and to heal old wounds. As we learn to forgive ourselves and others, we can heal the past: reconciliation.

SCOTS PINE Wisdom. Helps us find direction in our search for answers to our questions. By being open we can be guided from within by the all-knowing self and the inner teachers: truth.

SEA PINK Harmony. Aligns and infuses our being with Spirit. Blending and melding our life-force with divine will helps to balance the flow between all the energy centres: unity.

SNOWDROP Surrender. Allows us to surrender to the end of past events and attachments in life. In the death of the old we find the seed of our eternal inner light and behold new vistas: immortality.

SYCAMORE Softness. Recharges and uplifts body and soul when we are stressed, allowing the emergence of a soft yet powerful new energy supply: revitalization.

VALERIAN Humour. Lifts our spirits and helps us to rediscover delight and happiness in living. Taking ourselves lightly helps us to be at peace: mirth.

❋ GREEN MAN TREE ESSENCES ❋

Our relationship with trees is as old as time itself. For centuries humans have regarded certain trees as having healing qualities, and have revered and cared for them as sacred or even magical beings.

Trees are among the most ancient living organisms on this planet. They are protectors and regulators of their surroundings, offering food and shelter to many other forms of life. We now realize that our existence is totally dependent on the great forests and woods that cover the earth. They not only regulate the atmosphere ensuring a life-sustaining balance of oxygen and carbon dioxide, but also control weather systems and enrich the soil.

Trees flourish and survive by adjusting their form to harmonize with the prevailing conditionings, succeeding in maintaining this balance for hundreds, sometimes thousands of years. This ability to be balanced and flexible, to absorb and let go, is a lesson from which we could all benefit.

Each species of tree shows different characteristics and you can sense their particular energies when walking in ancient woodlands or forests. Integrating this energy into our own system helps us to act more responsibly towards nature.

The Green Man essences were created by Simon Lily and his partner Sue as an aid to meditation and self-healing. In traditional British folklore the Green Man is the perfect blending of human and plant life. He is the spirit of nature, an embodiment of fertility, and is celebrated every May Day.

The Green Man range comprises 74 tree essences (34 of which are included here; for further information, *see* Useful Addresses). The first essence made was from the flowers of the hazel tree, whose qualities encourage the growth of new skills and information.

ALDER 'Release'. Reduces nervousness and anxiety, eases stress, brings clarity of mind and increases life energy.

APPLE 'Detoxification'. Helps to eliminate toxins and bring in spiritual energies. Transforms negative emotions.

ASH 'Strength'. For feeling in harmony or in tune with your surroundings. Brings flexibility and security.

BAY 'Energy'. Releases blocked and suppressed emotions. Brings deep-rooted vitality and spiritualizes the physical level.

BLACK POPLAR 'Solidity'. Creates a powerful sense of peacefulness, security and inner clarity. Very comforting. Blends all energies.

BLACKTHORN 'Circulation'. Stabilizes emotions, brings hope and joy. Strengthens the blood supply and helps the absorption of nutrients.

BOX 'Clarity'. Strengthens the mind and will, clears the head, eases irrationality and confusion. Links us with the Higher Self.

CATALPA 'Joy'. Stabilizes emotions, helping us to find peace of mind. Reduces anxiety and increases self-confidence in what we can achieve.

CRACK WILLOW 'Spiritual sun'. Permits us to let go and allow things to happen. Brings a sense of oneness with the world. Stimulates communication with the Higher Self, the planet and the energies of the sun.

ELDER 'Self-worth'. For times of transformation and change. Good for fretful children. Calms aggression and brings stability, love and forgiveness. Balances self-image.

GEAN, WILD CHERRY 'Soothing'. Focuses energy in the physical body and stimulates self-healing. Calms the heart and mind, creating a smooth flow of energy. Helps reduce pain.

GLASTONBURY THORN 'Out of the woods'. A clearer direction is found. What feels right to do and be emerges from indecision and chaos. This brings immediate relaxation and release from tension, increasing subtle information and intuition. Good for claustrophobia.

GREAT SALLOW 'Soul'. For understanding the purpose of life. Allows the mind to expand and link with the soul. Energizes and links us to the earth's energy.

HAWTHORN 'Love'. Stimulates the healing power of love. Brings trust and forgiveness. Helps cleanse the heart of negativity.

HAZEL 'Skills'. Encourages the flowering of skills and the ability to receive and communicate wisdom, helping all forms of study. Clears away unwanted mental debris. Brings more stability and focus in order to help us integrate useful information.

HOLM OAK 'Negative emotions'. Relieves restlessness and emotions such as guilt, jealousy and anger that arise when expression is thwarted. Activates personal creativity. Balances emotional and mental energy.

JUDAS TREE 'Channelling'. Access to completely new thought-patterns and ideas. Brings openness and acceptance of very subtle levels of energy and the ability to communicate these to others. Confers the ability to discriminate and discern the validity of given information.

LAWSON CYPRESS 'The path'. Helps identify correct action and one's true needs. Initiates change in the right direction. Increases communication between mind and body. Brings the discipline to attain one's goals and true spiritual direction.

LEYLAND CYPRESS 'Freedom'. For those who dislike being themselves. Helps to ease hidden fears and anxieties and increase positive attitudes and a sense of humour, bestowing a sense of freedom to grow and feel comfortable.

LILAC 'Spine'. Eases all aspects of the spine, easing tension in the back and improving posture. Activates all chakras. Lilac is closely aligned with many different types of nature spirit.

LUCOMBE OAK 'Creative energy'. Brings life-supporting creativity, inspiration, ideas; increased mental focus; the commitment to act and bring change; wisdom and compassion.

NORWAY MAPLE 'Healing love'. Brings love and acceptance, healing, nurturing energy for emotional shock and trauma; lightness, happiness, relaxation. Helps you take back control of life and power for yourself.

OSIER 'Spiritual void'. To contact the Higher Self. Brings the energy to adapt, change and grow. Useful when everything seems empty and useless. Leads to energy and understanding.

PINE 'Insight'. Helps activate the third eye chakra and develop subtle awareness in a balanced way. Brings penetrating insight and increases tenacity and patience. Broadens one's outlook.

PLUM 'Empowerment'. Helps the highest spiritual energy enter into the material world. Brings practical solutions to problems. Increases awareness of surroundings and effective use of personal power. Confers self-worth, self-motivation.

ROWAN 'Nature'. For attuning to the energies of nature, particularly wood and earth. Enlarges perspectives to a cosmic level, allowing deep understanding of the universe.

SILVER BIRCH 'Beauty'. Helps us to experience beauty and calmness. Brings tolerance of ourselves and others. Also helps those who find it difficult to express themselves.

SILVER MAPLE 'Moods'. Helps to balance the flow of energy through the body; regulates mood swings. Realigns the meridians, so ideal for using in conjunction with acupuncture.

SWEET CHESTNUT 'The now'. For focusing and centring in the present moment. Releases guilt, particularly alienation with the physical world. Creates detachment and understanding so as to regain a wider perspective and find ways out of difficult situations.

SYCAMORE 'Lighten up'. Increases energy levels, so helps with lethargy and lifts heavy moods. Brings an awareness of the sweetness of life, harmony and relaxation.

TAMARISK 'Fire of transformation'. For finding spiritual direction, freeing up energies for personal expansion and growth. Deeply cleansing and uplifting, purging you of age-old dross so that your true self can emerge.

TREE LICHEN 'Wisdom'. For accessing past knowledge and ancient wisdom. Brings a sense of independence and detachment without isolation. Helps us to let go of things no longer needed, in order to grow.

WHITEBEAM 'Fairies'. Stimulates finer levels of perception and an understanding of the animal and plant kingdoms. Opens the heart and mind to the finer levels of creation.

YEW 'Protection'. Protects us from harm by activating the higher spiritual values of survival. Aids memory and powers of discrimination. Helps the immune system and increases energy.

❋ HAREBELL REMEDIES ❋

These essences are made from traditional British flowers by Ellie Webb in Scotland. They are prepared mostly in the Spring and Summer sunshine (sometimes during showers) and occasionally by moonlight.

ALKANET An alchemical uniting of opposites within us. Deeply centring, to prepare us for transformation.

BINDWEED Helps us to see that life makes sense, to acknowledge the spiral pattern of growth and be aware that each stage of life supports growth.

BLACKBERRY For an understanding of growth, vitality and fertility. Good against lethargy and depression or fear, especially about death. Brings the realization that everything is alive, that even death is just life in a new form.

BLUEBELL Cools, calms and brings a feeling of contentment and joy – just like being in a bluebell wood.

BORAGE Brings courage, cheer, confidence and joy. Defends and strengthens the heart, eases the emotions. A good tonic.

BROOM For despair. Helps us persevere through difficulties. Sweeps clean and renews our faith. Restores a strong, calm will to start afresh.

BUDDLEJA For those who feel alienated in but inevitably part of a dying urban culture. Also for those who sense the loss of artistic, magical expression. Gives us the strength to flourish in the wasteland.

BUTTERCUP Encourages relaxation and the feeling of being grounded, childlike, patient and appreciative of the earth's riches. Grants us the safety to experience pleasure, joy and abundance now, in the present.

CHAMOMILE For highly strung, over-responsible, churned-up states. Releases tension, anxiety and fear, helping deep relaxation, meditation and acceptance of our situation. Calms and soothes.

COMFREY For mending nerves, healing emotional bruises and enhancing memory and natural rhythm cycles. For feeling relaxed, integrated, in rhythm, united and whole.

CORNFLOWER Promotes self-love and a happiness to be different. Heals damage resulting from institutionalization (in schools, hospitals, prisons, etc.). Protects our psychic gifts.

COURGETTE For openness and security about sexual issues and your sexuality.

CYMBIDIUM For defiance in the face of undermining influences. Helps us to overcome frustration and fear of disapproval. Brings confidence and strength.

CYTISIS For self-motivation. Helps us to keep busy and active in spite of difficulties, distractions or lack of help and encouragement. Fosters an abundance of energy.

DAFFODIL For 'Spring cleaning': replaces depression and low self-worth with love and trust for ourselves.

DAISY For easy and clear understanding; helps deep breathing, organizational skills, uniting thoughts and integrating ideas around a central focus.

DANDELION For constantly tense people. Brings relaxation of mental stress and muscle tension. Helps with the letting go of fear and trusting in one's ability to cope with life.

DILL Helps us to process material and assimilate experiences when we feel overwhelmed. Good in intense urban environments or temporarily stressful situations. Grants us the time to digest experiences and make good use of what happens to us.

ELDER For protection from abuse, invasion, psychic obsession (feeling invaded). Gives us the strength to confront fears and learn to say no.

EYEBRIGHT For getting things into perspective. Eases the pain of seeing; encourages the release of fears. Good for weak brain and memory.

FLOWERING CURRANT For warming and opening the heart, expanding and softening the lungs and strengthening the free flow of energy.

FORGET-ME-NOT For remembering reality. Brings emotional balance and the release of negative thoughts (often through dreams). Restores the knowledge that there is wisdom in the subconscious, that there lies an explanation for all your fears.

FORSYTHIA For accepting and absorbing energy. Brings the realization that there is an abundance of available energy.

FOXGLOVE (PURPLE) For sharp pain, wounds in the heart, feeling betrayed. Helps us to accept pain as an essential part of self-growth.

FRENCH MARIGOLD For ears, hearing, listening and understanding the truth on all levels.

FUCHSIA For understanding the perfection of things as they are. Helps you to change a low opinion of yourself or others.

GERANIUM For bringing a project – such as giving up smoking or starting a business – through its first stages (so that it is well thought out and grounded). Allows all plans to manifest.

GYPSY ROSE For channelling spiritual energy. Clears your focus and purpose. Makes you feel centred in the source so that you know where you came from, what you are doing and where you are going.

HAREBELL For feeling a part of nature, enabling you to acquire gentleness, clarity and strength from living close to nature.

HAWKWEED For clear sight, visionary qualities, the ability to see the truth – the gift of sight and the discipline to use it wisely.

HAWTHORN Brings hope, protecting the spirit in extreme stress, pain or grief. Strengthens the immune system. Bestows the knowledge that your spirit is free, your body strong and your heart resilient.

HEARTSEASE Eases hurt and loneliness, bringing comforting thoughts to broken or damaged hearts.

HEATHER For fear of darkness and empty spaces. Helps you to find the strength to be alone, to allow some space in your life and accept the darkness as a friend. Brings acceptance of all aspects of the self.

HONESTY For confusion or lapses in consciousness. Fosters openness with others and honesty with yourself. Helps you to honour the truth and be clear about what is real.

HYSSOP For helping to acknowledge and release guilt, to confront the true cause of your feelings and forgive yourself.

JACOB'S LADDER For being open to receiving help when you need it.

LADY'S MANTLE For those who need the protection and inspiration of the Goddess. Helps with problems of infertility.

LADY'S SMOCK (CUCKOO FLOWER) For regulating sensitivity in those who need more or less. Helps us achieve the appropriate degree of sensitivity.

LAVENDER Calms, cleanses, soothes, creates space and brings a clear overview. Good for meditation and balancing the emotions, for feeling at peace.

LILAC For inflexibility and rigid posture. Relaxes, opens and connects the chakras.

LUNGWORT For cleansing and protecting a clear air space in the body (upper respirator) and mind (psychic airways) when we are feeling 'zapped'.

MAIZE For deep grounding, a sense of being in the right place and at the centre of things. Brings feelings of belonging.

MALLOW For fears of ageing. Helpful for mid-life crisis, puberty stress, for the prematurely elderly and sometimes younger children. Brings feelings of ease concerning the processes of growing up or getting old.

MARJORAM Calms, soothes, comforts and protects from harm. Supports life in times of danger or attack. Helps release emotions, especially fear, which in turn leads to trust in the life-preserving force.

MARSH WOUNDWORT For letting go of old hurts and fretfulness, being open and ready to heal, releasing the past and welcoming the future.

MEADOWSWEET For tight, tense heads and necks. Bestows the ability to relax, rest and let your head float.

MONK'S HOOD Offers strong spiritual protection (crown chakra) from the poisons of the world. Brings the knowledge that one's true identity and purpose cannot be harmed.

MOUSE EAR CHICKWEED For trance work and creative dreaming, astral travel, changing form. Allows you to feel safe to 'fly'.

MUGWORT For letting out stored up 'negative' emotions. Releases the bitterness of the past.

NASTURTIUM For vitality, sensitivity and broadmindedness. Good for the eyes, meditation and vision on all levels. Makes you feeling alive with vital energy.

NETTLE For cold, angry states. Promotes fiery, righteous anger and fearlessness in those who feel apart or hurt or who have been 'stung' by life. Restores the ability to connect to others through anger.

ORIENTAL POPPY For escapists. Helps us to find the strength to be in the here and now without needing to forget, 'switch off' or pretend.

PANSY Hardy resistance for anyone feeling low or vulnerable, or susceptible to frequent viral illness. Balances the immune system. Encourages, strength, resistance and the will to overcome illness.

PETUNIA For focusing on priorities. Helps some behaviour problems such as hyperactivity, stuttering, mild senility, as well as those worried about their behaviour. Makes you feel calm, sure and aware of what is most important.

PLANTAIN For turning resignation into acceptance in those who are heavy-hearted. Allows you to find strength in being grounded, to enjoy work and life.

POPPY (FIELD) For joyful pride, allowing sharp, bright, hot, angry feelings, the courage to shine and assert yourself.

POTATO For calming down over-excited and over-charged people. Allows you the freedom to be ordinary, to feel safe and centred.

PRIMROSE For lightness and cleansing, opening and relief. Helps with post-winter depression, tight, held-back feelings and toxic ailments.

RAGWORT For relaxing into the body, letting go of writhing thoughts and the need to understand. For quietening the mind and surrendering all thoughts that are not helpful to wisdom and intuition. Centres all our separate selves. Brings trust in and love and respect for the body.

RED CAMPION For those who disappear or who are not there when needed. Develops the ability to avoid feeling overpowered and running away from others' needs.

RED CLOVER For shock and anyone with a tendency to panic or react in an inharmonious way. Calms and soothes. Brings trust that the world will take care of itself, if you take care of yourself.

RED TULIP For overcoming shyness, for birthing or those who don't trust their fire (that is, who can be daring, vibrant and outgoing but tend to lose their centre). Balances and strengthens.

RHUBARB For exhibitionism and extrusive behaviour such as talking too much. Also for those who are vulnerable to being way off-centre, unaware of their own or other people's boundaries. Restores feelings of fulfilment and wholeness.

ROSE BAY WILLOW HERB For old defensive patterns that are hard to change; for numbness or feeling cut off from others. Releases and heals past injuries.

ROSEBUD (RED) For opening up to love and loving; for puberty; to help you to feel safe (and not too serious) about giving and receiving a little gentle, tender love.

ROSEBUD (WHITE) For infants and for babies in the womb to help them grow and keep their sense of heaven on earth.

ROSEMARY For remembrance. Good for fear of the loss of love and the autonomy of the sexes. Brings strength to heart and mind, trust in friends, strong bonds, common purpose. Opens you to receiving strength from the love of friends and from always being loved.

ROSE (RED) Fosters boldness, passion, being true to your desire. Dispels shame. Balances the base chakra. Allows you to feel proud of your sexuality and to see fertility as sacred.

ROSE (WHITE) For grace – the regenerating, inspiring and strengthening influence in your life.

ROSE (WILD) For feeling soft, warm, contented, sensual, easy-going and independent.

SAGE For the wisdom of accepting that you do not understand everything and of not taking yourself too seriously – the essential secret of longevity. Allows you to relax and enjoy life.

SAINT JOHN'S WORT For overly-worried or frightened people, paranoia and children's night fears. Brings protection and guidance. Seals the aura and helps bring sound sleep, which allows the release of subconscious fears. Frees you to trust that all is well and to feel protected by the light.

SALPGLOSSIS Encourages attentiveness to the healing sound of silence. Fosters meditation, calms mental chattering.

SCARLET PIMPERNEL For developing and opening a strong, loving heart. Bestows an intelligent and compassionate understanding of one's own strengths and weaknesses. Fosters 'dream harmony' and helps you know when to meditate.

SELF-HEAL For taking control, knowing what you need, developing self-love and acceptance. Liberates our capacity to heal ourselves and receive nourishment from life energy. Helps the assimilation of nutrients – good while fasting.

SNAPDRAGON For allowing clear expression of negative feelings and knowing they are valid. Good for any irritation in the throat or voice, or tightness in the face (lips and jaw).

SNOWDROP For simplicity, innocence and trust. Also for pelvic cleansing.

SPEEDWELL For safe and easy travel, crisis periods, more-haste-less-speed situations. For seeing your new direction clearly. Benefits the eyes and liver.

STAR JASMINE For low self-esteem. A general stimulant, helping you to process and absorb the good in life and eliminate the bad.

SUNFLOWER For dealing with power issues and connecting to your will. For feeling your intuition is strong and that you have the power to act upon it. Good for the spine and posture. Balances the spleen.

SWEET PEA For socialization, helping us to overcome fear, alienation or confusion about relating to others. Good in overcrowded situations or for hermits.

THISTLE For honour, dignity, self-respect, keeping the faith, defending your integrity and upholding what you believe is right.

TORMENTIL For the strength to resist being crushed or oppressed. Eases inner torment and emotional turmoil so that you can endure and keep hold of your reality in the face of any threat.

WHITE NARCISSUS For letting go of the superego, moving from being 'in the head' to the feelings, to the child within; trusting yourself to do the right thing.

WINDFLOWER For recognizing and respecting tearful, fearful vulnerability, fragility, mortality; for admitting fears, allowing tears. Allows you to be gentle, caring and protective of yourself.

YARROW For strong protection against negative influences in the environment and in the thoughts of others. Enhances and strengthens the aura, leaving you surrounded by white light and protected from harm.

YARROW IN SEA-WATER For exposure to radiation. Cleanses and releases us from vulnerability to radiation.

❈ DEVA FLOWER ELIXIRS ❈

In France there exists a very strong tradition of healing with flowers and plants. The doctrine of signatures and principles of homoeopathy are widely accepted in this region of Europe, due largely to the influence of healers such as Goethe and Paracelsus.

Deva Flower Elixirs were started by Philippe Deroide and Dominique Guillet after they had discovered the Flower Essence Society essences (*see pages* 129-38). The Deva essences are made from the blossoms of flowers in full bloom growing in the French Alps and Mediterranean region. Only the healthiest flowering plants growing in unpolluted environments are chosen; the garden essences are prepared in creative gardens tended according to organic principles.

At the Gaia Institute (the Deva laboratories) the research is being conducted by homoeopathic doctors into the ways in which flower essences exert their benefits. Around a thousand therapists contribute to the work that is being done at this Research Institute, where scientific methodology blends with the intuitive approach to glean information about the healing properties of flower essences.

ALMOND For those who fear growing old. Strengthens and regenerates the physical body, joy of living, vitality. Helps us to accept the ageing processes and perceive the beauty beyond superficial physical appearances.

ANGELICA For emergency situations and each time we feel that our lives are at stake. Offers spiritual protection. Strengthens trust and reinforces resistance in difficult moments. Helps us to face the unknown.

ARNICA To be taken after any physical, mental or emotional trauma. Regenerates and consoles. Repairs damages due to shocks or deep traumas. Re-establishes or maintains our contact with the Higher Self.

BASIL For those who fear and conceal their sexuality – especially when sexuality and spirituality are perceived as opposing forces. Brings sexual integration, helping us to harmonize our emotional and sexual desires with our spiritual worth. Eliminates conflicts of sexual or emotional origins within a relationship, by helping us to understand their roots.

BLACKBERRY For those who cannot materialize their projects, who have difficulties putting their ideas into practice. Also for those hampered by inertia, lethargy and mental confusion. Helps us to overcome confused mental states and develop our hidden talents. Recommended to those who meditate, who practise creative visualization and who work on dreams.

BLACK-EYED SUSAN For those who fear looking deeply within themselves and who resist all transformation processes. Aids understanding of hidden emotions and repressed aspects of the self, particularly when the mind censors or disassociates itself from certain aspects of the personality.

BLEEDING HEART For those who go through a painful experience of separation: loss of a loved one, break-up of a relationship. Fosters the emergence of intense emotions which lie heavy on the heart. Brings harmony and detachment.

BORAGE For depressive temperaments. Fosters courage and self-confidence. Helps us to overcome sorrow, sadness and discouragement when facing trials and danger.

BOX For those who lack will, who are shy, perhaps weak and let themselves become dominated by their nearest and dearest. Helps us develop individuality, detaching ourselves from the domination of others by bringing strength, courage and tenacity.

BUTTERCUP For those who are shy and reserved and have doubts about themselves, who don't know how to appreciate their true worth and underestimate themselves. Brings open-mindedness and trust, and promotes self-esteem.

CALENDULA For those who listen only superficially and who are often hurtful in what they say. Brings receptivity and understanding beyond words, the real meaning of others' messages. Confers warmth, sensitivity and mellowness in all communications.

CALIFORNIA POPPY Particularly for those who focus on outer means of spiritual development rather than harmonizing with the inner source of spiritual experience. Encourages awakening and recognition of one's qualities and personal abilities. Helps us in our spiritual search by developing attention and inner listening. Safeguards against over-fascination with spirituality.

CAYENNE A powerful catalyst for overcoming inertia, indecision and immobilization. Develops will-power, brings motivation and enthusiasm. Triggers dynamic transformation when 'stuck' in situations so we can move forward.

CHAMOMILE For nervousness, emotional instability and insomnia. Releases emotional tensions felt mainly in the stomach area. Good for hyperactive children prone to mood changes and to extreme emotional reactions.

COMFREY Strengthens and tones up the nervous system. Releases nervous tensions and improves memory. Develops conscious control of physiological processes and improves reflexes. Good for athletes.

COSMOS Allows shy, introverted or hesitant people to express their ideas more clearly and easily, allowing them to express themselves with calm and composure when facing the public. Helpful for public speakers, actors and writers.

DAISY Helps the mind to synthesize information coming from different sources and integrate them into a global perspective. Useful for those who must plan a project or organize an activity.

DANDELION For those who do too much and need to learn to release their tensions. Frees muscular, mental and emotional tension. Fosters spiritual openness by relaxing the physical body. Advised for athletes and those doing body work such as masseuses.

DILL For those who feel overwhelmed by the pace of life. Helps us to face up to stress caused by excessive stimulation. Brings liveliness and clear thoughts. Promotes assimilation and understanding of complicated or unusual situations.

EYEBRIGHT Helps healers develop perception of a patient's condition, and increases their sensitivity.

FIG TREE For coping with the complexity of modern life in a calm, assured manner. Encourages self-control. Develops mental clarity, confidence and memory. Frees hidden fears and helps in resolving relationship conflicts.

FIREWEED Liberates tensions and worries caused by traumatizing events. A transformation catalyst which leads one towards a new progressive phase. Promotes regeneration and purification.

FORGET-ME-NOT Releases repressed tensions; stimulates memory, quick-wit and insight. Develops our connection with the extrasensory spiritual world. Strengthens the mother–child bond during pregnancy.

FUCHSIA For freeing deep feelings of anger and sorrow, or feelings linked to sexuality which lead to tension, psychosomatic problems or false emotionalism. An emotional catalyst that encourages the emergence, understanding and elimination of repressed emotions, which often stem from childhood.

HAWTHORN MAY Frees one from outer influences, especially those induced by emotional attachments. Relieves emotional stresses linked to relationship problems. Eases the pain and sorrow of separation. Brings inner freedom.

HIBISCUS For women who have lost all contact with their sexuality. Allows the soul's warmth and feelings to permeate one's sexuality. Frees psychological blocks of sexual origin.

IRIS For eliminating the frustration caused by a lack of inspiration or feelings of imperfection. Brings creative and artistic inspiration.

LAVENDER For those whose nervous problems arise from having difficulties integrating spiritual steps to their daily life. A harmonizing essence for those subject to nervous tensions caused by excess stimulation. Brings purification, emotional equilibrium.

LEMON Stimulates and lightens the intellect by pushing aside emotional interference and co-ordinating thoughts. Fosters analytical reasoning.

LILAC For balancing the flow of energy in the back. Good for those who are fed up. Regenerates the spinal column, corrects posture and brings flexibility.

LINDEN Develops receptivity to love and imbues all communication and exchanges with respect and cordiality. Brings out qualities of protection, nourishing warmth, softness and calmness. Strengthens the relationship between mother and child.

LOTUS A universal essence for all aspects of the human being. For blossoming and spiritual harmony. Dynamizes and amplifies other remedies. Encourages reception and spiritual openness. Harmonizes the soul forces and purifies the emotions.

MALLOW For accepting the transformation processes that occur in life. For overcoming insecurity and introvertedness. Good for those who feel ill at ease socially. Eliminates the tensions and stresses that arise from a fear of ageing. Develops trust and heartiness in shy people.

MARTAGON LILY Recommended to women with fears linked to sexuality, as well as warlike, aggressive, dominating and authoritative individuals. Develops co-operation, solidarity and the ability to listen to others. Helps group work and the search for a joint success.

MORNING GLORY For liberating oneself from harmful habits such as dependence on alcohol, coffee, tobacco. Balances vital strength and tones the nervous system. Regularizes the rhythms of daily life.

MULLEIN For those in doubt about which moral values to follow. Encourages awareness of the 'inner voice'. Facilitates and promotes group work by creating unity and developing harmony.

NASTURTIUM To be used during 'funny spells', such as when overloaded by work or in a pre-influenza state. Also for those who tend to over-indulge the intellect to the detriment of their physical well-being. Stimulates vitality.

NETTLES For resolving psychological problems encountered in perturbed homes. Relieves emotional stress and brings calmness and courage after a family split or break-up. Strengthens family unity.

ONION For women who have suffered domestic violence or sexual abuse. Eases the process of introspection and the emergence of repressed emotions in psychotherapy. For emotional liberation and 'letting go'.

PASSION FLOWER Frees physical tensions, allowing us to consider life's events calmly and serenely. Brings stability and eliminates emotional confusion. Opens us up to higher levels of consciousness. For spiritual balance.

PENNYROYAL For those disturbed by others' negative thoughts. Reduces the mental confusion provoked by the ill-will of others. For protection.

PEPPERMINT For those who tend to be dull-minded due to excess mental activity. Helps us to overcome mental laziness and psychic lethargy. Develops mental clarity and a quick wit; encourages active and awakened thought processes. Good for students and intellectuals.

PINK YARROW For those who are too emotional or who identify with the emotions of others. Protects against emotional tension emitted from the surrounding environment. Reinforces the emotional structure of those who are over-sensitive and easily influenced.

POMEGRANATE For emphasizing all the feminine qualities. Helps women to resolve conflicts whose origin is an imbalance between career and family life. Balances feminine creativity.

QUINCE For women confronted with power conflicts who have difficulty integrating their outer ambitions – such as professional ambitions – with maternal love. Balances the feminine aspect of the personality.

RED CLOVER For keeping one's psychic equilibrium. Recommended in emergency situations such as disasters, conflicts. Allows us to remain calm and centred while facing fear, panic or the collective hysteria generated by certain groups or certain collective states of mind.

RHODODENDRON For those inclined to sadness, melancholy and discouragement when confronted with a difficult and harsh environment. Brings warmth, consolation and a sense of joy; encourages emotional liberation in the thoracic area (linked to breathing).

ROSEMARY For those who are disorientated, prone to forgetfulness and drowsiness, find it difficult to be present in their body. Develops clarity of mind and sensitivity. Helpful for introverted and sullen temperaments. For inner peace.

SAGE Promotes reflection on the meaning of life's events. Brings understanding, inner peace and consciousness of our spiritual dimension. Allows us to look more objectively at life's experiences.

SAINT JOHN'S WORT For children prone to restless dreams. Offers freedom from nightmares, nocturnal fears, night terrors, feelings of obscurity and the fear of death. For courage, protection and freedom.

SCARLET MONKEYFLOWER For those who repress powerful emotions linked to anger and aggressiveness, fearing a loss of self-control or the disapproval of others. Liberates these emotions, helping to resolve power struggles and angry situations in relationships. Frees the vitality that may be concealed by repressed negativity and resentment.

SCOTCH BROOM For pessimism, discouragement and despair. Helps us to consider life's hardships as opportunities for growth and evolution. Brings tenacity and perseverance to those who are continually confronted by obstacles.

SELF-HEAL A catalyst for inner healing and transformation, enabling us to develop our inner power of healing. Supports us when we are fasting or convalescing. Helps the body assimilate most nutritional substances. Good for those who try many therapies unsuccessfully.

SNAPDRAGON For those who find it difficult to express their feelings. Encourages us to give voice to our repressed emotions. Encourages verbal 'letting go' and the expression of truth.

SPRUCE For those suffering from tenseness, austerity and coldness, who lack flexibility and refuse to make compromises or concessions. Brings grace and harmony.

STICKY MONKEYFLOWER For integrating love and sexuality, discovering the sacred meaning of all life's aspects. Frees fears and resolves conflict or confusion linked to sexuality and intimacy. Balances out sexual energies.

SUNFLOWER For resolving conflicts linked to parents or parental images. Balances the ego when it is excessive (vanity) or lacking (low self-esteem). Develops the harmonious expression of our spiritual nature, helping us to work in a creative manner. Encourages our individuality.

SWEET CORN For those who live in an artificial environment and need to re-establish contact with the earth (city-dwellers). Also for those who tend to shut themselves away when feeling hostile or alienated. Develops the harmonious and balanced relationship between one's social and natural environment.

VALERIAN To overcome insomnia, stress and nervous irritation. Brings tranquillity and peace.

WATERMELON For birth: the development of a harmonious and correct attitude before, during and after conception in couples wishing to have a child. Eliminates emotional stress during pregnancy.

WHITE YARROW For those who feel too vulnerable and those who, through their professions, are confronted with the problems of others. Reinforces the energy structure of the individual and protects against disturbing environmental influences (radioactivity, electromagnetic and the electronic radiation of computers).

WILD GARLIC For eliminating fear, anxiety, insecurity and nervousness. Releases tension around the solar plexus. Strengthens any part of us that is prone to repeated infections and to general weakness.

ZINNIA Cheerfulness and joy: For those who are depressed, restless or hypersensitive and need to laugh. Helps us to accept that laughter is a very effective therapy. Releases tensions. Helps adults who have communication problems with their children to rediscover the child within them.

ZUCCHINI For a harmonious pregnancy: Helps pregnant women balance out their emotions and eliminate physical tensions. Generally stimulates and increases feminine creativity, especially when it has been smothered and repressed due to difficult social and cultural environments.

INDIA

India has a very rich floral heritage.
The country boasts wide variations in climate, from the icy north to the
tropical south, which support the growth of a great variety of
flowering plants.
In India flowers are traditionally associated
with various deities and with ceremonies, pujas, prayers and other
occasions. There are also mythological stories regarding various flowers,
clearly indicating the effect of flowers on day-to-day life. Flowers still
have a role to play in Ayurvedic medicine, a tradition of healing whose
principles date back at least 2,000 years. Regarded throughout
the world as one of the most spiritual of flowers, the
Lotus is India's national flower.

The Himalayan mountains in particular exhibit a spectacular floral show every year. Here the land is still relatively unpolluted and uncorrupted by human activity. It pulses with a vibrancy and life-force that is fast fading elsewhere on this planet. Each year the peaks grow a few centimetres, a tell-tale sign of the tremendous upward thrust generated from deep within the earth.

Pilgrims have traditionally journeyed to the Himalayas to mediate and seek enlighten-ment. Many sages of old lived in the Himalayas, while others (including the famous Chinese philosopher Lao Tzu) trav-elled there to end their days having reached a higher state of consciousness, knowing that their final impressions or images of earth were these eternally snowy peaks. Reaching through the clouds towards the heavens, the Himalayas symbolize the peak of conscious-ness; the flowers that grow here reflect the extraordinary energies of this land.

☀ HIMALAYAN ADITI FLOWER ESSENCES ☀

Aditi is the Sanskrit word for 'earth'. It is also the spiritual name given to the white Lotus flower, representing divine consciousness. For this reason Drs Atul and Rupa Shah chose Aditi as the name of their collection of flower essences.

This husband and wife team are both allopathic doctors who became increasingly interested in complementary medicine. They researched various different therapies before they came across the Bach Flower Remedies. Particularly impressed by the results they achieved with the Bach Remedies, they were prompted to prepare remedies from flowers growing wild on the slopes of the Himalayas and from other particularly verdant spots in this colourful country.

The Shahs have invented a method of preparing essences *in situ*, so that they can avoid cutting the flowers' stems. This technique involves placing a glass bulb around a flower and pouring water through it. With the intervention of sunlight they have their 'mother tincture'. They try to determine the most auspicious time to do their work and always pray first for permission to collect the essences. The essences are preserved in Ganges water (from the source) as well as brandy. Aware that some people are unable to tolerate alcohol, they are currently looking into making essences with honey.

At their two health centres, where both orthodox and complementary methods work in synergy, the Shahs carry out in-depth research into the properties of their essences. Medical techniques such as X-rays, cardiograms and blood tests are employed to assess the benefits flower essences are bringing to their patients. The Shahs claim to have had much success in treating a broad spectrum of health problems related to stress and tension including infertility, hypertension, breast cancer and arthritis using their own essences as well as others from around the world.

ASHOKA TREE For those who have gone through great trauma such as a bereavement, disease or failure and are suffering from deep-seated sorrow, sadness, grief, isolation and disharmony. Brings a profound inner state of joy, harmony and well-being. Especially good for elderly people.

BOURGAINVILLA For evoking meditation when we need to reaffirm our connection with our higher spiritual destiny when anxiety, fear or mediocrity swamp us. Rekindles enthusiasm, interest and emotional well-being, promoting our sense of the sacred in life.

BUTTERFLY LILY For those who exercise great power over people in an evil or negative way. For seeing clearly what has been done, wishing to be forgiven and making amends. Brings true remorse for wrong-doing, and inner peace.

CANNON BALL TREE For overcoming frigidity in women caused by deep fears in the mind concerning sexual expression. To use in sexual therapy for women when a strong desire to conceive is blocked by inexplicable frigidity.

CHRIST'S THORN For those in a constant state of internal turmoil for no obvious reasons. Relieves the state of negativity in the psyche and resolves conflicts from the consciousness. A redemptive essence.

CURRY LEAF For healing ulcers and hyper-acidity caused by mental tension and an imbalanced diet (which may include a lot of meat and alcohol). Produces greater relaxation as well as a balanced awareness and concern about diet and lifestyle.

DAY-BLOOMING JESSAMINE For those going through great suffering from painful, debilitating diseases. Brings acceptance and transformation of suffering into positive love, kindness and sensitivity to others. Relieves the burden of fear, nightmares and pain.

DRUM STICK For dispelling bitterness, resentment and other pains by building up positive feelings. Also for reducing the desire to smoke and resolving difficult emotions. Good for bronchitis.

GOLDEN ROD For those who feel insecure and seek negative attention from others in social situations by being naughty, bad or repulsive. Brings real humility, love and mental realism about others and our relationship with them. Eases internal emotional disharmony.

GUL MOHAR Spiritual healing for those who have committed acts of sexually-related violence in past lives. Restores deep peace and harmony, letting the sexual energy flow so lovemaking becomes fulfilling once more.

INDIAN CORAL For bureaucrats and those holding positions of power over society who are self-interested, power-seeking, generally arrogant and insensitive. Brings a transformation of consciousness for those wielding political power and gives them wisdom, enlightenment, understanding and peace. Dissolves the blockages of selfishness and impure intentions.

INDIAN MULBERRY For groups of people in conflict who are antagonistic and hate one another. Alleviates long-held prejudices, hatred and deep disharmony. Good for dealing with the legacy of negative patriotism and social conflict. Brings reconciliation.

IXORA Relationship enhancer for couples lacking direction or suffering a loss of interest and vitality in their sexual energy. Revitalizes and enhances sexual energy and activity. Enhances and brings responsibility, wisdom, calmness and balance into sexual expression.

KARVI For changing distorted attitudes towards sex and the expression of sexuality. For problems of sexual performance, or seeing sex as purely for financial gain. Guides us away from pornography and selfish sexual gratification towards more loving, sensitive and equal sexual relationships and practices. Helps with the problems of frigidity or impotence.

LOTUS A spiritual elixir and aid to meditation. Calms the mind and improves concentration. Gently releases negative emotions, correcting imbalances. Hastens recovery from illness. Aligns and balances the chakras by releasing, adding and directing energies to them. Clears the entire system of toxins. Balances, cleanses and strengthens the aura. Harmonizes interpersonal relationships. Amplifies the effect of other flower essences when used in combination with them.

MALABAR NUT FLOWER For those who feel superior to others because of nationality or class. Deals with prejudice, deep-seated pride and snobbery. Enhances love and tolerance and understanding of others.

MEENALIH For religious or self-righteous people who repress their sexuality, feeling it is wrong or sinful. For impotence caused by guilt about one's body and the pleasure that sexual urges bring. Transforms old fearful attitudes of guilt. Teaches us that true virtue lies in real love, which embraces everything, and that we have the right to a pleasurable and enjoyable sex life.

MORNING GLORY For addiction to opiates and nicotine, benefiting those trying to give up drugs at any stage of treatment. Eases nervous discomfort and physical withdrawal symptoms.

NEEM Essence of the heart. For bringing overly cerebral people into their hearts, making them more loving, intuitive, understanding and giving and less judgmental.

NIGHT JASMINE (Newara) For those who find it difficult to make love successfully. Can be used to foster long-term synchronization between two people or as an instant tonic prior to love-making. A sexual enhancer for attuning and integrating lovers' sexual energies. Produces the state of real pleasure, fulfilment and ecstasy in love-making. Revitalizes sexual relationships when taken by both partners.

NILGIRI LONGY/ST JOHN'S LILY/CAPE LILY Specifically for teachers and professionals who are too strict and rigid with students. Helps teachers to make learning more creative and fun.

OFFICE FLOWER For those who work in modern, high-tech offices sitting in front of video display screens the whole day, resulting in mental and nervous stress, frustration and associated skin problems.

OLD MAID (Pink) For women who are too promiscuous as a result of mistaken attitudes towards sex, seeing men as playthings for their own sexual gratification and ego, neglecting love and responsibility in sex. For women who have become brutal and insensitive towards men after being used or abused. Brings a loving, caring attitudes towards sex and love-making.

OLD MAID (White) For men who are too promiscuous through mistaken attitudes towards sex. Helps men change egotistical, self-centred, insensitive attitudes which make them emphasize their own pleasure above all else. Promotes love, caring and greater control over sexual urges. Stimulates deep concern about a partner's experience of the quality of the shared relationship.

PAGODA TREE For those who treat sexual partners as mere objects to satisfy their desire and fantasies, putting their own power and satisfaction above love. Dissolves illusions about sex, corrects channelling of sexual energy and cultivates a loving, caring attitude in love-making.

PARROT (Flame of the Forest) For public speakers who wish to improve the timing of their elocution and co-ordination between thought and speech. Synchronizes thought, will and speech to improve pronunciation and enunciation. Helps the mind to gain control over the delivery of speech, so enhancing confidence and vocal expression.

PARVAL For hard-hearted people. Opens up the emotions, harmonizing and rekindling compassion and sensitivity towards others. Makes us more spontaneous and joyful.

PEACOCK FLOWER For overcoming the effects of long debilitating illnesses or of physical and mental torture. Valuable for any rehabilitation process, such as overcoming drug addiction. Restores the nervous energy flow.

PILL-BEARING SPURGE For those who are accident-prone, going through a bad patch or feeling powerlessness to control their own lives. Alleviates the effects of cyclical misfortune and the consequent bitterness.

PRICKLY POPPY For men who mistreat women sexually, seeing them merely as objects. Brings a caring responsibility and love back to sex without diminishing physical arousal or pleasure. Steers a man towards seeking a fulfilling and caring relationship by teaching that sex can be more fun when responsibly and lovingly undertaken.

RADISH For anyone suffering from bereavement and from a sense of being unable to cope. Specifically strengthens and reorders the mind, affording mental objectivity, well-being and comfort following the death of someone very close. Integrates the mind after shock and trauma or bereavement.

RANGOON CREEPER (Madhumalti) Frees those who are captured in soul and will by very powerful gurus or cult leaders.

RED HIBISCUS For enhancing compatibility between people in one-to-one relationships, thus evoking warmth and responsiveness. Restores mental harmony and emotional well-being, and indirectly improves sexual interaction.

RED-HOT CAT TAIL For those who have been abused and wronged in past lives. Opens the heart centre, bringing a warm and loving transformation. Dissolves deep-seated blocks of hard-heartedness and unforgivingness in the psyche. Restores faith in a universal spirit.

RED SILK COTTON TREE For those drawn to spiritual paths. Cleanses and transforms the inner intention of such people. Liberates them from spiritual glamour and power-seeking by bringing a purity of spiritual intention,

humility, love and appreciation for all people.

RIPPY HILLOX For those who are negative and fearful about sex because they have had difficult or traumatic sexual experiences in the past; for victims of rape or sexual perversion who find the thought of sex too painful to bear.

SITHIHEA For those who are self-centred in business and their dealings with others. For anyone whose vanity and insensitivity creates a mental block in his or her awareness of others. Evokes qualities of patience, reasonableness, compassion and integrity. Enhances, sensitizes and balances external, financial and material relationships.

SLOW MATCH For those who feel badly treated in one-to-one relationships such as a marriage or parent/child relationship, resulting in bitterness and resentment towards the other person. Brings real love, openness, trust and understanding of the other person and a will to keep the relationship good.

SPOTTED GLICIRIDIA (Rikry Rorshia Flower) For oppressive political leaders. Reforms those who imprison others for their political beliefs, bringing a change of heart as well as enlightenment and wisdom.

SWALLOW WORT For those in a state of torment, disharmony and fear in their subconscious minds giving rise to disturbed sleep, nightmares, panic attacks and general restlessness. Alleviates deep disharmony so that peace, well-being and courage return.

TASSEL FLOWER For deep emotional wounds and disharmony with members of one's own family, particularly for parent/child but also for distant relationships. Fosters forgiveness and aids the reconciliation process.

TEAK WOOD FLOWER For vagueness, irrational and confused thinking, mental tiredness. For anyone over 60, especially those with senile dementia. Revitalizes and refreshes the mind, enhancing concentration and keeping the mind alert and interested.

TEMPLE For deepening and strengthening the experience of worship; helpful to anyone who has totally rejected religion. Restores true awareness of the universal spirit.

TORROYIA RORSHI PLANT For those living in urban and industrial cultures. Encourages environmental sensitivity and awareness.

TULIP For those who are aloof and disinterested in their day-to-day lives and in those around them. For anyone unable to wake early due to the intensity of his or her dreams. Brings a willingness to work and an ability to open up to and interact with others joyfully. Promotes early rising and applying oneself more completely to work and daily tasks. Reduces dreaming and astral travelling, helping one to be earthed and to accept physical life fully.

UKSHI For elderly women who used to be glamorous or beautiful but who feel rejected, depressed and resentful in their old age. Helps dissolve resentment, bitterness and isolation. Rekindles self-esteem and a sense of *joie-de-vivre*.

VILAYATI AMLI For mild envy of those close to us, making us unable to open up to or share/communicate with family and friends because they seem better than us or due to our own inferiority complex. Brings real pleasure in others' success, encouraging us to love and help others with warmth and caring. Improves relationships, particularly those within the family or among close friends.

WATER LILY The Kama Sutra among flower essences. A powerful tonic for those with psychological inhibitions about intimacy and sex. Enhances enjoyment of love-making by heightening sensuality.

WHITE CORAL TREE For narrow-minded religious people who tend to be dogmatic, critical and simplistic in their assessments of others, seeing the world in black and white. Liberates us from a state of ignorance, broadening understanding and making us more flexible, loving and real in our religious faith.

WHITE HIBISCUS For anyone who feels blocked, tense and out of tune with his or her spiritual nature. Increases responsiveness to the spiritual world and our own spirituality. Increases our psychic and sensory ability to respond to the higher planes of being – the first step towards self-discovery.

YELLOW SILK COTTON TREE For those who long to be free of a subconscious craving for spiritual power. Brings a pure, clear will to do spiritual work selflessly, humbly and without the desire for spiritual power over others.

❈ HIMALAYAN FLOWER ENHANCERS ❈

These essences are made from flowers that grow 10,000 ft (3,000 m) above sea level in the Parati Valley of the Khulamen area of the Indian Himalayas. Their creator is a man called Tanmaya, a former landscape gardener who left his native Australia to spend the next 20 years as a nomad and spiritual seeker in India.

He has always been passionate about flowers, and discovering these flower essences marked a turning point in his life for they brought him out of his reclusive lifestyle.

Tanmaya calls his essences 'enhancers' because of their ability to empower each of the body's main chakras or energy centres. The enhancers shine their light into these centres, dispelling any blockages or stored negativity.

The first enhancer he created was for the crown chakra; he named it 'Flight'. Unlike many other prepared essences, the names of Tanmaya's enhancers derive not from the plants themselves but from their therapeutic qualities, such as 'Let Go' or 'Ecstasy'.

Tanmaya believes we can learn a great deal from the flowers growing in the Himalayas:

They push up through the earth and rocks with such determination and courage...
[they] are a celebration and a gift from the earth which share their beauty, individuality and uniqueness willingly with us.

He makes his 'enhancers' by placing the blossoms directly into pure locally-produced alcohol – made from wild white roses, mountain spring water, wheat and sugar. The same white rose is the source of his Happiness essence.

FLOWERS OF THE WORLD

GODDESS Enhances the goddess, the wise woman. Provokes beauty, grace, receptivity, feminine strength. Connected to the energy of the Moon and Venus.

ISAN (Neem) Made from the flowers of an old neem tree beside the temples of Khajuraho. Helps integrate body, mind and spirit, creating wisdom. Good to take after meditation sessions. Strengthens the ability to live one's truth.

LOTUS Symbol of enlightenment. General tonic and cleanser for the entire system. Activates the crown chakra and enhances all forms of healing; acts as a booster for other flower enhancers, herbs and gem elixirs. Excellent to use in conjunction with meditation.

MORNING GLORY Helps you get up and greet the morning with enthusiasm. Enhances vitality and tones the entire nervous system, thus reducing nervous behaviour. Helps break addictive habits such as smoking. Good for restlessness at night.

VEIL OF DREAMS Enhances ability to dream consciously and step through the veil of dreams, so that you can understand the mysteries behind dreams. Excellent to take before going to sleep. Use in conjunction with 'Clarity' and 'Blue Dragon' (see below) for psychic work.

WARRIOR Enhances masculine strength, grounding, courage, male sexuality, strength of purpose. Best taken in conjunction with the flower enhancer 'Ecstasy' (see below). Connected to the energy of the Sun and Mars.

THE SEVEN CHAKRAS

FIRST/BASE: DOWN TO EARTH For low libido and psychological wounds surrounding sexuality, anxiety around material existence, subtle or hidden fears, anxiety and stress, sluggishness, lack of drive. Enhances sexual, life energy, the connection with the earth.

SECOND/HARA: WELL-BEING Enhances the connection with our inner power and centre, stimulating creativity and integrating emotions. Helps diffuse internalized anger, birth traumas, fear of death, imbalance of emotions. This chakra is the storehouse and focal point for transforming basic energy.

THIRD/SOLAR PLEXUS: STRENGTH For insecurity, lack of personal power, direction and motivation in life, hopelessness, depression, oppression. Enhances individuality, personal creativity, sincerity, honesty, feelings of self-worth, love and identity; the power of manifestation. Releases early conditioning patterns. Helps us overcome self-doubt, lack of self-esteem, the inability to express our innate creativity.

FOURTH/HEART: ECSTASY For cases of rigidity, constriction, bitterness, jealousy, feeling unloved or undernourished, being over-critical of others, being too reserved, disillusionment, lack of truth, irritability. Enhances love, compassion, sincerity, truthfulness, depth of feeling, expansiveness, universal love, service, sharing. Promotes empathy with all living things, transpersonal love.

FIFTH/THROAT: AUTHENTICITY For timidity, shyness, fear of speaking one's truth, difficulty communicating, stress, tension, apprehension, claustrophobia, lack of conviction, stage fright, frigidity or unwillingness to change. Enhances expression, verbal communication, appreciation of pleasure and beauty, refined experience, questing and seeking, singing, sharing ideas, stimulating dreams, creativity, imagination, conviction, self-authority, embracing humanity.

SIXTH/THIRD EYE: CLARITY For poor concentration, unawareness, lack of clarity, direction. Enhances clarity, awareness, sharpness of intellect, perception, intuition, sense of spirituality, insight, clairvoyance, meditation, concentration, understanding, dominion, ability to see into heart of things, bliss. Sense of universal self. Dispels feelings of isolation, alienation, meaninglessness. Helps headaches.

SEVENTH/CROWN: FLIGHT For feelings of separateness, isolation, lack of meaning and insignificance. Enhances oneness, powers of meditation, prayer; fosters a sense of the formless, Higher Self, the union of mind, body and spirit – the ability to experience nothingness.

OTHER HIMALAYAN FLOWER ENHANCERS

AURA CLEANING Cleans and refreshes the aura, adding a lightness and sparkle to the energy field. Excellent for use in the bath or spraying over the body.

BLUE DRAGON Enhances single-mindedness. Pierces straight into the heart of any matter. Excellent for meditation.

CHAMPAGNE For celebration – particularly good at night. Take with the Floral Enhancer 'Ecstasy' for a night of celebration, 'Clarity' for a more mysterious night, or 'Down to Earth' and 'Ecstasy' for a night of passionate love-making.

EXPANSION For the chest and breasts; brings relaxation, expansion, the experience of letting go.

GATEWAY Assists in periods of transition, rites of passage, the dark night of the soul. Gives strength and resilience in times of inner turmoil.

GRATEFULNESS Enhances universal brotherhood and sharing, wonder, awe. Catalyst for all essences. Helps counter egocentric and selfish attitudes.

HAPPINESS Provokes radiance from within that sends a smile and a soothing glow throughout the whole body and relaxes the mind. Very supportive for inner-smile meditations.

HEALING For healers. Helps them to be in touch with the basic life-forces in nature; especially helpful to healers working in cities or heavy urban environments. Clears channels for the healer, centring and bringing them back to their natural relationship with existence. Encourages an instinctive relationship between healer and client, particularly if taken in conjunction with the Heart Essence and the essence most suitable to the client. Of great help where the life-force is weak. Apply directly onto the hara or wherever there is a marked absence of energy.

HEART OF TANTRA Creates a circle of light between the sex chakra and around the heart chakra. For men particularly, this bridges the solar plexus with the heart, thus moving sex from being about power to being about love.

HIDDEN SPLENDOUR Brings forth the splendour within. For reclaiming your birthright: your inner glory. Helps combat feelings of worthlessness, constriction, insignificance, smallness.

LET GO A Pisces flower – letting go into the flow; relaxation. Good for hypnosis and guided fantasy work.

LONGEVITY Supports youthful vigour and vitality; slows down the ageing process.

NIRJARA For deconditioning and deprogramming. Erases outmoded imprints from the cells where there is a conscious intention to change conditioned attitudes and behavioural patterns. Supports change.

SOBER UP For alcoholic excess and related problems such as the spins and hang-over.

VITAL SPARK Enhances vitality and life-force, especially in situations of shock, fear and extreme emotions. Helps you relax, let go and surrender to the moment, thereby providing space for healing to take place.

✳ HIMALAYAN INDIAN TREE AND ✳ FLOWER ESSENCES

These essences have produced in India by Dr R. Nadhu and Tulsi (a healer and flower essence practitioner) for the last 20 years. At present they do not wish to reveal any more information about their work.

ASHOKA TREE Brings colour and spice into your life, lifting depression and negativity.

Develops attachments and promotes a sense of well-being through communication with others.

BANYAN TREE For those needing shelter and protection of any kind, including that of a spiritual nature (over-sensitivity and nervousness). For weak people needing strength.

BOURGAINVILLA Spreads the joy of life, bringing spiritual abundance and uplifting feelings to those following their path in life. Promotes universal love and compassion for others.

CANNON BALL TREE For people who find it difficult to make decisions in life; for those who make mistakes and are then reluctant to try again.

CASTOR OIL PLANT Helps in many areas where there is sluggishness and inactivity. Brings vitality.

CHRIST'S THORN For those who understand humility through suffering and who reach out to comfort and heal others. For compassionate people who need a cloak of protection.

COCONUT PALM For those who find it hard to make decisions and keep to them. For picking up the strands and weaving life's pattern together.

COMMELINA Helps to reduce all pain physically, emotionally and mentally. Calms the nervous system and brings a sense of tranquillity.

CURRY LEAF TREE For bringing warmth into the lives of those who feel alone in this world. Brings a glow to the aura which helps to attract the right people.

DAY-BLOOMING JESSAMINE For those who cannot face the day ahead. Gives strength of mind to overcome all kinds of negativity.

DRUM STICK TREE Opens up the chakra centres, bringing a new spiritual awareness. Opens up the psyche for those with mediumistic tendencies.

GREEN ROSE For those who are resentful and intolerant of others, wanting to cut themselves off because of an inability to communicate, only accepting their own way of thinking. Helps us to become more outgoing and aware of other people's opinions.

GUL MOHAR Helps escapists who live in a world of fantasy and daydreams to come down to earth gently and face up to reality and responsibility.

HIBISCUS For healing all traumas connected with psychic and spiritual shocks. Restores balance and realignment to the body. Brings love and warmth to women who have been abused in any way.

INDIAN ALMOND Brings relief from grief and sadness. Helps to overcome the fear of water. Good for easing water retention.

INDIAN GOOSEBERRY When feeling lost and that life has no meaning. Brings in the light, dispelling the shadows and illuminating another, brighter pathway.

INDIAN MULBERRY For those who have not been shown love. Warms the heart and helps communication with others.

IXORA For those going through different levels of change and finding it difficult to accept and understand why these adjustments have to be made for life to progress forward.

JACK FRUIT TREE For those who seek and explore new ventures. Brings zest and the ability to reach out in all directions. An uplifting remedy for the underdog, bringing joy.

JUJUBE TREE For those prone to nervous stomach disorders. Helps to strengthen this area and to relieve anxiety and nausea.

LOTUS For those who wish to reach out to the higher realms through the crown chakra. Also for those who have reached understanding of spirituality through meditation.

MALABAR NUT FLOWER For those who have experienced disappointments in life and find it difficult to know which direction to take. Helps us stop and assess life; to listen to the inner voice and find balance.

MAST TREE For those unable to bring action or movement into their lives. Rekindles enthusiasm and get up and go, making it possible to look forward to the future.

NEEM For those who have difficulty concentrating. Helps in times when there is great need to focus, such as when for taking exams, tests and so forth.

NIGHT QUEEN For those who only come alive as dusk falls, finding it hard to communicate during the day because they are drained by the humdrum way of life.

NILGIRI LONGY PLANT For those in authority who do not want others to be better than themselves and therefore suppress them. Helps release us from the fear of other people's progress.

PAGODA TREE For those wishing to join the spiritual way of understanding life by reaching out to meet soul-mates. Helps us to love and grow together with caring and nurturing, attaining a state of union and joyfulness.

PARROT TREE For those who do not think before they speak and cannot retract what they have said, causing pain and suffering to all. Encourages forethought and calms the tongue.

PARVEL For dissolving deeply rooted convictions of a religious nature. Allows us to look further and show sensitivity to other spiritual pathways.

PEACOCK FLOWER Helps to restore and rekindle the flow of energy to the nervous system, especially after severe illnesses and for those who are receiving treatment after taking drugs.

PEEPAL TREE For enhancing the sense of smell which has been blocked by mucus or shock. Brings back the joy of being able to communicate through all aromas such as those of flowers, herbs, perfumes and oils.

PILL-BEARING SPURGE For accident-prone people who seem thrown into all sorts of situations, who always seem to be in the wrong place at the wrong time. Helps to align the mind and alleviate misfortune.

THE PONGHAM TREE For those whose minds are hyperactive. A cooling remedy which rests the brain and calms the mind.

PORTIA TREE For becoming more carefree. Brings lightheartedness into life, dispersing dullness and changing greys into white to enhance the aura.

RAIN TREE For those who feel bruised by life's ups and downs. Instils strength and brings the patience to wait for better times.

RANGOON CREEPER For restless wanderers who cannot settle but want to put down roots. Conversely, bestows the courage to cut loose on those who are rooted and have the urge to wander.

RED HIBISCUS Promotes spontaneity and brings harmony to the mind, so creating an emotional sense of well-being and the feeling (in mind, body and soul) that it is good to be alive.

RED-HOT CAT TAIL For impulsive people; stops them jumping into situations that only bring remorse and regret later. Soothes and helps control the emotions and balance the energies.

RED SILK COTTON TREE Helps you think before exploding into verbal abuse which you always regret later. Quietens the mind and brings out your softer nature.

RIPPY HILLOX PLANT Rebuilds self-esteem after childhood trauma and abuse. Restores dignity and gives you the strength to follow your pathway in life. A rebuilding and reshaping remedy.

SCREW PINE Helps those with great feelings of remorse and regret, sometimes more imaginary than real, which need to be released so they can find total harmony and self-love. Helps them make up for time lost on self-deprecation so that they can move forward.

SLOW MATCH TREE For those who are detached and alone due to feelings of jealousy, envy and even bitterness which can destroy the soul. Helps to repair damage caused by these destructive feelings and restore feelings of self-love.

SOAP NUT TREE For opening the heart in the sense of opening up to others. Brings love where there is despair and loneliness. Fosters togetherness.

SUN PLANT Bring out the warmth of the soul, to radiate personality especially when self-esteem is low. Allows understanding of a father figure.

SWALLOW WORT For those always having to battle with the subconscious, bringing a feeling of inner disharmony. Bestows peace and greater self-understanding.

TAMARIND TREE For selfishness. Enables people to become more giving of themselves, encouraging new ideas and more stability in life.

TASSEL FLOWER Helps repair rifts where there is disharmony in close relationships – that is, family discord. Brings reconciliation and forgiveness.

TEAK WOOD TREE Restores energy for concentration when the brain begins to tire and the way of thinking becomes muddled. Brings renewed clarity to focus on all things.

TEMPLE TREE For those wishing to connect to the higher energies through meditation, wanting to become teachers of spirituality for the right motives: to help humanity.

TORROYIA RORSHI PLANT Brings a new awareness of all environmental issues, a desire to help throughout the world and to see new horizons through mother nature.

TULIP TREE For enhancing awareness of your inner voice, so as to receive guidance through insight (whether this comes from dreams, meditation or just connection through your thought-forms). For communication with the higher levels.

UKSI For those who are very cynical and deeply angry with everyone and everything in life, causing hardship to themselves and others. Brings a more objective attitude and softens the character.

VINCA ALBA For leaving past lives behind in order to live this life to the fullest. Brings you to the here and now.

VINCA ROSA For those with deep spiritual understanding who have been unable to heed the call to religious vocation because of crossed pathways in life. Allows you to come to terms with what cannot be spiritually.

WATER LILY For those who are so intensely shy that living becomes quite painful. Breaks down the barriers of fear, encouraging a more outgoing nature and enjoyment of life.

WHITE CORAL TREE For those who are dog-matic and see things from their own viewpoint. Brings out their softer nature and a sense of humility, helping them see all sides of every issue or situation.

WOOD APPLE TREE A cleansing remedy that clears away imperfections. Brings acceptance of the way you are. Helps allergies and alleviates psychosomatic illness.

YELLOW CANNA For those with overactive minds who find it hard to concentrate and who suffer lack of energy because the mind cannot relax. Quietens the mind, bringing peace and promoting concentration.

YELLOW CHAMPA For those who allow themselves to be dictated to by others, to be the underdog. Brings the strength to rise up, be noticed and do battle in such situations.

YELLOW SILK COTTON TREE For those who have a deep affinity with their God, enabling them to work not for power and ego but with a deep sense of caring for humanity.

USA AND CANADA

For hundreds of years before
the arrival of European settlers, the vast and colourful North American continent was inhabited by peoples who knew it as Turtle Island.
These Native Americans regarded themselves
as caretakers or keepers of the land who were responsible for safeguarding
its fertility. They saw themselves as belonging to the natural world and also
saw it as their duty not to disturb the balance that exists in nature. The idea
of splitting up and owning various bits of land was alien to them. The
whole of Turtle Island was their home and they regarded it as sacred.
Native American legends talk of Gentle Giants who once walked upon the
earth in times when all was peace and harmony. These 'Giants' were
reputedly a highly spiritual people, such was their awareness of the Great
Spirit – Gitchi Manitou – in all living things and their deep connection with
the nature. They are said to have possessed the gift of talking with the
energies of animals, flowers, the wind, water and thunder. They also had
the ability to utilize these energies for healing purposes.
Native American traditions live on
and are an inspiration to many of those who seek to explore the healing
powers of nature.

❋ ALASKAN FLOWER AND ENVIRONMENTAL ❋ ESSENCES

The Alaskan Flower Essence Project was founded by Steve Johnson in 1984 to co-ordinate the collection of new flower essences from the extensive ecological regions of Alaska.

Johnson was born and raised in the mountains of Idaho where he developed a deep connection with the natural environment. He spent his childhood playing in the gardens and orchards, walking in the forests and swimming in the nearby lakes and rivers. After graduating from high school he began his career working as a fire-fighter and he was stationed near the largest wilderness area in the United States where he learned the names and uses of all the local plants. He then transferred to Alaska, a land of vast, unspoiled forests and tundra regions which are home to many unusual species of plants.

Johnson's interest in flower essences was kindled in 1980 when he was given two Bach Flower Remedies and experienced a notable change in his health and emotional being. As a result of this experience he decided to find out as much as he could about flower essences and their mode of healing. During the next three years he trained in auric energy balancing, polarity, reflexology and massage before specializing in using vibrational energies for emotional, mental and spiritual healing.

He began making Alaskan Flower Essences in the summer of 1983, preparing them from the native plants of Alaska which have adapted and flourished over many aeons in a vibrant ecosystem, an environment of extremes from frigid cold to sweltering heat, from long dark winters to summers of perpetual light. These flowering plants reflect the special strength, power and vitality of this land.

Because they have evolved freely, without human intrusion, this community of plants embodies a unique range of vibrational energies and healing qualities that are especially relevant to the growth and evolution of human consciousness.

While the Alaskan Kits 1 and 2 are composed primarily of the essences of flowering trees and plants, and aim to balance the core or fundamental life-energy patterns, Kit 3 features essences from unique and rare plants which work on the subtle or spiritual levels of our being. The majority of essences in these kits come from wildflowers growing in healthy thriving plant communities at the peak of their blossoming stage, while the garden remedies come from blossoms growing in a co-creative garden (nature and the nature spirits co-creating together).

Encapsulating the special energies of Alaska, these flower essences provide significant levels of support for the process of conscious change and transformation and work on issues related to unfolding one's future, opening to higher levels of perception and understanding, and living life in alignment with divine purpose. They are also unique in their orientation towards healing the heart and therefore healing our relationship with each other and all forms of nature.

KIT 1

ALDER For clarity of perception on all levels, allowing our seeing to become knowing, recognizing truth in personal experience. Empowers us to move beyond limited mental programming and respond to higher learning.

BALSAM POPLAR Releases the pain and emotional tension associated with sexual issues (which block the circulation of energy in the body); synchronizes sexual energy with earth cycles and rhythms.

BLACK SPRUCE Allows integration of the eternal into awareness and experience in the present; opens us up to information contained within the archetypes of nature. Helps us to learn the wisdom of the Ages.

BLUE ELF VIOLA Helps us to understand the seeds of our anger and frustrations; releases the energy surrounding unresolved conflicts, bringing the whole process to completion.

CHIMING BELLS Peace through understanding one's true nature; joy in physical existence; awakens a spiritual awareness of nature. For regeneration and renewal.

COTTON GRASS For letting go of pain held in the body; restores equilibrium after injury or trauma; shifts our focus from pain to healing. Can be applied topically.

DANDELION Brings awareness and release of emotional tension and stress held in muscle tissue; increases one's level of body–mind communication. For use both internally and externally.

FIREWEED Helps us ground and cleanse old energy patterns from the body so that new life may enter; restores a nurturing flow of energy after a traumatic or transforming experience. Useful in emergency situations especially for releasing physical pain and trauma.

FORGET-ME-NOT Opens our hearts for the release of pain held deep in the subconscious; helps us to remember our original innocence. To regain true respect for ourselves, others and the earth.

FOXGLOVE Releases tension centred around the heart; allows us to see through perceptual constrictions to the 'heart' of the matter.

GOLDEN CORYDALIS Creates a focus for positive growth of the personality. Restores full communication between the soul and the personality; re-integrates our identity after an experience of deep transformation.

GREEN BELLS OF IRELAND For opening our perceptual awareness to the various levels of energy and intelligence that exist in nature; helps us to reconnect with the energy of the natural world and to feel at home on the earth.

ICELANDIC POPPY For reflecting one's inner radiance to all aspects of life. Opens us up to and helps us maintain a spiritual focus in life.

JACOB'S LADDER Helps to bring awareness of our attempts to control the events of our lives and be open to receiving the creative impulses of the soul; allows mental control to evolve into a disciplined acceptance of spirit.

LABRADOR TEA Centres energy in the body and calms extreme imbalances of physical, emotional and mental energy; relieves the stress associated with the experience of extremes. Useful in times of emotional catharsis or after traumatic experiences.

LADY'S SLIPPER Helps us to gain awareness of subtler energy flows in and around the body; fosters the collection, focus and release of energy for healing. Works on the chakras and central nervous system and spine – a gentle catalyst.

MONK'S HOOD 'Fearlessness.' For those who feel vulnerable through lack of well-defined boundaries and have difficulty allowing others true access. A powerful and precise essence which increases our ability to interact with others through a stronger identification with our divine nature; strengthens and defines our energy fields so we can create and maintain our physical, emotional and mental boundaries so that we can function in accordance with our higher purpose.

PAPER BIRCH Helps us gain a clear perspective of our true purpose; reveals the underlying true and essential self present within. Useful when facing important life decisions, or when lost or uncertain how to proceed.

PRICKLY WILD ROSE For openness, courage and renewed interest in life in the face of adverse circumstances. Allows the heart to open in response to conflict. Brings our hopes to fruition.

SPIRAEA To overcome resistance to conscious growth and expansion. For unconditional acceptance of support, regardless of the form it comes in. To learn to nurture and be nurtured by living things.

TWINFLOWER For those who have difficulty expressing themselves or listening to/understanding others. Improves communication skills, helping us to listen and speak to others from a place of quiet and focused neutrality.

WILD IRIS Brings a focused release of creativity; for sharing one's inner beauty and creative energy freely.

WILLOW Brings mental receptivity and resilience; for creating positive reality from the quality of one's thoughts.

YARROW For strengthening the overall integrity of the energy field; knowing and being the source of one's own protection. Used to strengthen the aura and build a protective shield against environmental hazards, such as electro-magnetic radiation from computers and fluorescent lights.

KIT 2

ALPINE AZALEA Releases old patterns of self-doubt. Opens your heart to the spirit of love; for living in total unconditional acceptance of yourself.

BOG BLUEBERRY For abundance – dissolves patterns of limitation held in the mind; encourages receptivity towards the even exchange of life-force in our lives and relationships to others.

BOG ROSEMARY Nurtures through the process of trust. For deep cleansing and healing of the experience of Life, helps one let go of any resistance to being healed. Strengthens one's connection with the infinite life-force.

BUNCHBERRY For focusing and directing the power of the will; for mental steadfastness and emotional clarity in demanding situations. Strengthens the boundary between the emotional and mental body.

CASSANDRA Quietens the mind; increases the depth of perception so that we can sense the currents of life. Acts as a catalyst to improve the quality of our relationship with nature. An aid to meditation in order to receive inner guidance.

COLUMBINE For self-appreciation, cherishing our unique and personal beauty regardless of how it differs from others'. For projecting a strong sense of self.

COW PARSNIP For those who feel powerless to direct their lives. Helps us to thrive wherever we are; brings awareness of inner strength, contentment with present circumstances and peace of mind during times of change.

GRASS OF PARNASSUS Brings a high and pure quality of light into the aura for cleansing, purification and protection; attracts nourishment from nature. Helpful for those living and working in crowded, polluted surroundings.

GROVE SANDWORT Strengthens the bonds of communication and comfort between mother and child; opens us up to support from our earth mother and encourages share this nurturing support with others.

HORSETAIL For feeling connected; enhances communication with our different levels of consciousness. Through this we are better able to make true contact with others.

LACE FLOWER For appreciation of all nature and of ourselves; realizing the importance of our contribution to the whole, however humble.

MOUNTAIN WORMWOOD For healing old wounds; helps us by releasing unforgiven areas in our relationships with others and with ourselves. Helps to bring all our relationships into balance.

OPIUM POPPY Integrates previous experiments in order to live fully in the present. Balances extremes of activity and rest, being and doing.

PINEAPPLE WEED Encourages freedom from injury and risk through harmony with our surroundings; builds affinity between mothers and children. For active young children, mothers and mothers to be. Promotes sense of well-being during pregnancy.

RIVER BEAUTY Regeneration; to help you start over after a devastating experience and to see adverse circumstances as potential for cleansing and growth.

SINGLE DELIGHT For those suffering feelings of isolation. Links us energetically with other members of our soul family. Opens the heart and reminds us of the support we have always had.

STICKY GERANIUM For getting out of a rut, or 'unstuck'; frees the many aspects of our potential; helps us to go beyond previous stages of growth. Encourages us to move from procrastination and lethargy to decisive and focused action.

SUNFLOWER Strengthens our radiant expression; harmonizes the active, masculine aspect of energy in both men and women. Teaches us to accept the authority of the Higher Self, without imposing our will on others.

SWEETGALE For the deep integration and release of emotional pain and tension; heals the core of our emotional interactions with others. Aids completion of unfinished emotional experiences, enabling us to respond to the present with strength and clarity.

TAMARACK Builds self confidence through a deeper understanding of one's abilities. Helps us remain centred in the knowledge that our abilities will carry us through challenging times.

TUNDRA ROSE Love of life: allowing the power of life to be communicated through our living of it; for combating fears of living and dying. Releases deep resistance that has blocked the dynamic expression of spirit in our lives.

WHITE SPRUCE Unification: balances intuition, thought and emotion together and unifies them, in the present moment. Native Alaskans considered this to be 'the gentle grandfather healer' – a touchstone to our higher knowledge. Brings us to a place of balance and stability. Opens us up to that internal wisdom that will illuminate our current situation.

WHITE VIOLET Opens our hearts to the essence of purity; connects us with the highest in ourselves and in others. For highly sensitive people who find contained environments intolerable. Supports creation of new energetic boundaries, allowing trust and relaxation to develop.

YELLOW DRYAS Support for those who explore the edge of the unknown; for the expansion and clarification and maintaining awareness of self and family throughout dynamic cycles of growth and change. For the pioneer in us.

KIT 3

BLADDERWORT Brings awareness of truth and shattering illusion through clear internal knowing so that we see only truth.

BLUEBERRY POLLEN Releases deep patterns of limitation from the mind so we can attract and be open to receive all we need to live life to the fullest.

CATTAIL POLLEN For standing tall in one's truth; helps you to find the courage even during pain and trauma to follow your chosen path.

COMANDRA For clearing disharmonious energies from the heart that limit one's ability to be open to and aware of subtle energies in nature.

GREEN BOG ORCHID Releases pain and fear held deep in the heart; for coming into true balance with the natural kingdom so that we can fulfil our divine co-creative potential. Expands one's awareness, sensitivity and ability to perceive life from a place of openess and neutrality.

GREEN FAIRY ORCHID For accepting oneness through total internal balance. Balances the inner male/female at the deepest level of the body and being – releases duality.

HAIRY BUTTERWORT Ascension: helps one access support and guidance needed in order to move through threshold points of transition with grace, ease and deep understanding without creating crisis or illness.

HAREBELL Removes self imposed mental and emotional limitations, allowing one to receive and give unconditional love.

LADIES' TRESSES Deep internal alignment: for releasing deeply-held traumas held at the cellular level and realigning with one's soul purpose in this lifetime.

LAMB'S QUARTERS Heals separation between the heart and mind. Helps to assimilate information through the heart before interpreting it through the mind. For those who tend to be highly intellectual. Brings the power of the mind into balance with the joy of the heart.

MOSCHATEL Opens our intuitive connection with the plant kingdom; for those wishing to work with the growth and evolution of plants on a subtle level.

NORTHERN LADY'S SLIPPER Reconnects body and spirit. Allows one's being to be touched and healed by infinite gentleness. A positive catalyst for adults who need to heal the core traumas of their inner child. Good for children and babies with birth traumas.

NORTHERN TWAYBLADE Opens the heart and perceptions to the spiritual consciousness that resides in nature. Attunes our perceptions to very subtle levels of physical manifestation. For grounding this awareness into the physical body and life experience.

ONE-SIDED WINTERGREEN For creating and maintaining functional boundaries that are in alignment with one's highest truth and life purpose.

ROUND-LEAVED SUNDEW For merging with the source of life; relinquishing identification with your ego, blending ego and divine will. Letting go of resistance to change and attachment to the known.

SHOOTING STAR For developing our connection to inner spiritual guidance for understanding cosmic origins and earthly purpose.

SILKA SPRUCE POLLEN A 'grandfather' essence which acts as a catalyst by supporting the right action for the present moment, fostering a positive relationship with one's power. Clears and expands our energy channels so that we can accept a strong flow of energy in the body. Connects us with ancient archetypes of mastery, male and female power perfectly joined together. Balances power and gentleness in men and women supporting the balanced partnership with nature.

SITKA BURNET Healing the past on all levels; completion on all levels – a facilitation essence which helps one identify issues that are contributing to internal conflict, bringing forth the potential in any healing process.

SOAPBERRY Release of constrictions around the heart associated with a fear of the power of nature; for understanding and integrating intense experiences in nature. Harmonizes both personal and planetary power.

SPHAGNUM MOSS Releasing judgement from the heart; learning to see with unconditional love.

SWEETGRASS For the cleansing and rejuvanating of the etheric and physical body. Helps to bring one's lessons and experiences to completion on all levels.

TUNDRA TWAYBLADE Supports the release of trauma held at the deepest level of one's being. Opens the heart to allow unconditional love complete access to areas of the body that need healing – especially dysfunctional patterns held within the collective consciousness (abuse being the most prevalent form of these patterns today).

WHITE FIREWEED For deep emotional healing of shock and trauma. Calms the emotional body, releasing the energetic imprint of the past emotionally painful experiences from our cellular memory so rejuvenation can begin.

WILD RHUBARB Promotes mental flexibility, clearing and expanding the channel of communication between the heart and mind. As a result, new thoughts, plans for action and solutions to problems come about.

NEW ESSENCES

ANGELICA For effortless acceptance of spiritual support in all situations; letting the light into your life, experiencing the protection that comes from within.

CLOUDBERRY Opening to the true source of your being and reflecting this outwardly for others to see; helps you see the light of purity deep within yourself; recognizing the 'angelic' level of your being.

COMBINATION POPPY For balance at the core levels of your being; unification of all energies in the body.

COMFREY Supports healing on all levels; heals the etheric body when there has been injury.

CRYSTAL SAXIFRAGE For blending the creative power of thought, intuition and divine will within the heart to accelerate your healing process.

DWARF FIREWEED Helps transform unresolved issues that are held at the core of your being; helps you release pain and trauma from the past so you can reconnect with the original joy of living, with the feeling of 'I have my whole life to live.'

INDIAN PAINTBRUSH Helps you release emotional frustrations and feelings of self-limitation that block your outward expression; helps to open and cleanse the heart so that it may act as a focal point for the expression of creative energies.

LAPLAND ROSEBAY For penetrating insight into the self and all of nature; seeing without distortion.

LILAC For raising energetic vibration in the body; aligning the chakras to receive and embody light energy fully.

PALE CORYDALIS Balances addictive and conditional patterns of loving; helps you see relationships as catalysts for spiritual growth and enlightenment; helps you follow the divine plan in relationships.

PINK-PURPLE POPPY Purity in form; helps you embody and project universal love through your heart.

POTATO Physical release: helps you 'thaw out' incomplete cycles of experience that are being held in the body; allowing love to penetrate into every cell and into all manifestations of your being.

PURPLE MOUNTAIN SAXIFRAGE Grounding wisdom from the Higher Self; helps you tune in to higher frequencies of information.

PURPLE POPPY Balance during rapid phases of evolution; helps you open up to and experience deeper levels of integration and rest while allowing the transformation process to continue.

RED ELDER 'Grandmother' wisdom (Native American for wisdom of the ages) helps one view life from the centre rather than from the periphery; helps you open up to your future potential. Also helps one contract over-expanded states, i.e. feeling frazzled and over-whelmed.

RED-PURPLE POPPY For balancing extremes between earth and the etheric levels; blending the survival and spiritual aspects of life together in a balanced way.

SELF-HEAL For raising self-esteem; the expan-sion of love and compassion for yourself. Strengthens belief in the body's ability to heal itself. Relaxing and calming, slows one down in order to gain perspective on priorities, especially under pressure to do and decide.

VALERIAN Harmony in relationships; finding a peaceful common ground.

WILD SWEET PEA Increases your sense of your own inner strength and stability; helps bring these qualities to the surface to be offered in balance to others; promotes confidence and ease in your interactions with others.

❁ DESERT ALCHEMY FLOWER ESSENCES ❁

The desert is an environment of extremes, with an abundance of heat from the sun and little water. Throughout history people wishing to strengthen their sense of spirituality have spent time in the desert. Key words to describe the energy of the desert are adaptability, individuality, expansion and inner security.

The plants inhabiting this place have evolved amazing strategies for adapting to the formidable climate in order to survive. Some only bloom at night, while others can produce leaves within six hours of a rainfall although they can continue to photosynthesize without foliage at all if necessary.

Desert Alchemy was founded in 1983 by Cynthia Athina Kemp with a view to researching and making essences from desert flowers.

The inspiration for making a flower essence from desert plants came to Cynthia while driving through the Arizona desert one day. She found herself in the midst of a whole forest of Saguaro cacti, some standing 15 m (50 ft) tall with great arms that seemed to reach towards the heavens. She felt as if the Saguaro cacti *was communicating* with her and giving her a message to make flower essences, though at the time she did not even know what flower essences were.

Out of this experience grew the Desert Alchemy essences, which capture the extraordinary qualities of the plants growing wild in this harsh environment. With an emphasis on survival, these essences are perfect for crisis situations, helping us to adapt and cope in extremely demanding situations. They encourage shifts in our perspective which enable us to deal with and embrace any emergency as an opportunity for change and growth.

AGAVE For those holding back their gifts, abilities or power out of fear. Helps you to own your level of mastery and manifest inner beauty and strength in daily life.

ALOE VERA For surrendering to the healing process with a sense of joy; feeling supported from within oneself.

ARIZONA WHITE OAK Changes feelings of nostalgia, depression or fear of change to comfort, stability, rest and strength.

ARROYO WILLOW For restoring a consciousness of will. Helps us to create our life's experiences responsibly while remaining true to ourselves.

BEARGRASS For fear of aggressiveness or of someone else's intentions overpowering your own. Helps us to be centred in heart energy, knowing that no outside influence can overpower our deeply-held intentions. Makes us aware of simplicity in any situation.

BIG ROOT JATROPHA Excellent for 'growth spurts'. Encourages a feeling of security as great inner expansion takes place. Helps one to feel safe enough to allow change to happen without the need to control. Excellent for sexual abuse issues.

BISBEE BEEHIVE CACTUS Especially for sexual abuse issues. Helps one to go to the core of an issue and to feel grace and healing energy at a cellular level.

BOURGAINVILLA Relaxes the body and deepens breathing, encouraging feelings of peace and ease, self-reflection and inner listening. Helps us to feel sadness without suffering, and to meet crisis with stillness and without overreacting.

BOUVARDIA Fortifies the will to confront life directly and consciously, changing emotional over-reaction and avoidance patterns into positive response and action.

BRIGHT STAR For those who become entangled in situations or others, unable to say 'no'. Brings protection, feelings of safety and security by encouraging healthy boundaries. Fosters trust that we deserve what we want.

BUFFALO GOURD For feeling out of balance, erratic, frazzled, depleted. Brings emotional stability and equilibrium. Helps maintain a deep inner place of healing and calm while participating in external activity. Restores inner balance, knowing that 'I am the centre' in all situations.

CAMPHORWEED For feeling scattered, ungrounded, caught up in confusion. While gently diffusing old patterns, it brings a sense of purpose and appropriateness, helping us to feel grounded and to bring projects to manifestation.

CANDY BARREL CACTUS For feeling agitated within, worth less than others. Fosters mental clarity and emotional calmness, flexibility in thinking and relating to others. Allows recognition of the wisdom within, thereby tapping long-stored abilities.

CANE CHOLLA CACTUS For an overly rigid attitude or perspective about a situation, defensiveness, impasse. Brings a leap to a new point of view, embracing apparent duality. Allows us to be with others joyfully without defensiveness or pretension.

CANYON GRAPEVINE Helps us to appreciate other energies as interdependent rather than competing; good for issues of autonomy, finding a balance between alienation and a sense of being trapped, to overcome dominance and dependency. For seeing obstacles as opportunities.

CARDON CACTUS For self-effacement, shame. Releases powerful energies as repression is unlocked; the shadow side becomes a source of strength and confidence. Brings the impetus to change, determination and deep energy reserves to move ahead in life.

CHAPARRAL For intense inner desolation, feeling totally alone, sadness. Dispels unconscious dark states by releasing, on a cellular level, what is unexpressed or held in. Confers a bright sense of being freed. Also for those who are self-involved, enclosed in their own magical world.

CLARET CUP HEDGEHOG CACTUS For clarity and focus. Excellent for meditation, manifestation or any situation requiring mental steadiness and acuity.

CLIFF ROSE For those who are unfocused, unable to follow a creative idea or project through to fruition. For uniting will, intention and the power to act. Connects us to the source of energy and brings spiritual energy into everyday situations.

COMPASS BARREL CACTUS For those who grumble, complain or hold on to anger or resentment. Helps us move beyond the emotionally 'stuck' space by letting us lighten up and let go, trusting inner wisdom to point the way.

CORAL BEAN Helps to overcome a drug-like dulling of the survival instinct. Stimulates focus and will in facing or recovering from dangerous situations.

COW PARSNIP For feelings of insecurity, responsibility for everything and an inability to handle life. Transforms insecurity into a deep sense of self, of relaxation and surrender to divine will; for allowing the universe to handle the details.

CROWN OF THORNS For anyone ascetic or self-punishing, holding back from life and relationships. Also for those who believe they must suffer or pay a price for love, that everything worthwhile is difficult to obtain. Helps us to know that abundance is our birthright.

DAMIANA For feelings of inadequacy, weakness, emotional neediness, detachment from the flow of vital life-force. Relaxes and restores radiant fullness of energy and sensuality.

DESERT CHRISTMAS CHOLLA For anyone stressed, overextended, facing too many demands, taking on other people's emotional problems. Facilitates communication of our limitations with humour and ease.

DESERT HOLLY Helps us to live in a heart-centred state, opening easily to love rather than working at it.

DESERT MARIGOLD A solar plexus essence for owning one's power, taking responsibility and transforming victim consciousness.

DESERT SUMAC For those who feel they are on the outside looking in on social relationships. Helps us transform the pain of loneliness and separation between ourselves and others. For seeing beyond the superficial differences in people.

DESERT WILLOW For a sense of being driven, of rush and clutter. Helps one to be flexible, 'in the flow of life', soothed, sheltered, aware of beauty, surrendering to the reality of abundance.

DEVIL'S CLAW For those who use their attractiveness or personal magnetism to manipulate others, or for those who fall prey to another's persuasions. Enhances a sense of responsibility for one's charisma.

EPHEDRA Stimulates the awareness of self-healing and ability to escape damaging situations; activates will and innate resources, giving direction, vision, determination and confidence.

EVENING STAR For issues of dependency, emerging identity, doubt, inner questioning. Helps us to shift from outer dependence to self-reliance with confidence and quiet surety.

FAIRY DUSTER Balances the tendency to swing between high and low energy states; for those with inflated expectations, builders of castles in the air. Excellent for nervous excitability and over-reaction to stimuli.

FIRE PRICKLY PEAR CACTUS For those with an obsessive concentration on one aspect of life or the body, neglecting the whole. Helps us find alternative avenues of expression when the current pathway is no longer rewarding.

FISHHOOK CACTUS For those who are uncommunicative, refusing to discuss or negotiate an issue for fear of losing face. Dissolves defensive barriers to communication; encourages trust and risk-taking.

FOOTHILLS PALOVERDE Deals with issues of shame and self-judgement. Brings the mind to a quiet place so as to be in touch with one's own perfection.

HACKBERRY Encourages one to feel grief, especially unresolved grief.

HEDGEHOG CACTUS Helps one be clear as to the difference between self-nurturing and over-indulgence. Intensifies empathetic perceptions, bringing one closer to nature and to others.

HOPTREE For anxiety at losing sight of one's true purpose, trying too hard to control.

Strengthens the ability to stay focused on what is essential, dispelling distractions.

IMMORTAL For deep depression, shame, victim consciousness, feeling stuck or having a problem that cannot be solved. Helps us surrender to the grace of transcendence and to realize our own magnificence.

INDIAN ROOT Shows us the value of simplicity, of overcoming the tendency to try too hard, making things complex. Helps with deep-seated fears that block our free-flowing creative expression.

INDIAN TOBACCO For perceiving growth processes as opportunities, not hindrances. Encourages a heightened perception of depth and meaning, as though seeing below the surface of things. Fosters peace.

INDIGO BUSH Helps anchor our spiritually-achieved ideas into daily life; it warms the heart and brings the light of clear vision or inner sight to an area that needs it.

JOJOBA For grounding; helps participation in daily life and relationships. Also for the overly sensitive individual who finds it hard to cope with the mundane.

JUMPING CHOLLA CACTUS An antidote for obsessive worry, frenzied rushing around, reacting rather than responding. Brings inner balance, being in the moment.

KLEIN'S PENCIL CHOLLA CACTUS Encourages creativity and growth in dealing with a relationship that is stagnating and holding you back emotionally.

MALA MUJER For those who are crabby, venomous, shrewish, grouchy. Helps the positive expression of feminine qualities, releasing emotional tensions and bringing a lighter, more honest quality to overall self-expression.

MARIOLA For those who hide behind a false persona, pretending to be what they are not. Restores the congruence of inner experience and outer expression; brings essential honesty and feeling of being at ease with who you are.

MARIPOSA LILY For desolation and isolation. Brings joy and freedom through self-mothering, healing the feelings of separation and alienation. Encourages receptivity to human love, connection to the source of energy.

MELON LOCO Brings the emotions into closer alignment with the body; quietens over-zealousness, strengthens emotional responsibility. Brings calmness, balance and honesty.

MESQUITE Opens us to abundance and pleasure. Amplifies compassion and warmth. Good for loners.

MEXICAN SHELL FLOWER Supports the willingness to confront life and its possibilities. For 'coming out of one's shell'.

MEXICAN STAR Fosters strong self-contained individuality, enjoying one's uniqueness rather than feeling isolated by it.

MILKY NIPPLE CACTUS For our 'inner mother'. This weaning essence calms, gives us a sense of belonging to the earth and transforms dependence into self-nurturing autonomy.

MORNING GLORY TREE For becoming conscious of issues of ancestral addictions. Facilitates a conscious chance to change an ancestral pattern.

MOUNTAIN MAHOGANY For those who push and try aggressively to make things happen; for those who feel 'stuck'. Provides a gentle but firm push toward the next state of development.

MULLEIN For feeling joyfully full of self; helps us to observe the dark side without threat, to be emotionally self-nurturing, especially when external support isn't available. Brings a sense of security, purpose and protection.

OCOTILLO For subconscious or unexpressed feelings that erupt in uncontrolled ways. Gives insight into and acceptance of our emotions without leading us to becoming victimized by them.

OREGON GRAPE For self-criticism and judgement, self-dissatisfaction, bitterness, feeling unloved and left out, paranoia. Helps us to overcome fear of hostility; transforms self-criticism and judgement into self-love and acceptance.

ORGAN PIPE CACTUS Asks no questions, accepts and comforts like a mother, soothes away worry, pressure and preoccupation, strengthens the emotional bond with humanity. Heals and energizes body and emotions by calming the mind.

PENCIL CHOLLA CACTUS For those feeling overwhelmed by details who are easily distracted and panicky because of confusion. Enables us to focus continually in a specific direction; balances energies, brings clarity and surrender into and through obstacles.

POMEGRANATE For scattered energy, trying too hard but getting nowhere because the commitment is not right or is not total. For those who have difficulty giving or receiving mothering. Kindles fire energy, the primal urge to produce, create, procreate and care for others. Brings energy and clarity to choose commitment.

PRICKLY PEAR CACTUS For inner turmoil, feeling frazzled, wanting to give up or give in to something that is not right for you. Brings adaptability, so we no longer push to make things happen. Helps us to find strength in surrendering to the flow of life's events.

PURPLE MAT For those who secretly harbour feelings or needs for fear of being rejected if they are openly exposed. Helps us to risk in order to stay true to ourselves and others.

QUEEN OF THE NIGHT CACTUS For those who are fearful, scattered, frantically searching, pushing or trying but feeling inadequate. Also for any distortion or blockage of the female receptive principle. Helps us to be deeply intuitive, understanding, feeling, sensual and receptive. Allows a feeling of spiritual wholeness, radiance.

RAINBOW CACTUS A searchlight to illuminate something dark or held in. Helps us to release petrified emotion without becoming entangled in it, emerging bright, free and whole; for meditation or regression work, facilitating easy movement from one state of consciousness to another.

RATANY For the conflict of love, being pulled between two choices. Enables one to recognize, follow and communicate the heart's desire or truth.

RED-ORANGE EPIPHYLLUM Facilitates the grounding of feminine (goddess) energy into worldly existence. For manifestation.

RED ROOT For prejudice, vulnerability to fear, feeling guilty because you choose not to suffer while others around you do. Also for those who are motivated by superstitions or other unconscious forces. Brings clear, mature discrimination, perceptions free from cultural conditioning. Helps us to release entanglements with others.

SACRED DATURA For those who feel detached from reality, disorientated, spaced out, who fear because their identity, situation or perception is threatened. Helps us to see beyond our present view of reality to a more comprehensive, visionary state; encourages us to let go of the known and familiar without feeling threatened.

SAGUARO CACTUS For those who are sentimental, complaining, making excuses. Foster the feeling of 'I can.' Brings human dignity, endurance, compassion, acceptance of who and where we are. Restores the will to live and to heal, to be the best that we are, allowing us to trust inner wisdom and authority.

SCORPION WEED For those who see obstacles as unapproachable monsters. Brings the strength of innocence and direct confrontation; overcomes fear and paralysis.

SENITA CACTUS Help us simply to 'be', without bitterness from the past or expectations for the future. Grants us the wisdom of the sage, allows us to see the pain and hurts of life as a necessay part of the soul's development so that opening our perspective opens the flow of emotion without pain. Soft and sweet, with an ancient strength.

SKULLCAP For those who are frazzled, disconnected, preoccupied. Brings relaxation, being present in the moment, allowing contemplation, gently dissolving old thought-patterns or ways of perceiving.

SOAPTREE YUCCA For keeping sight of one's long-term goals with faith, perseverance and endurance.

SOW THISTLE For anyone who feels intimidated by dominating personalities. Helps us to deal appropriately with obnoxious behaviour, whether our own or others'.

SPANISH BAYONET YUCCA For indecisiveness, hesitation or fear in facing challenges. Brings unification of will and intention.

SPINELESS PRICKLY PEAR CACTUS For those who feel lacking or needful of something else to be able to handle life and its situations. Brings a deep sense of purpose and power, and the realization that you don't need anything outside yourself – whatever *is* at a given moment is your tool for survival.

STAGHORN CHOLLA CACTUS The self-organizing principle of life; reconstruction after disintegration and change.

STAR LEAF Helps you to be simply and purely yourself, without the need for external approval. Frees self-expression.

STAR PRIMROSE For those with a poor self-image, or who are self-critical, feeling awkward, angry or resentful, blaming negative feelings on an outside source while simultaneously denying such feelings exist. To help with confusion about spirituality/sexuality. Also for those who want to repress sensuality and put their energy into occult, mystical or mental pursuits. Brings purity and clarity of purpose. Allows you to experience the joy and beauty in yourself.

STRAWBERRY CACTUS For those who take life too seriously, never having fun and always expecting things to go wrong. Emotionally soothing and calming, allowing you to let go and let your heart transmute difficult emotions. Brings joy and a sense of fun.

SYRIAN RUE An energetic 'truth serum'; helps to bring up and release any issues about telling the truth either to oneself or others; for knowing and trusting in one's own truth regardless of external pressures.

TARBUSH Strengthens inspiration and motivation to change something that has been accepted as a limitation or condition of life; it works with stubborn or addictive attitudes.

TEDDY BEAR CHOLLA CACTUS Brings perseverance and patience with your growth processes; helps with deep fears of intimacy, allowing others close enough to see your perfection.

THERESA CACTUS For those who hide behind serving others. Fosters a deep sense of caring for yourself. Helps you to change conditional into unconditional service.

THISTLE For those who lack trust or faith in their own spiritual connection. Helps us to let down intense defensiveness so we can recognize grace in our lives.

THURBER'S GILIA For those who are in a state of 'limbo' when the old sense of 'self' has dissolved and the 'new you' is not yet born. Helps to dissolve fear and limitations.

VIOLET CURLS Helps you recognize and express emotional energies as they arise to prevent a backlog of unprocessed emotions building up; eases emotional tensions, relieves congestion in the emotional body; restores harmony in the emotional, mental and physical bodies.

WHITE DESERT PRIMROSE For self-doubt or confusion about discerning what actions or expression are in harmony with your essential nature. For trusting, valuing and believing in yourself, and discerning your unique soul pattern.

WHITETHORN For those who feel driven and exhausted, overextended, nervous, burnt out. Helps you to be more gentle with yourself. Brings a sense of newness and optimistic freshness, helps your thinking move in new, innovative directions; calms the buzz of adrenaline excess.

WINDFLOWER For those who feel energized at one moment and depleted the next. Facilitates a more even and balanced distribution of energy. Excellent for those with a tendancy towards adrenaline addictions.

WOLFBERRY Releases deep sadness from the past, for those who try to avoid past experiences that seem too painful, feeling overwhelmed. Allows emotional processes to take place without conscious involvement.

WOVEN SPINE PINEAPPLE CACTUS For those who feel over-burdened, tired, as if they have had enough; for victim consciousness. Loosens old emotional tensions in the body and revitalizes at the core of your being. Restores self-confidence and self-esteem. Encourages a lighter, more courageous attitude; to be our own best friend.

❋ FES AND CALIFORNIAN ❋ RESEARCH ESSENCES

These essences are currently in the process of being fully researched. From my own personal experience and diagnoses I have found them helpful and appropriate for certain conditions. With a few essences already researched I have indicated some possible further use.

ANGELICA For integrating the whole energetic system. Helps nerve-related skin conditions. Used to get to the root of alcoholism problems.

APRICOT For mood swings linked to blood sugar imbalances (i.e. hyperglycaemia). Cleanses the lymphatic system, soothing inflammation and allergic reactions.

AVOCADO Clears the lymphatic system and blood. Good for elimination.

BO-TREE Used in anti-smoking mix.

BOTTLEBRUSH Helps when there is insufficient clearing of toxic waste products giving rise to toxaemia.

CEDAR For colon problems, poor assimilation, ulcerous conditions and toxin build-up.

CHAMOMILE Calms the nervous system – for restlessness, insomnia, stress affecting the stomach. Brings emotional objectivity; clears stress and unprocessed emotions out of the solar plexus and nervous system.

CHERRY Enhances basic energy levels. Clove Combats tension and stress leading to headache.

COMFREY Invigorates the nervous and muscular systems. For relaxing and releasing stored nervous stress and tension. Especially good for

healing nervous breakdown. Acts as a preventative where nervous conditions are indicated: a 'safety valve' remedy.

EUCALYPTUS Clears congestion and soothes inflammation in the lungs, sinuses and nasal passages. Helps combat colds and flu as well as asthma and breathing difficulties.

EVENING PRIMROSE Balances the hormonal cycles in women.

FEVERFEW For headaches, particularly those related to hormonal fluctuations during the menstrual cycle.

GOOSEBERRY For menopausal problems such as hot flushes, panic attacks, lack of self-worth and tension during this time. Also helps with problems accepting hysterectomy and infertility.

GRAPEFRUIT For stress. Relaxes tension in the facial muscles. Used in my complexion cream (*see* page 211).

GREEN ROSE For hayfever. Also good when there has been a suppression of the psycho/spiritual aspect in childhood which has manifested as an allergic condition, such as asthma, migraine-type headache, ulcers and colitis. Heals past-life trauma in the heart chakra, which blocks the advancement of spiritual development.

JASMINE For mucous congestion associated with colds in the lungs, sinuses, throat and nasal passages. Excellent for pneumonia.

KOENIGN VAN DAENMARK Booster for the immune system. Affords better mental control

❋

over immunity.

LICORICE Calms restlessness that causes sleeplessness. For treating insomnia.

LUFFA Treats most skin conditions such as eczema and dry skin. Good for adding to skin creams.

LUNGWORT Cleanses and heals the lungs and throat.

MORNING GLORY Used as a liberating remedy for drug abuse and addiction (ranging from opiates to tobacco), its key purpose being to break destructive habits and cleanse the body of associated side-effects (restlessness and nervous hypertension). Restores the nervous system to its original balance and vitality.

PANSY Antiviral. Helps to clear any viral or bacterial infection from the body. Also effective for relieving the painful itching of cold sores/herpes.

PEANUT Fights stress and tension.

ROSE DAMACEA For conquering addiction and dependency patterns.

SAGE As an aid to digestion disrupted by nervous conditions. Used by the Native Americans for energy protection.

SKULLCAP Clears effects of toxins and eases withdrawal from drug addiction, especially morphine. For giving up caffeine/coffee.

SPIDERWORT Clears pollutants from the system, especially environmental pollutants and radiation.

SPRUCE For general detoxification; also prevents the side-effects of anaesthetics.

VALERIAN Promotes relaxation. Treats restlessness and insomnia, releasing mental and physical stress to aid pain relief, sedation and control of physical pain.

WATERMELON Balances male/female hormones. Helps fertility problems and the birthing process.

YLANG YLANG For emotional upset, stress and tension. Treats insomnia and jet lag.

(N.B. Some of this information was supplied by Eric Pelham.)

ADDITIONAL FES AND CALIFORNIAN RESEARCH ESSENCES

BANANA For blood sugar imbalances.

COFFEE For clearing the blocking effects of caffeine out of the system. Conquers the addiction to coffee and other forms of caffeine (cola drinks, chocolate, etc.). Has a cleansing and stabilizing effect on the parasympathetic nervous system, reducing physical and nervous instability which leads to a craving for caffeine.

HYSSOP For respiratory conditions, especially those linked to stress and nervousness. Cleanser for the lungs.

KHAT Provides support for the immune system.

LEMON For stimulating greater mental acumen. Cleanser for the system.

NETTLE A tonic and blood cleanser. Releases stress.

PAW PAW For anorexia and anaemia. Aids the absorption of nutrients.

PEACH A catalyst for kicking the self-healing process into gear.

PENNYROYAL For protection on the subtle energetic level – physically, emotionally, mentally and psychically. Excellent for mending damage to the aura such as holes caused by addictions.

ROSE BEAUTY SECRET For city stress.

SAGUAGO For inflammation of the skin and cleansing the lymphatic system.

SUGAR BEET For depression, see-sawing energy and moodiness accompanying hypoglycaemia. Balances blood sugar.

TOBACCO Helps to clear the effects of nicotine from the body. Re-balances the system.

❈ FLOWER ESSENCE SOCIETY ❈

The Flower Essence Society has been in existence longer than almost any other flower remedy organization (the exception being the Bach Flower Centre). It was established in 1979 by Richard Katz with a view to gathering together information and research into newer flower essences and educating the public through classes and publications. In 1980 he formed a professional partnership with his wife, Patricia Kaminski; together they not only run the Flower Essence Society but through their company Flower Essence Services prepare an extensive range of high-quality North American flower essences known as the 'FES Quintessentials'. They are made from flowers wildcrafted from pristine natural habitats in California and other parts of North America, and from organic gardens and wild areas on their 17-acre centre, Terra Flora, located near Nevada City in the foothills of California's Sierra Nevada, a place of granite peaks studded with golden quartz and sparkling rivers.

Katz and Kaminski have devoted particular attention to researching their essences thoroughly, using extensive case studies and clinical reports by practitioners, and by studies of the essence plants, including morphological and botanical characteristics. They also conduct seminars and practitioner training and certification programmes, write and publish newsletters and books, including their comprehensive *Flower Essence Repertory*. Flower Essence Society membership provides a communication network for those teaching, researching and practising in this field.

The FES essences are currently being used by thousands of practitioners and lay people in more than 50 countries around the world.

As Katz and Kaminski have said,

Flower essences are not panaceas, but catalysts *which stimulate and energize the inner transformative process, while leaving us free to develop our own innate capacities. Just as food nourishes the body, so can flower essences nourish and heal the soul.*

They are a harbinger of a new alchemy of the soul, one which incorporates ancient widsom with a modern awareness of the human psyche and of Nature.

PROFESSIONAL KIT

ALOE For who have an abundance of fiery energy but tend to overuse it and literally burn out – workaholics who neglect their emotional and physical needs. Brings a sense of renewal and rejuvenation, restores nourishment. Balances creative activity and centres vital life energy.

ARNICA For deep-seated shock or trauma which may become locked into the body and prevent full healing recovery. For accidents and violent experiences where the soul or Higher Self dissociates from the physical body. Brings conscious embodiment, especially during shock or trauma, and aids recovery. Helpful for treatment of psychosomatic illnesses which do not respond to other treatments.

BASIL For those who have a tendency to separate the experience of spirituality from that of sexuality. They may be secretive about sex, regarding it as sinful while finding illicit sexual practices attractive and compelling. Integrates sexuality and spirituality into a sacred wholeness.

BLACKBERRY For those who have lofty visions and desires but are unable to put them into action, lacking the ability to organize their intentions into specific goals and priorities. Also for poor circulation and sluggish metabolism. Directs will-power and enables you to take decisive action.

BLACK-EYED SUSAN For those who avoid or repress parts of their personality or traumatic episodes from the past, for instance rape or incest, often experiencing emotional amnesia and paralysis. Enables you to acknowledge all aspects of the self, and to achieve penetrating insight.

BLEEDING HEART For a tendency to form relationships based on fear or possessiveness; for emotional dependence which leads to a lack of freedom in the relationship. Sufferers may feel tremendous pain and broken-heartedness by loving someone who is emotionally distanced or no longer present. Brings the open-hearted ability to love others unconditionally, and emotional freedom.

BORAGE For heavy-heartedness, or lack of confidence in the face of difficult circumstances. For those who feel discouraged or disheartened in times of grief, sadness or other adversity. Uplifts the heart, gives buoyant courage, rekindles a sense of optimism and enthusiasm.

BUTTERCUP For those who feel humbled and lack self-worth, unable to acknowledge or experience their uniqueness and inner light. Brings recognition of the inner light which is a source of healing and peace. Relieves you from the need to judge yourself by conventional standards of achievement and success. Helpful for children who may be physically handicapped or impaired.

CALENDULA For those prone to being argumentative, who have a tendency to use cutting or sharp words and lack receptivity when communicating with others. Gives warmth and benign compassion; encourages receptivity in conversations.

CALIFORNIA PITCHER PLANT For those who fear their instinctive desires; they may lack strength and physical vigour, be anaemic, or be unable to assimilate nutrients properly. Restores earthly vitality, balancing instinctual desire so these energies can strengthen physical vitality.

CALIFORNIA POPPY For those seeking false forms of light or higher consciousness, 'spiritual glamour' or psychic experiences. Balances the forces of light and love, encouraging more self-responsibility and quiet inner development.

CALIFORNIA WILD ROSE For apathy or resignation, not wanting to take full responsibility or to experience the pain or challenge of life. For those who recoil from relationships which may involve taking emotional risks, or who feel socially alienated. Brings the ability to care for and give oneself to life and to others. Kindles enthusiasm for doing and serving.

CAYENNE For those prone to stagnation, complacency, feeling stuck or immobilized, unable to make any progress or change, caught in a pattern of procrastination and resistance. Ignites and sparks the soul, encouraging our capacity to initiate and sustain spiritual and emotional development.

CHAMOMILE For those easily upset, moody, irritable and unable to release emotional tension, often leading to insomnia. Releases tension, encouraging serenity, emotional balance and a sunny disposition. Also good for children's stomach complaints, which are often emotionally based.

CHAPARRAL For disturbed dreams or psychic toxicity when over-exposed to violent or chaotic images. Important remedy for modern civi-

lization. Important psychic cleanser which works especially through the dream life to cleanse the psyche.

CORN For disorientation and stress, particularly in urban environments; helpful for those who feel uncomfortable living in congested, chaotic environments, preferring rural or uncrowded areas. Helps you stay centred and in alignment with the earth, with your feet firmly on the ground.

DANDELION For those who have a natural intensity and love for life but who tend to over-stretch themselves, making themselves overly tense, especially in the muscles. Encourages listening to bodily messages. Allows release of tensions from the body and emotions, bringing dynamic, effortless energy.

DEER BRUSH For mixed or conflicting motives, deceiving ourselves by lack of honesty in our relationships with others and in the affairs of daily life. Brings gentle purity, clarity of purpose and sincerity of motive. Helps the soul attain purity so that it radiates truth and harmony.

DILL For when the senses are overwhelmed and over-stimulated; for hypersensitivity to the environment, sensory congestion. Enables us to absorb and experience the fullness of life, especially sensory impressions.

DOGWOOD For emotional trauma stored deep within the body – often springing from physical or sexual abuse or harsh physical living circumstances – which can cause the body to feel awkward and ungainly. Also for those with self-destructive, accident-prone tendencies. Evokes a sense of gentleness, grace and inner sanctity.

FILAREE For disproportionate worry and those who become too enmeshed in/overly concerned with the mundane affairs of daily life, wasting energy on small problems. Helps give a cosmic overview and puts life into perspective, unleashing inner strength and reserve.

FUCHSIA For those who mask their true feelings (such as pain and deep-seated trauma) with false emotions and psychosomatic symptoms. Brings genuine emotional vitality. Allows expression of deep feelings and enables emotions such as grief, deep-seated anger or rejection to be encountered and transformed.

GARLIC For those who are fearful, weak, or easily influenced, prone to low vitality. Brings a sense of wholeness which imparts strength and active resistance. Good for poor immune response and vulnerability to infection.

GOLDEN EAR DROPS For those who suppress painful memories and trauma from the past (especially childhood) which affect present emotional life. Encourages the ability to be in touch with one's inner child as a source of spirituality. Stimulates remembrance and release of these traumatic memories so the past can become a source of strength, wisdom and insight.

GOLDENROD For those easily influenced by family or others, subject to peer pressure or social expectations, unable to be themselves or to establish their own values and beliefs. Conforming to social norms to win approval and acceptance, such people may one day resort to anti-social or obnoxious behaviour as in adolescence. Encourages well-developed individuality, greater strength and inner conviction.

HOUND'S TONGUE For those who tend to see the world in materialistic terms, becoming weighed down or dulled by an overly worldly view. Promotes holistic, balanced thinking; restores a sense of wonder and reverence for life. Stimulates the ability to perceive the physical world with/spiritual clarity.

INDIAN PAINTBRUSH For creative people who suffer from low vitality, exhaustion and other forms of physical illness during their work because they are unable to stay grounded and energized, unable to bring creative forces into physical expression. Helps the physical body to be lively, exuberant and healthy while using creative potential.

INDIAN PINK For those who take on too many activities at once, becoming tense, emotionally volatile, depleted and unable to see the self as a centre of activity. Assists in becoming centred and focused even under stress, so as to manage and co-ordinate diverse activities.

IRIS For those unable to feel inspiration, lacking creativity and feeling weighed down by the ordinariness of the world. Encourages perception of beauty, making everything seem alive and vibrant, and a deep soulfulness which is in touch with the higher realms.

LARKSPUR For those in positions of leadership who feel over-burdened by duty or inflated with self-importance. Encourages charismatic, contagious enthusiasm and joy in serving others.

LAVENDER For nervousness and over-stimulation of spiritual forces which deplete the physical body; for those who are highly strung and wound up, typically suffering from headaches, vision problems, neck and shoulder tension. Soothes and teaches moderation.

LOTUS For spiritual pride – those who regard themselves as 'spiritually correct'. An all-purpose remedy for enhancing and harmonizing the higher consciousness.

MADIA For those who are easily distracted, unable to concentrate, and having trouble living in the present. Also for seasonal distress, when hot weather can make you feel listless and distracted. Brings precision thinking, disciplined focus and concentration.

MALLOW For insecurity/an inability to trust others and radiate warmth. Removes barriers and helps us trust our inner feelings. Encourages open-hearted sharing and friendliness.

MANZANITA For those who have an aversion to their body and the physical world. Often drawn to punishing dietary regimes, such people often feel ill even if they are following perfect health programmes. Softens attitude to physical matter and encourages positive involvement in the world.

MARIPOSA LILY For those alienated from their mother or the mothering instinct due to abandonment, abuse or trauma in childhood. Heals the trauma and encourages our ability to nurture and show caring attention to others. Strengthens maternal instincts and the mother–child bond. Restores the inner child.

MORNING GLORY For 'night owls' with erratic eating and sleeping rhythms who have difficulty getting up in the morning, perhaps making them susceptible to nervous depletion and poor immunity. Also for addictive habits. Encourages attunement with rhythms to restore natural energy and sparkling life-force, so that we are refreshed and in touch with life.

MOUNTAIN PENNYROYAL For difficulty thinking clearly and making rational decisions because of the negative thoughts of others – psychic contamination. Cleanses the mind to promote clear, positive thinking.

MOUNTAIN PRIDE For fear and withdrawal when faced with challenges, making us unable to take a stand for what we believe in. Cultivates a courageous warrior-like attitude for taking positive action.

MUGWORT For those prone to irrational, hysterical, over-emotional behaviour, out of touch with reality. Balances dream experiences so we can glean greater insight into the affairs of daily life.

MULLEIN For those feeling weak and confused, unable to tune in to their inner voice and lacking in decisiveness, who are prone to lying or deceiving themselves and others. Develops a strong sense of inner conscience, truthfulness and moral fortitude.

NASTURTIUM For intellectuals who think too much and deplete their life-force. Restores warmth, vitality and radiant energy.

OREGON GRAPE For paranoid, fearful people who see others and the outside world as hostile and unfair. Helps cultivate trust in the goodness of others. Good for tension and ill-will that predominates in many urban environments.

PENSTEMON For those who feel persecuted or victimized, or who pity themselves for having been dealt an unfair hand in life – they may be disabled or may have lost a loved one, their home or possessions. Develops inner strength, courage and resilience in the face of hardships. Fosters a persevering attitude.

PEPPERMINT For mental dullness and lethargy, craving stimulation or food only to feel sluggish afterwards – unbalanced metabolism. Imparts mental clarity and vibrancy.

PINK YARROW For those who are overly sympathetic towards others and excessively vulnerable to their emotional influence, giving rise to emotional confusion. Imparts greater objectivity and containment, teaching how we can radiate love.

POMEGRANATE For women torn between career and home life, feeling confused and compromised. Such psychological tension can affect sexual organs. Enables women to see their destiny and choices more clearly, encouraging active productivity and nurturing.

QUAKING GRASS For those who have difficulty finding their place in the work or family setting. Helps individuals maintain their identify without being subservient or over-exerting their ego.

QUINCE For difficulty in combining nurturing and gentle qualities with discipline and objectivity. Helps us to use our loving nature in a way that does not compromise our essential dignity and strength.

RABBITBRUSH For combining focus and attention to detail with wide-ranging perspective. Encourages our capacity to integrate details while simultaneously being aware of the total situation.

RED CLOVER For those whose individuality is challenged by mass consciousness, feeling swept away on a tide of mass hysteria and anxiety, easily influenced by panic around them. Encourages awareness of our behaviour,

helping us to maintain calm and steadiness, especially in emergencies.

SAGEBRUSH For those who cling to proof of their existence by over-identifying with illusory parts of the self, needing to purify and cleanse the self and release dysfunctional aspects of the self and surroundings. Encourages us to become more aware of our essential identity, to be true to ourselves – thus capable of transformation and change.

SAGUARO For rebellious tendencies – conflict with authority – reacting against your past. Brings awareness of what is ancient and sacred, and an understanding of your culture, lineage or tradition, in order to embrace and understand the past.

SAINT JOHN'S WORT For those sensitive to light/fair-skinned/easily burned/adversely affected by heat and light/prone to environmental stress including allergies/vulnerable to psychic attack at night leading to bed-wetting and night sweats. For psychic and physical vulnerability, deep fears and disturbed dreams. Gives protection and strength, illuminated consciousness, light-filled awareness and strength.

SCARLET MONKEYFLOWER For fear of intense feelings/repression of powerful emotions/inability to resolve issues of power or anger/fear of exploding in a blind rage. Gives courage to acknowledge and confront such feelings. Imparts emotional depth and honestly, direct and clear communication of feelings – integration of our emotional 'shadow'.

SCOTCH BROOM For those anxious and depressed by uncertainty and upheaval in the world/pessimistic and despairing of your role in larger events. Gives tenacity and strength, cultivating hope and a positive view of the world's future.

SELF-HEAL For those unable to take responsibility for their own healing and well-being, lacking in spiritual motivation for good health, overly dependent on external help. Encourages belief in your own capacity for recovery and an awareness of your own healing potential: a vital and healthy sense of self.

SHASTA DAISY For over-analytical people who have a tendency to see information as separate pieces rather than parts of a whole. Gives insight into the larger patterns of mental and emotional experience and helps us to synthesize these patterns into a living wholeness. Helpful for those involved in writing, teaching, research and other intellectual professions.

SHOOTING STAR For feeling profoundly alienated, not at home on earth/obsessed with extra-terrestrial existence. Brings the ability to find the right earthly connection and to be warmed with caring for all that is human and earthly.

STAR THISTLE For socially reclusive, lonely people who find it difficult to trust and be generous; those who tend to hoard or guard their material possessions due to feeling malnourished at a deeper level. Brings feelings of security and a sense of abundance. Encourages the ability to give and share.

STAR TULIP For men who deny their softer, receptive side, or women who have built a shell of protection around themselves. Increases sensitivity and receptivity. Encourages quiet inner listening.

STICKY MONKEYFLOWER For fear of sexual intimacy and contact, often compensated for by seeking superficial sexual encounters. Encourages ability to express warmth and deep feelings of love in sexual relationships.

SUNFLOWER For inflated ego and vanity or low self-esteem and self-effacement resulting from a distorted sense of oneself. Encourages sense of individuality, balancing receptivity and nurturing self-expression and outgoing qualities.

SWEET PEA For wanderers who have difficulty with caring, committed relationships. Also for a sense of homelessness which may stem from moving around frequently as a child as well from as living in urban and suburban environments, disconnected from the natural world. Kindles feelings of being at home. Encourages commitment and forming connections with others and the earth.

TANSY For sluggish, lethargic people who are indecisive, prone to procrastination, appearing lazy, indifferent and nonchalant. They may often be exposed to much chaos, confusion, emotional instability and even violence in childhood and respond by withdrawing and restricting their energy. Encourages straightforward responses to others and life. For being purposeful and decisive.

TIGER LILY For over-aggressive, hostile, competitive people who strive against others rather than working for the common good. A feminine flower which makes inner peace and harmony the basis for relationships with others, encouraging co-operation.

TRILLIUM For excessive ambition, greed and lust for possessions, power and material wealth. Cultivates altruism, balances energy and brings inner purity.

TRUMPET VINE For lack of vitality, an inability to be assertive or speak clearly due to feeling intimidated and shy. Also for speech impediments. Encourages lively, colourful free-flowing speech, an ability to express feelings verbally, dynamism in social situations.

VIOLET For those who are profoundly shy, reserved, aloof and lonely. They may long to share themselves with others but hold back for fear of being overwhelmed. Allows interaction with others while protecting individuality.

YARROW For extreme vulnerability to thoughts or the negative intentions of others, easily affected by surroundings and prone to environmental illness or allergies. Protects with a shield of light. Rebuilds vitality and solidity by repairing the aura.

YERBA SANTA For internalized grief and melancholy, deeply repressed emotions, feelings constricted in the chest. They may appear to be wasting away and are susceptible to chest congestion, pneumonia, tuberculosis, addiction to tobacco. Lightens the heart. Allows the emotions to flow freely.

ZINNIA For those who are over-serious and sombre, too earnest and lacking humour. Encourages childlike qualities of playfulness, laughter and humour.

RESEARCH KIT

ALPINE LILY For women who have difficulty accepting their femininity, who may be susceptible to reproductive and sexual problems.

ANGELICA For those who feel cut off, bereft of spiritual guidance and protection. Encourages feelings of being protected, guided and cared for, especially in times of crisis. Good for birthing, dying, festive celebrations and other major life passages.

ANGEL'S TRUMPET For those who fear death, who resist letting go of physical life. Brings surrender at death and times of deep transformation or transition.

BABY BLUE EYES For those who are unsure of themselves and unable to trust in the goodness of others and the world – defensive, insecure, with a cynical mistrust of the world. Restores innocence and childlike trust, and a recognition of goodness in others and the world.

CALLA LILY For confusion or ambivalence about sexual identity or gender. Brings acceptance of sexuality and clarity about sexual identify.

CANYON DUDLEYA For those who exaggerate the relevance of psychic experiences; attracted to mediumism, channelling and experiences which spark off psychic fantasies; prone to neglecting daily activities. Encourages inner contentment which dispels the necessity for psychic excitement.

CHRYSANTHEMUM For fear of ageing and mortality, over-identification with youthfulness or with fame and fortune, the material world. For mid-life crisis. Brings a shift towards identifying with what is truly eternal.

COSMOS For those who find it difficult to organize their thoughts into words. Overwhelmed by too many ideas, their speech is rapid and inarticulate. Harmonizes thinking and speaking patterns to bring more coherency.

ECHINACEA For feeling shattered by severe trauma or abuse, loss of dignity, profound alienation. Restores a sense of true identity and dignity. Maintains self-integrity.

EVENING PRIMROSE For feeling rejected and unwanted due to past abuse or childhood neglect; avoiding commitment in relationships; fear of parenthood; sexual and emotional repression. Brings emotional warmth and presence, and the ability to form committed relationships.

FAIRY LANTERN For immaturity, helplessness, dependency – the eternal child, delicate and needy, lacking inner strength to face the world or shoulder responsibility. Brings about a mature, independent adult. Use during childhood and adolescence for retarded phases of physical or emotional development.

FAWN LILY For withdrawal, isolation, self-protection; those who are highly developed spiritually who find it difficult to cope with the stress and strain of modern society. Encourages acceptance and involvement in the world, and the ability to share spiritual, healing gifts with others.

FORGET-ME-NOT For feelings of isolation, lack of awareness of spiritual connections with others. Encourages awareness of our relationship and responsibility to everyone. Good for maintaining a conscious link with lost loved ones.

GOLDEN YARROW For those with a tendency to withdraw from society or artistic involvement due to profound sensitivity, avoiding the limelight or performance, becoming hardened to cope with vulnerability. Shields and protects, allowing you to stay open and balanced without compromising your integrity and health.

HIBISCUS For when sexual expression becomes cold and unresponsive – often due to prior sexual exploitation or abuse. Particularly for women profoundly affected and offended by stereotyped images of female sexuality. Kindles sexual warmth and vitality, the integration of the soul's warmth and the body's passion.

MILKWEED For extreme dependency on drugs, alcohol, food as a means of escaping from self-awareness. Brings independence, strength and a healthy ego; nourishes at the deepest level.

PINK MONKEY FLOWER For shame, guilt, unworthiness, fear of exposure and rejection, masking feelings and hiding your real self from others. For fear of anyone seeing your pain, possibly due to childhood trauma or abuse. Brings self-acceptance and forgiveness, the ability to let go of the past as well as emotional openness to experience the love and affection of others.

POISON OAK For fear of intimate contact, being violated. For those who put up a hostile front, so driving away intimacy. Brings emotional openness and vulnerability so others can make close contact. Especially for men who fear being too open.

PRETTY FACE For those feeling ugly and rejected because of their physical appearance, such as those born with deformities or whose features are ungainly. Allows inner beauty to radiate within; brings acceptance of our own appearance.

QUEEN ANNE'S LACE For those who close their eyes to what is really happening, denying the subtler levels of reality. Helps clear the vision, bringing spiritual insight while keeping both feet on the earth.

ROSEMARY For those who tend to be forgetful and absent-minded because their spirit feels insecure about being here. Their feet and hands may often be cold and devitalized. Brings the ability to feel warm and secure. For feeling vibrant.

SAGE For a tendency to see life as ill-fated or undeserved, unable to perceive the higher purpose and meaning in life events. Enables you to learn and reflect about life experience which brings insight, wisdom and inner peace. Helpful during transitions and phases in life when you need to step back and consider the events that are unfolding.

SNAPDRAGON For energetic people with powerful wills and libidos who tend to repress these tendencies – prone to sarcasm, lashing criticism, tension around the jaws (teeth-grinding). Encourages a lively, dynamic, healthy libido and communication which is emotion-ally balanced.

YELLOW STAR TULIP For insensitivity to the feelings of others, and lack of awareness of the consequences of your actions. Brings compassion and caring. Encourages empathy with and sensitivity to the suffering of others.

SUPPLEMENTAL KIT

BLACK COHOSH For those caught in relationships and lifestyles that are abusive, addictive or violent. Gives us the courage to confront rather than shrink from abusive or threatening situations – transforming the negativity – gaining power and balance in destructive circumstances.

EASTER LILY For those in conflict about their sexuality, leading to an imbalance towards either prudishness or promiscuity. Cleanses the conflict, conferring the ability to integrate sexuality and spirituality; enhancing the inner purity of the soul.

LADY'S SLIPPER For those estranged from their inner authority, unable to integrate their higher spiritual purpose with real life and work, leading to nervous exhaustion and sexual depletion. Calms and restabilizes the nervous system, helping to regain inner composure and spiritual strength, integrating spiritual purpose with daily work, bringing spiritual power into the body.

LOVE-LIES-BLEEDING For intensification of pain and suffering due to isolation; profound melancholia due to the over-personalization of one's pain. Brings transcendent consciousness, the ability to move beyond personal pain, suffering or mental anguish by finding larger, transpersonal meaning in such suffering; compassionate awareness of and attention to the meaning of pain or suffering.

NICOTIANA For numbing of the emotions accompanied by mechanization or hardening of the body; inability to cope with deep feelings and finer sensibilities. Brings peace which is deeply centred in the heart; integration of physical and emotional well-being through harmonious connection with the Earth.

PURPLE MONKEYFLOWER For fear of the occult, or of any spiritual experience; fear of retribution or censure if one departs from religious conventions of family or community. Brings inner calm and clarity when experiencing any sprital or psychic phenomenon; the courage to trust in one's own spiritual experience or guidance; love-based rather than fear-based spirituality.

YARROW SPECIAL FORMULA For exposure to nuclear radiation and other forms of noxious environmental or geopathic stress including radiation from VDUs, X-rays, radiation therapy and other invasive electromagnetic fields. Originally developed in response to requests after the Chernobyl nuclear plant disaster in 1986. Directly counters the destructive effects of radiation on the human energy field by acting as a shield, so imparting powerful vitalizing and restorative properties.

❋ MASTER'S FLOWER ESSENCES ❋ YOGA FLOWER REMEDIES*

These essences are made exclusively from the blossoms of flowering fruits and vegetables from local organic fruit orchards and vegetable gardens. Date, avocado, pineapple, coconut and banana are prepared on the Hawaiian island of Kaui. They arise from the idea that we are not drawn to foods purely for their nutritional benefits but because they possess inherent psychological strengths, providing us with relief from stress, anxiety and emotional unrest.

This is the philosophy of Parmahansa Yogananda, a well respected master teacher of spirituality and metaphysician who came to the United States from India in the 1920s to share his practical techniques for self-improvement. He proposed, for example, that cherries signify the psychological quality of cheerfulness while apples encourage good health, hence the saying 'an apple a day keeps the doctor away'. Yogananda's autobiography is now considered a spiritual and psychological classic.

Inspired by Yogananda's teachings, Lila Devi reasoned that if foods have such powers, surely their blossoms (which contain 90 per cent of the plant's energy) would bring even more direct and potent benefits. After spending 18 years research in this field initiated in 1977, she developed the Master Flower Essences (at the foot of the Sierra Nevada Mountains, in California) to help people to become 'masters of their own lives'. She proposes:

They help us manifest those qualities which we already possess in our own delightfully unique way. This process is accomplished through the supportive interaction of the essence with our own readiness and willingness to make needed changes in our lives and attitudes.

They are particularly recommended for children as well as during pregnancy and childbirth; also they are invaluable for animals, pets and humans.

ALMOND 'Self-control.' For over-indulgence in activity, foods and other substances, immoderation of body and mind, sexual excess, uneasiness, nervousness. Calms the mind and nerves. Use when you need to be more inward, less affected by environment and circumstances. Good in times of activity and high demands on your energy reserves. Promotes

* This material is reprinted with permission.

synchronicity of body/mind/spirit, restoring balance and moderation.

APPLE 'Healthfulness.' For inharmonious states of mind, including hypochondria, worry and doubt, and recurring negative emotions such as anger and fear. Helps bring clarity, receptivity and joy. Restores a sense of well-being to one's thoughts and outlook on life. Unlocks the spring of true health and vitality, providing the motivation to take better care of oneself.

AVOCADO 'Good memory.' For forgetfulness, absent-mindedness, dullness, mental fuzziness, going along without purpose and direction, 'missing the boat'. For when greater awareness is needed to deal with an issue. Brings mental focus, recollection of details, inspiration for new projects and challenges for the mind (such as exams), as well as a greater awareness of life's purpose.

BANANA 'Humility.' For when anxiety upsets perspective, clouding judgement. For those burdened by responsibility, feeling nervous, quarrelsome, proud. Instils a calm, non-reactive attitude to negative attachments, so that you can step back and observe rather than get too involved. Lightens one's mental load.

BLACKBERRY 'Purity of thought.' For negativity, pessimism, sarcasm, cynicism, focus on dark or unkind thoughts, fault-finding, nitpicking. Brings kindness, mental clarity, optimism, seeing the good within oneself and others. Helps us to be inspirational, incisive and direct yet gentle, offended by the mistreatment of living things. Encourages true friendships and harmony in the environment.

CHERRY 'Cheerfulness.' For moodiness, grumpiness, contrariness, unhappiness, despondency, hopelessness, feeling mildly to moderately out of control emotionally – whether these moods are from a known or unknown origin. Encourages seeing the good in every situation, being hopeful, inspiring to others, optimistic, positive, light-hearted, even-minded. Helps whenever there is lack of energy, enthusiasm and interest in life.

COCONUT 'Uplifting.' For shakiness, lack of endurance, escapism, avoidance of tests; for those who make excuses, foresee problems, give up easily. Brings endurance and perseverance for completing tasks, living up to one's greatest potential. Helps us to see solutions, welcoming and offering support for meeting any kind of challenge.

CORN 'Mental vitality.' For sluggishness, blocked energy, unresponsiveness, procrastination, unwillingness, resistance, lethargy. Brings initiative to projects, rekindling enthusiasm and providing unlimited energy to accomplish anything you desire.

DATE 'Sweetness and tenderness.' For those who are judgmental, critical of others, intolerant, easily irritated, unpleasant to be around, inhospitable. Encourages sensitivity to other's feelings, discrimination, receptivity, open-mindedness; allows us to be easy to talk to, welcoming, magnetic, warm-hearted.

FIG 'Flexibility.' For those who are too hard on themselves, showing only rigidity, an uncompromising nature, difficulty with change, unrealistic expectations of self, fanaticism, a too-strict sense of discipline, self-limitation. Brings a sense of humour, fluidity, self-liberation, going with the flow, being relaxed and at ease with oneself and others.

GRAPE 'Love, devotion.' For envy, greed, lust, jealousy, neediness, cruelty, loneliness, feeling disconnected, alienated and vulnerable, being unwilling to commit. For states of abandonment such as separation, divorce or death. Brings a realization of the source of love within, purity, loving without condition, demand or expectation, patience with others' shortcomings. Transcendence.

LETTUCE 'Calmness.' For restlessness, inability to concentrate, excitability, repressed and troubled emotions, anger, indecision. Brings a quality of profound stillness, dispelling emotional turmoil, replacing it with even-mindedness. Confers the ability to speak one's truth, restores clear communication skills, and creates a productive, clear-thinking environment for highly creative people. Freedom to experience the more subtle states of relaxation.

ORANGE 'Joy.' For mild to severe depression or melancholy, hopelessness, despair, self-pity, for present and past abuse issues – physical, sexual or emotional. Brings energy, resolution of conflict, lightness, banishing melancholy, for cultivating an inner smile.

PEACH 'Selflessness.' For selfishness, self-involvement, thoughtlessness, and constrictive smothering, exploiting others and being unable to relate to their realities. Brings concern for the welfare of others, maturity, nurturing, consideration, deep compassion, sensitivity and empathy.

PEAR 'Emergency use.' For accidents, illness, surgery, childbirth complications, physical and/or emotional crises, shock, extreme grief and any situation which throws us off balance; uncontrollable thoughts and non-productive habit patterns; minor to monumental auric disturbances. Restores peace of mind, a sense of rhythm and proportion, for living fully in the present moment; an ability to handle crises.

PINEAPPLE 'Self-assured.' For those with an inferiority complex, comparing themselves to others, unhappy in their jobs, unable to choose a career and stick with it. Encourages confidence, wisdom, a strong sense of identity and contentment with career.

RASPBERRY 'Kind-heartedness.' For those feeling easily hurt, touchy, over-reactive, insensitive – who lash out, lack understanding and judgement, are clouded by emotions, blame others and feel resentful and bitter. Fosters responsibility for one's actions, sympathy, forgiveness, benevolence, generosity and the desire to help others heal their hurts. Releases old wounds.

SPINACH 'Simplicity.' For stress, feeling burdened or overwhelmed, from mild distrust to paranoia. For an unhappy or dysfunctional childhood. Brings childlike joy, trust, a sense of wonder, a free spirit, a playful nature and love of adventure. Allows us to be uncomplicated, straightforward and easily understood.

STRAWBERRY 'Dignity.' For those who are guilt-ridden, self-blaming, feeling unworthy, undeserving, irresponsible, ungrounded, unsure of themselves, with low self-esteem. They may have a history of emotionally abusive parents, psychic over-sensitivity. Brings strength, grounding, poise, grace, stateliness, self-worth, reliability. Allows us to leave a dysfunctional childhood in the past.

TOMATO 'Strength, courage.' For fear, nightmares, withdrawal, defensiveness, addictions, shyness (from minor hesitation to sheer terror), defeatist attitude. Allows us to know there is no failure, only another chance to succeed. Encourages belief in oneself, invincibility, psychic protection and immunity from the effects of crowds or negative environments.

❋ PEGASUS ESSENCES ❋

Fred Rubenfeld, the owner of Pegasus products, was introduced to the world of vibrational healing when he went to work in the diamond industry in New York. While surrounded by gemstones and crystals he began to learn about and experience the healing effects of the stones he worked with. In 1983 he was among the first to open a mineral and crystal store, selling Gem Elixirs in New York. He then expanded into the world of flower essences when he took over the Pegasus company. Fred has now created a phenomenal 'remedy bank' which offers a vast range of over 500 flower essences and more than 300 gem elixirs, as well as Star Light elixirs from the stars and planets.

The Pegasus range is made up of contributions from all over the world: Lily from Africa, Holy Thorn from Glastonbury, Creeping Thistle from Scotland, and many flowers from Tahiti etc. The company is based in the Rocky Mountains in a town called Love Land, near Boulder, Colorado, a sparsely populated area with an abundance of wildlife and rich gold and quartz deposits. Geographically it is the centre of North America. People living here seem to derive a great deal of energy from the land, which is conducive to good health.

Fred believes the secret of making good essences and elixirs is to welcome participation from all kingdoms – floral, mineral, elemental, planetary, extraterrestrial – while detaching ourselves mentally and emotionally from the process of making essences.

To make his flower essences he uses a special quartz crystal bowl and sunlight that is filtered through xenon gas before hitting the water. The gas acts as a filter, reputedly eliminating any harmful effects of the sun's rays.

The essences are potentized by a geometric shape called a metaform, an aquarian pyramid filled with crushed quartz. This process is carried out after the essence is made, again after it is bottled and once again prior to shipping, to clear any negativity and ensure a safe journey and long shelf life.

At this particular time these essences aim to deal with and provide the energy needed to cope with issues, destruction, change and disaster. Flowers and crystals in particular, Fred Rubenfeld maintains, can assist with these issues. He feels there is something quite unique about the urban flowers that push themselves up through the sidewalks of New York. They show a determination to move through obstructions, a strength of spirit that is appropriate for dealing with the issues of today, and indicative of the tenacity needed to work through the kinds of obstacles we face daily.

He also feels that at this time there is greater awareness of the higher realms, as there was in biblical times and even earlier. At a time when so much life on earth is in jeopardy, flowers and gems are providing some possible solutions. Elephants, for example, are now being saved thanks to the discovery of a new substance that comes from a bean plant and can be worked to look like ivory. Its qualities are captured for the first time in Fred Rubenfeld's Tagua essence.

AGAVE YAQUINANA Affects the unconscious decisions people make based upon deep-seated beliefs about separation, loneliness, aloneness, etc. that are often the legacy of past-life information and experiences. When taken repeatedly

❋

it helps loosen the hold of these hidden or unconscious belief-patterns.

ALOE ERU Helpful in closing holes in the etheric body due to other entities and, to a lesser extent, due to an individual's own experiences. Soothes after severing an association with a negative entity.

ALYOGYNE HUEGELLI Increases the capacity of the crown chakra to assimilate and work with information. For accessing the 'cosmic computer'. Can increase understanding of the nature of kundalini energy as it moves through the spine.

BIRD OF PARADISE For understanding flight, movement. Brings a realization of the interconnectedness among people and communities. Useful in people-management and for the appropriate use of new technology and its impact on freedom – for humour created around relationships and freedom.

BLAZING STAR Can awaken expressive energies felt as a build-up of energy in the heart which then pours through the hands and fingertips, especially the middle finger. Useful in utilizing the energy of love for healing.

BLUE WITCH Has the ability to create energy shifts in chakras 4–9 (the 8th and 9th chakras reside in the subtle bodies), beginning at the heart and extending upwards before returning. May provide a deeper understanding of the higher dimensions.

BUTTERFLY LILY For attuning to the process of transformation as symbolized by the butterfly; increasing awareness of this transformation for the human race. For those involved in group work when they are faced with insurmountable obstacles. Brings encouragement, strength of purpose and the ability to let go of stress.

CALIFORNIA BAYLAUREL Opens the mind and gives a feeling of flexibility to the mind and nervous system. Helps overcome rigid mindsets, ideas and body armour, bringing wisdom. Soothes and relieves.

CALIFORNIA BUCKEYE Strengthens one's ability to understand and work with vision. May provide attunement to one's purpose as well as to ecosystems, agriculture and nature spirits. Increases third-eye abilities.

CALYPSO ORCHID Helps one climb through several spiritual levels simultaneously. Enhances the ability to communicate with the Higher Self or one's guides; encourages teachers to be drawn to you. Cleanses and opens the crown chakra.

CAPE HONEYSUCKLE Can bring co-ordination between the physical body and chakras 4–8. May intensify psychic abilities and a shift in the emotional body. Balances the energies of grief, loneliness and other difficult emotions.

CATERPILLAR PLANT Brings encouragement to access and receive spiritual gifts that one is not aware of. Makes it easier to assimilate and integrate psychic abilities when they start to appear.

CHOKE CHERRY Brings illumination to an lack of clarity in ourselves and our relationships. Sheds light when we needs to see the problem, chasing away the darkness, ending confusion and clarifying motivations.

CLARKIA Brings some affiliation with the energies of forgiveness, especially in relation to physical aspects and the influence of our genetic structures. Brings greater awareness of genetic structures and our ability to work with them.

CORALROOT (SPOTTED) Brings greater awareness of the role of disease in our lives, the need to recognize and understand the lesson of disease on subtler levels so that the disease no longer needs to manifest physically. It may reduce the influence of antibiotics which can last for a long time after taking them.

CREEPING THISTLE Produces tendrils of light and energy from the 7th chakra, causing a temporary blending or bringing of new energies in many different forms and directions. Can make a bridge from the seventh to the heart to the base chakra. Brings clear internal healing energy to the physical body and steps up vibrational transference from other subtler levels to the physical, which can be a joyful experience.

CURRY LEAF TREE A catalyst for things already happening in one's life. Spiritual practices become clearer. Encourages synergy in relationships, especially within the family. Brings playfulness and a sense of relaxed purpose.

DAYFLOWER Allows access to greater light, which is especially helpful for the physical body and those using light therapy, and for a greater awareness of the connection between the sun and the earth. Benefits those seeking to reduce their food intake and increase their attunement to light.

DEER'S TONGUE Awakens psychic gifts of an expressive nature. Working with the 6th chakra, these gifts can project mind-energy. The accelerated and enhanced ability to project energies of love from a group to many beings will assist the earth at this time.

DESERT BARREL CACTUS Assists those seeking to understand boundaries, where they begin and end, where their relationship to someone begins and ends, where and how they relate to the whole of humanity. Helps us to confront the sadness and separation sometimes felt during our spiritual journey between ourselves and our soul family.

DRAGON FLOWER CACTUS Assists the capacity to apply spiritual principles to the physical realm. For balancing the physical aspects of the body properly. Especially helpful in movement and exercise.

DUTCHMAN'S BREECHES Enhances the release of emotional residues into the aura which can then be cleansed easily by movement, water or air. Can also clear away residues from negative environments.

EASTER LILY CACTUS For deeper attunement to chaos and the balance of perfect symmetry. Improves communication through gesture and movement.

ELEPHANT'S HEAD Creates a vibrational link to the energies of the angelic kingdom and those associated with humanity's own development. Strengthens the ability to perceive and work with earth energy. For deeper attunement and awareness of angelic or spirit guides; for wisdom.

EVERLASTING Helps to moderate a shift in consciousness which contains repressed memories from childhood or past lives. Increases self-esteem and self-recognition of spiritual progress. Encourages positive energy.

GARDENIA For emotional shifts from accepting one's consciousness in a new way; greater attunement to knowledge received in the recent past. Excellent for student/teacher relationships. Creates a sense of peace, caring and compassion.

GENTIAN Improves the ability to communicate on many levels. Improves speaking abilities for deeper insights and connection with others. For future expression.

GILIA-SCARLET Gives deep strength to those seeking an understanding about how they populate the earth and share it with others. Enhances the possibilities of the spiritual aspects of sexuality. May assist in treating mysterious skin complaints. Enhances empathy with the plant and animal kingdoms. Encourages harmony.

GREEN REIN ORCHID For seeing the continuity of patterns of emotions – a common thread running through lifetimes – particularly for understanding one's parents and early upbringing. Benefits both therapist and patient when used for depressive states or co-addictive energies.

HELICONIA Creates energy spirals which can influence the left and right balance of the subtle bodies. The brain and spine are positively affected. Helps to gain ideas and put them into from, accepting the results and making the necessary internal changes. Strengthens the 7th–10th chakras.

HOLY THORN Opens the crown chakra, bringing a greater willingness to work with a universal energy connection. Allows a deeper attunement to any particular spiritual avenue. It is best to have a specific being or ideal in mind when taking this essence. Forms a bond with the essential energy behind the spiritual idea or ideal. Best used by itself.

HOODED LADIES' TRESSES Maintains higher states after peak experiences, catalytic change or catharsis so they continue in a constant but less intense fashion. Brings a slight strengthening of psychic gifts.

HYDRANGEA (GREEN) Works in many ways to combine energies of the chakras, balancing them and allowing them to intermingle and transmute energies in useful ways. For visualizing and awakening the different chakras.

INDIAN PIPE Balances the flow of energy between chakras, so enhancing movement. For establishing a clear contact with higher vibrations in channeling. Releases stress/strain in the back.

KINNICK-KINNICK Allows one to connect consciously more easily to others and to break any unnecessary connections. Assists one to move with ease and more freedom and to alleviate unwanted past-life connections.

LEMMON'S PAINTBRUSH May bring a deeper level of connection to our higher energies. Especially useful in creating a deeper understanding of our interaction with society or communities. For social interaction.

LEOPARD LILY Strengthens our ability to improve self-image. For expressing ourselves clearly and allowing our inner nature to shine through. Especially helpful for public speakers and writers who have an alternative viewpoint.

LOBIVIA CACTUS For attuning the heart to an awareness of the Christ principles manifest in your relationship to the earth. May bring a feeling of deeper groundedness and awareness of another, enhancing the interchange of energies between you both.

MILKMAIDS Dissolves critical attitudes towards oneself and others. Brings sweetness, love, acceptance and self-esteem. Helps the heart understand and appreciate goodness and positive qualities so one can let go of judgements and move back to spiritual love.

MOCK ORANGE Increases the ability to co-ordinate in deep states of relaxation and meditation. Useful in forming new ideas. Reduces stress.

MONKEYFLOWER Helps emotional clearing, especially with issues of denial and addictive states. Enhances ability to absorb light directly, providing deep nurturing for the 2nd and 3rd chakras.

MONVELLEA CACTUS For attuning to and understanding the symbolism of the breast and genitals. Brings attunement to moonlight and the unconscious.

MOUNTAIN MISERY Increases the ability to stick with a task. To modify old ways so new energies can be brought in. Assists in discovering additional inspiration and deeper understanding of a project.

MOUNTAIN PRIDE Brings awareness of base chakra energy and understanding of the emotional connection with spirituality. May bring greater acceptance of sexuality and sexual feelings. Restores a clearer sense of one's connection to the earth energy.

MYRTLEWOOD TREE For projecting healing capacities across long distances. Useful in transferring information about healing work.

NEOPORTERIA CACTUS Strengthens your higher potential by assisting a deeper contact of the soul with incoming energy. Clarifies and focuses the soul's energy for understanding how to put this into action. For overcoming procrastination and getting going when you see where you wish to go. May create a deeper and stronger connection to and awareness of your soul group. Enhances motivation.

NOBLE STAR FLOWER CACTUS For blending of love energies and an awareness of the consequences of eating meat. Assists in giving up meat and adopting a lighter, vegetarian diet out of love and willingness to assist all animals. Brings a sense of love and compassion for the animals that are consumed for food.

OLD MAID (Pink/White) Brings greater understanding of and clarity about what is truly important in life. For working with the inner child. Brings acceptance and forgiveness of parents and of older plaguing patterns. Increases our connection with all things.

ORANGE FLAME FLOWER CACTUS Assists in understanding and releasing anger, to enable us to see how it can improve relationships by creating greater enthusiasm. For understanding our deliberate attempt to be alone and separate in ways that are self-forgiving. Aids an understanding of the differences among people and brings a willingness to release negative attitudes.

OWL'S CLOVER Brings out joy and an appreciation of artistic expression and talent. Endeavours to develop self-expression, especially those of the dream state. Brings optimism to those out of touch with, depressed about or lacking confidence in their artistic expression.

PEGASUS ORCHID CACTUS For evolving a new creation of destiny and purpose which affects this life and future lifetimes. May bring a shift in the way we create new kinds of relationships, which allows the chance for a deeper connection and intimacy between both partners. For future relationships.

PINE DROPS For a clearer perspective on the entire nature of difficult relationships. To realize the higher aspects within any relationship. For increased understanding of the genetic structure and code for individuals. Combines well with alternatives to antibiotics.

PLUMERIA Brings a deep awareness of one's roots, connection to the human family and attunement to one's ancestors. Useful in group meditation, especially across great distances, in world peace meditation and harmonic convergence.

PRICKLY POPPY Increases the ability to love in the face of various obstacles, creating a love bond that transcends time and space. Enhances past-life recall in those consciously seeking it. Can increase forgiveness of our own past-life actions and those of others. Assists absolution of those creating war, famine and disease.

PROTEA (Pink Mink) Helps to focus energy in one particular direction. Aids in receiving information from past lives, especially concepts and ideas, integrating them into current ways of thinking. Increases telepathy.

PURPLE NIGHTSHADE Calms and relieves irritation, especially that brought on by trying too hard. Soothes jangled, burned-out nervous states and relieves the emotional disturbance brought on by coffee and other stimulants.

RATTAIL CACTUS Enhances the capacity to reach into multi-dimensions, across time and space to extract information including a new knowledge relating to one's cultural heritage. Assists in transcending time and creating a deeper connection to time-flow in the future.

RATTLESNAKE PLANTAIN ORCHID For issues relating to aggressive or male-orientated tendencies. Helps men deal with anger and aggression issues. Helps women seeking a greater male/female balance in their manner of speech, approach to men, how they are seen and the way they see themselves.

RED GINGER Brings the ability to spiritualize many physical characteristics. Opens the base chakra to spiritual energy. Deepens understanding and acceptance of the male/female balance within. Useful for martial arts and dance. Enhances sexuality, Tantra and Taoist, the union of male/female with the earth.

RED MOUNTAIN HEATHER For improving the ability to perceive and work with different forms of sound such as music. Brings greater attunement to the inner voice and vibration of all kinds. Enhances our capacity to love and recognize ourselves in all things. Brings a deeper attachment to all forms of vibration.

SHASTA LILY Speeds up the etheric bodies. Promotes greater awareness of one's role in serving to heal the earth. Helps in understanding and utilizing the energies available in different power spots, like the site of the Joshua Tree and Sedona, which have in the past been a source of revelation to many.

SIERRA RED ORCHID Has an excellent capacity to transmute emotion, so that deeply buried or denied feelings can surface. Especially effective for depression or sadness.

SNOWPLANT Creates a deeper understanding of incoming light and energy, especially for hands-on healers. Strengthens the aura and subtle bodies; supports changes in one's life: new job, new home, new relationships.

SOURGRASS Increases the movement of substances in and out of the subtle bodies, especially the etheric. This allows greater physical ease and movement as well as calm and peace on many levels. Good to use in conjunction with physical therapies such as massage and aromatherapy.

SPIDER LILY (RED) Increases the nadis' ability to reach other dimensional areas. Helps the nadis in the base of the spine to transform and transfer energy from the interdimensional regions, especially the etheric body. Improves the ability to open and close the chakras at will, for taking in what is useful and rejecting that which is not beneficial. Benefits those seeking to strengthen the digestive organs, the sexual reproductive organs, the kidneys and skin.

STARFLOWER Assists those working with others to understand the truth better, even when it is blocked in their consciousness. Stimulates the 2nd chakra.

STAR THISTLE Helpful for radiating energy. Useful for therapists working with patients, encouraging a higher spiritual awakening in both. Activates the 9th and 10th chakras.

SULCOREBUTIA CACTUS Creates a vortex of energy within an individual to increase one's focus and alignment with one's own capacities – those associated with the soul, centre of the universe and universal purpose or earthly manifestation. Helps remove obstacles from one's path and may be useful to those who respond poorly to certain holistic treatments.

SWAMP ONION Brings a powerful cleansing, usually beginning at the top and working down through the body, from head to toe. Creates an awareness of higher energies associated with such cleansing – a powerful universal energy pouring lovingly through you. Especially useful for cleansing the subtle bodies of things like psychic debris which stand in the way of greater evolution.

SYCAMORE Eases stress and overcomes problems of too much or too little discipline. Gives us a handle on life, so we know when to let go.

TAGUA Encompasses the beautiful aspects of elephant ivory in plant form. Brings a sense of great power, longevity, increased memory, strength of purpose, kindness and a deep awareness. Allows direct connection to higher realms. For being aware of how we can release old ways and come to new ones.

TREE OPUNTIA Assists in maintaining a willingness to change, even when we are comfortable at certain levels of existence. Reminds us to shift and offers us the physical energy for the rapid change necessary at this present time.

TRILLIUM RED Assists in amplifying and grounding our natural healing abilities. Enhances our ability to understand another's life lesson, to recognize what may be beneficial to his or her change and how it may be our own learning experience. Assists those who are bored in their jobs, bringing new ideas into form.

WAIKIKI RAINBOW CACTUS For seeing our own self-expression act as a deeper connection to others. Enhances self-worth.

WASHINGTON LILY Increases our innate ability to love unconsciously and universally. Creates a deeper understanding and acceptance of spirituality in its different forms in those approaching difficult spiritual change in life. Strengthens the etheric and astral bodies. Brings spiritual perseverance.

WOOLY SUNFLOWER Benefits those working with the sun's energy. Represents the more gentle, subtle, female-related aspects of the solar principle. Strengthens the 3rd chakra.

❋ HAWAIIAN FLOWER ESSENCES ❋

Hawaii is renowned for its wonderfully exotic subtropical species of flowers, many of which were reputedly introduced by the migrating Polynesians when they discovered the islands and settled there some 1,600 years ago. Inspired by the beauty of these islands, some suggest they may be the remainder of ancient Lemuria/Oceania, a mythical land that is said to have existed some 50,000 years ago. They speculate that some of the endemic Hawaiian flower essences such as Koa and Hawaiian Sandalwood have properties which help to enhance spiritual awareness, and these species could date back to these times.

The Hawaiian people traditionally turned to herbs for healing wounds and easing digestive problems. Internal illness was believed to be induced by evil spirits which weakened the 'mana' or spiritual life-force in a person. Their medicine men or 'Kahunas' treated illnesses by holding a ceremony called a *ho'oponono* in which they used herbal potions with rituals to clear psychological disharmony within the family and so appease the spirits. The Hawaiians as a race of people recognized and were respectful of the spirit of life present in the plants, trees and rocks, referred to in the Western world as fairies or devas.

ALOHA FLOWER ESSENCE INC.

All the Hawaiian Tropical Flower Essences listed have been prepared on the volcanically active Big Island of Hawaii by Penny Medeiros, a therapeutic massage practitioner. She has always been enchanted by the wonder and diversity of flowers, plants and trees, and was drawn to the idea of preparing flower essences on discovering that they offer us a pure and natural way to live in health and harmony. On moving to Hawaii in 1986, she was inspired to develop essences from the exquisite flowers growing there. After carrying out in-depth research into their properties she founded the Aloha Flower Essence Company in 1988. She found these essences unusually potent and relective of the primal and volcanic forces of nature or *mama* which the plant life absorbs and reflects – a force that can still be experienced in this group of islands.

AMAZON SWORDPLANT To enhance free-flowing emotional expression which leads to improving one's relationships. Useful in past-life therapy to focus on the source of emotional blocks.

AVOCADO To alleviate fear of being touched by another, promoting relaxed acceptance, enjoyment and pleasure – and sensitivity to the joy of touch.

AWAPUHI-MELEMELE (Yellow Ginger) To increase sensitivity, magnifying our perceptions of sight, hearing and touch. Brings one into the here and now, aiding relaxation. Can be used with hypnotic regression to release repressed subconscious mind traumas.

BAMBOO ORCHID To inspire self-reliance, faith and trust in oneself. Taken consistently to clear karmic blocks it gives clarity to one's higher destiny path.

BOURGAINVILLA (Orange and Pink) Rekindles awareness to the magic, beauty and wonder of life. For mystical and higher inspiration, enthusiasm and purposefulness.

CHINESE VIOLET For restoring close family relations when alienation, hostility and separation has been brought about by strong religious/cult belief systems.

COFFEE For decisiveness and inspiration; stabilizes emotions and restores receptivity to flower essences when affected by caffeine. Taken consistently, helps to overcome the psychological cravings for caffeine.

COTTON For releasing fear and its accompanying stress. To sharpen one's visual perceptions and to enable us to face fearful life situations.

CUP OF GOLD For those following spiritual and religious disciplines who tend to be aloof, cold and superior to others. A heart-centred essence to open up and share abundance and knowledge with genuine warmth and love.

DAY-BLOOMING WATERLILY/AMERICAN BEAUTY To overcome mental negativity towards sex and become sexually fulfilled with one's partner.

HAU A calming, healing and balancing influence for those overcome by nervous stress.

HAWAIIAN TREE ESSENCE Realigns the mental, astral and physical bodies; also specifically energizes the physical body in a very particular way: It strengthens the blood-based immune system against diseases generally and in so doing enhances overall vitality.

HINAHINA-KU-KAHAKAI To empower women to fulfil their own life's purpose, restoring will-power and direction when clouded or lost due to male domination.

'ILI'AHI (Hawaiian Sandalwood) Deepens receptivity to aromatherapy oils and sensitivity to aromas. In meditation, the essence energizes the crown chakra, enhancing our awareness of bliss.

ILIMA To dispel inbuilt illusions and become open to the highest truths of spiritual reality and the true nature of the universal spirit. Brings a sense of freedom.

IMPATIENS To alleviate impatience, restoring tolerance and acceptance of situations and circumstances.

JADE VINE For overcoming negativity and opening up to others. For developing deep, heart-centred communication and sincerity.

KAMANI To protect the sanctity and integrity of a place from negative energies (use in a spray or bowl of water). Also heals trauma and disharmony by clearing the heart centre in a person who has become insensitive and unloving.

KOA An essence that affects the crown chakra to be used with meditation practices. Brings deep peace and light from the higher realms, promoting regeneration, transformation and healing.

KOU Stimulates the third eye chakra, giving clarity of perceptions; for psychic and clairvoyant abilities. Taken consistently it discourages astral possession brought on by excessive alcohol consumption.

KUKUI For inspiring understanding and calmness and to promote emotionally 'opening up' to others, dissolving fears, anger and anxiety. To heal relationships (especially those carried over from past lives).

LA'AU'-AILA/CASTOR BEAN A soothing, calming and strengthening essence for women who are overcome with deeply ingrained anxieties, fears and phobias.

LEHUA Strengthens the female aspect, bringing self-esteem by increasing sensuality and joy in femininity. This liberating effect restores balance to the psyche by enhancing activity of the sexual chakra.

LOTUS Symbol of spiritual enlightenment, its purpose is to accelerate spiritual evolution and enhance healing on every level in the human system.

MACADAMIA For those caught in contrary, delinquent behaviour. Dissolves such negative patterns and brings clarity for constructiveness and love.

MAMANE To bring illumination for understanding divine truth, dispelling erroneous, spiritual and religious beliefs that have governed one's life. Restores clarity and emotional well-being.

MANGO Increases one's ability to assimilate the higher frequencies of cosmic light energies, which assists spiritual growth and reduces the need for denser physical foods (such as meat).

MA'O For releasing fear and its accompanying stress. To sharpen one's visual perceptions and be able to face fearful life situations.

NAIO Strengthens the will-power to break the addiction of over-eating.

NANA-HONUA For attuning to the higher realms. For soul-level guidance, clarity of thought and sharpness of mind.

NANI-AHIAHI To resolve deep, overwhelming, emotional issues which have been repressed. Such emotional anxiety, tension and/or grief can be linked to cancer in the stomach area.

NAUPAKA-KAHAKAI Fosters a sense of responsibility for one's earthly action, especially when past lifetimes have been devoted to the pursuit of wealth, power and glamour. Heals negativity within the mind; encourages connection with the Higher Self and spiritual truths.

NIGHT-BLOOMING WATERLILY/H. C. HAARSTICK Fosters unconditional love in a close, sexual relationship, attuning on the mental level, and enrichment of the lovemaking experience.

NIU (Coconut) Stimulates the breastfeeding instinct in mothers. For balancing male and female energies, bringing clarity when confused by sexual issues.

NOHO-MALIE Instils calm and comfort to those who sense agitation, unrest and inner conflict, especially when stemming from past-life events.

NONI To prepare women for childbearing and motherhood. Purifies and cleanses the emotions, aiding the body to detoxify. For attuning to the Earth Mother, awakening instincts for nurturing, caring and love.

OHAI-ALI'I Dissolves blockages of long-term, rigid, inflexible thought-patterns, which can eventually lead to impairment of the skeletal structure.

OHELO To purify deep fears, darkness and isolation which have engulfed those who have been involved in the black arts, in this and/or past lifetimes.

OHI'A-AI Strengthens the mind's control over the immune system and enhances general vitality.

PANINI-AWA'AWA A specialist remedy for healing holes in the etheric body and resultant damage caused by excessive use of psychotropic drugs.

PA-NINI-O-KA/NIGHT-BLOOMING CEREUS Restores balance in those who shun daylight, 'night owls' who prefer darkness, wearing black and/or sunglasses. To relieve deep-seated fears of negative entities and fearful dreams.

PAPAYA Enhances relationships by focusing on spiritual love between individuals. Clears mental confusion and tensions, stimulates psychic abilities.

PASSION FLOWER For attuning with the Christ-consciousness; stabilizes spiritual focus; opens the heart and throat chakras; eases tensions in the dream state. Stimulates pure, divine and unconditional love, which in its wake heals negativity, pain and trauma.

PA'U-O-HI-IAKA For spiritual protection when encountering dark forces, for healing when the spirit is harmed and for establishing contact with higher realms.

PLEMOMELE FRAGRANS To bring positive attitudes into one's mental framework, releasing depression, anxiety and irritability.

PLUMBAGO For restoring love, caring and vitality to close interpersonal relationships within a family.

PLUMERIA/PUA MELIA Strengthens resolve and motivation to practise ethnic, spiritual traditions that are often weakened or lost by modern influences. Gives clarity and purpose to restore and maintain traditional lifestyles.

POHA For enhancing learning abilities in children up to 15 years of age, who are emotionally unstable from relationship problems with family, close friends and/or teachers. Promotes a vital and positive frame of mind and dissolves emotional blocks.

PUA HOKU For harmonizing and aligning one's individual will with that of the collective group or organization one is involved with – so aiding its successful 'outworking'.

PUA-KENIKENI For overcoming cravings for drugs and sexual promiscuity. Restores clarity and purposefulness.

PUA-PILO To overcome lethargy and become active and fulfilled in life. Can liberate those with weight problems who do not over-eat but who have a negative self-image, are lethargic and need to break free from this inertia.

PUKIAWE Revitalizes – to overcome inertia. For taking care and interest in yourself and the environment. Promotes realization of your interconnectedness with life.

SPIDER LILY For overcoming negative mental states. For men who feel alienated from women, fostering loving attunement, respect and true equality with them.

STENOGYNE CALAMINTHOIDES/STICK RORRISH PLANT For those who have a severely disintegrated personality, displaying deranged behaviour. Re-integrates orderliness to the mental body.

THANKSGIVING CACTUS Increases harmony with our Higher Self. This resonance can dissolve our lower energy attachments to glamour and power. Literally shakes out the pernicious toxins of the ego and of self-seeking and self-serving behaviours.

TI To relieve astral possession. When taken steadily it will rid us from the grip of an invading entity. Good to take in 'psychically stressed' environments and for lifting a curse put on a place (use spray atomizer).

'ULUA For restoring communication in a young child who has suffered an accident or trauma and cannot express feelings of shock, helplessness, frustration and anger. Restores emotional well-being so that full healing may take place.

ULEI For enhancing communication and receptivity to others. Improves the memory and facilitates past-life recall. To connect diversely minded people, resolving hostilities and promoting tranquillity of mind. Enhances interpersonal communication, balancing love and interest for others with reason and logic.

WATER POPPY For releasing egocentric mental conflict so that a harmonic equilibrium with oneself and others may be experienced. To promote a fluid balance between overactivity and lethargy.

WILIWILI Inspires positivity, courage and honesty to face major life issues. To re-evaluate belief systems and dissolve fears that can prevent clarity in relationships and dealings in life.

YELLOW GINGER Increases sensitivity, magnifying the perceptions of sight, hearing and touch (for masseurs and aromatherapists). It brings one into the here and now. Aids relaxation. Use with regression to release subconscious traumas.

❋ PETITE FLEUR ESSENCES ❋

The Petite Fleur essences are created by Judy Griffin, a master herbalist and professional gardener who has already written five books on these subjects.

She is a scientist with a PhD in nutrition from the University of Alabama who has also spent time studying various disciplines with Chinese, Indian, Native American and Mediterranean peoples.

These essences were developed in response to Judy's recognition that 80 per cent of disease prevalent in Western society is related to stress. This brought her to the realization that any treatment which focuses on just one aspect of illness will always be incomplete. A more holistic approach is needed which addresses mind, body and spirit.

The Petite Fleur essences are used internationally by progressive medical and chiropractic physicians as well as health care practitioners. The original 60 wildflower essences affect the attitudes connected to our emotions and fears and their related endocrine responses. The Native Texans strengthen the essential character – a form of fine tuning – and clear inappropriate models and, together with wildflower essences, focus on enhancing the immune system by correcting unstable emotional signals which trigger the 'fight or flight' stress response. Essences in the Antique Rose collection enhance the nervous system, while the Master essences awaken consciousness by aiding personality transitions and helping us to focus on the here and now so we can fulfil our destiny. They also work to harmonize all chakras. These can be used as enhancers in association with the Native Texans and Antique Roses.

In the words of Judy Griffin,

Mother nature awaits with open arms to transcend physical, emotional and mental limitations as we expand our conscious awareness and oneness with the Eternal Life Force.

AFRICAN VIOLET Promotes nurturing, love from within and the release of endorphins which bring feelings of elation and ease pain. Helps heal wounds.

AMARYLLIS For anxiety about the future. Brings clarity about the future, helps overcome fears of what may lie in store and enhances intuitive abilities. Also treats parasites.

ANEMONE For when life is hard, a struggle and you cannot experience pleasure. Also helps regenerate tissue damaged by scarring or burning.

AZALEA For those who are left-brain dominated and wish to be more creative. Enhances creativity and visualization, bringing forth latent talents.

BABIES' BREATH For those who reject new ideas by thinking 'it won't work.' Encourages childlike faith and innocence. Eases congestion in the lungs; benefits asthma and emphysema.

BACHELOR BUTTON For those who keep looking back and are afraid to release the past. Brings beginner's luck and an ability to complete projects. Helps release suppressed tears and eases oedema.

BAMBOO For those who are not sure what to

do next. Helps in planning career, setting goals, learning to have fun. Eases intestinal upsets, lack of colonic acidity.

BASIL For critical people, high achievers who feel they are not good enough. Encourages self-nurturing habits. Helps purify the blood.

BEGONIA For having a belief in limitations. Encourages letting go and the realization that even global problems can be solved. Acts as a diuretic for the kidneys. Helps the sensory nerves.

BOUQUET OF HARMONY For uncontrolled thoughts and emotions when the imagination runs riot. Helps discipline the mind, focusing attention and bringing a sense of direction.

BOURGAINVILLA For guilt, fear of reprisal. Helps others enjoy life and fulfil their desires. Eases local aches and pains.

CHAMOMILE For those who swallow their hurt, feeling misunderstood. Brings counsel. Good for indigestion and a sluggish gall bladder.

CREPE MYRTLE For those who are afraid to speak their mind or of seeming foolish by expressing themselves incorrectly. Brings the realization that rage often underlies such fears. Fosters the ability to release this anger in a creative way and to speak only words of kindness.

CROSSANDRA For people who are insecure and fearful of new ideas or any major changes in life, not wanting to rock the boat. This personality is prone to gastro-intestinal stagnation and toxicity, and also to catarrh. Helpful in any new situations over which we have no control – such as having a baby, moving to a new job or environment. Encourages you to 'go for it'.

DAFFODIL For quiet, timid, shy people who try to please everyone, placing themselves under constant tension and anxiety which causes symptoms like heart palpitations. Their aversion to anger and angry scenes may stem from being intimidated by explosive or violent parents. Helps you to feel more at ease with yourself and others, not needing to appease others all the time.

DIANTHUS For apathetic people who claim they 'don't care', feeling uncared for and separate from humanity, disinterested in life and having nothing to look forward to. They are withdrawn and often anaemic. Helps us to view life in a brighter way, rekindling enthusiasm and self-nurturing.

GARDEN MUM For critical, bitter thoughts which often affect the liver and gallbladder. Aids the flow of bile. For those secretly wishing the worst for everyone else and always looking for a scapegoat. Enhances love for mankind, and acceptance of people as they are. Brings compassion.

IRIS For mental strain that stems from being over-analytical and logical, left-brain dominated, having an explanation for everything, prone to violent behaviour. Releases latent creative abilities, allowing us to feel carefree and humorous. Encourages carefree feelings, promotes a sense of humour. Helps regulate blood-pressure, temperature and breathing.

JAPANESE MAGNOLIA For women who are unhappy, feeling dependent on men, vulnerable and used. Also for sufferers of pre-menstrual syndrome, headaches, fluid retention. Brings a sense of independence, equality and security. Eases physical problems.

JASMINE For loners, those who rebel against authority and find it difficult to get on well with others. They may be prone to accidents such as bone fractures due to a weakness in skeletal structure. Eases bursitis and cartilage/bone/tendon disease. Replaces feelings of alienation with diplomacy. Helps you to find peace in your environment.

LANTANA For those who are quiet, artistic, over-sensitive, easily hurt and shy. They may be sensitive to allergens – hayfever sufferers. Helps us to become more independent and assertive, feeling less threatened. For commanding respect.

LEMON GRASS For those who need nurturing, often rejected by parents, feeling that love hurts and being drawn to painful relationships. Eases pain and promotes self-nurturing, learning to trust and reach out to love. Enhances the absorption of vitamin A.

LIGUSTRUM For an inability to be assertive or express anger, leading to apathy or haughtiness, fatigue and lack of spontaneity. Also for energy leaks from the aura, internal bleeding, liver toxicity, weak eyes, immune deficiency, hypothyroidism. Releases repressive feelings, rekindles optimism and encourages self-expression. Eases physical symptoms.

LILAC For those with a tendency to hold grudges. Also for tumours, growths and cancers. Helps forgiveness of self and others, releases the past.

LILY For those who are anxious about the outcome of everyday affairs and the future, fearful of not being in control of their destiny. Typically such people bite their fingernails or demonstrate other compulsive behaviour. Also for colds, flu, auto-toxicity, skin diseases and allergies. Releases anxiety and fear. Helps to boost the immune system.

MAGNOLIA For those lacking self-appreciation or belief in themselves, feeling undeserving. For problems with the assimilation of nutrients and protein. Increases self-confidence and boosts self-image, so you can prosper and grow.

MARIGOLD For guilt about sexual permissiveness, sexual guilt, confusion about sexual role or identity. For impotence, hormone imbalance, prostate problems, sterility and frigidity. Balances male and female aspects of the self so we can accept both sides of ourselves without feeling threatened.

MORNING GLORY For those deluding themselves with the idea of a golden past, romanticizing better times and making the present seem unpleasant. Also for uric acid accumulation and bowel problems. Helps us to find faith in ourselves and in the future. Aids circulation and eliminatory systems.

MOSS ROSE For those feeling they need more of anything – money, possessions – giving rise to anxiety and the feeling that they lack something. They may also be prone to weight problems. Also helps problems of pancreatic function, irregular glucose absorption, poor digestion of starches and fats, and proteolytic enzyme production. Enables a change of outlook, seeing yourself as sufficiently providing for your needs.

MUSHROOM For feeling insecure about changes in life, leading to procrastination and resistance. Also for discomfort in the feet, ankles, calves, spine and neck. Helps you to become more independent and adaptable.

NARCISSUS For those who are withdrawn and introverted, living in their own world and reluctant to share themselves with others. Prone to migraine, tension and neuralgia. Enhances feelings of pleasure and security, promoting warmth and affection.

ONION For those who are narrow-minded, holding one-sided opinions and becoming critical of others' views and habits. Cultivates tolerance, compassion and ability to listen. Also helps treat viral infections and fevers.

ORCHID For those (often high achievers) who silently punish themselves for past failures. May suffer from numbness and nerve degeneration. Helps us to become less workaholic and more interested in loved ones and the community.

PANSY For those experiencing a deep-seated sense of grief over the loss of a loved one. Affects adrenal and kidney function. Brings transcendence over grief, pointing the way to new outlets for our loving nature and generosity. Helps in the elimination of toxins.

PENTA For selfish, self-reliant people who are inconsiderate of others, withholding love and thinking that love hurts. They often suffer from low blood-pressure. Also for vertigo, lack of oxygenation. Eases pain and promotes feelings of well-being and self-love, making for a more delightful partner or spouse.

PEPPERMINT For those who live in fear of losing loved ones, possessions, health, security, of having little control over their emotions. May suffer inner conflict related to an incomplete relationship with their mother. Builds confidence and a sense of control; fosters the ability to visualize a future in which their desires are fulfilled, making life feel safer. Also aids protein digestion and treats gastric ulcers.

PERIWINKLE For clearing past experiences. Clarifies goals, affords a greater overview of life and boosts energy levels. Heals and regenerates.

PINE For those who only remember mistakes of the past, experiencing guilt, punishment and pain. For fatigue brought on by poor absorption of nutrients; for aches and mood swings. Cultivates inner strength and perseverance, so we can learn positive lessons from past misfortunes.

PINK GERANIUM For those who appear tense, suppressing their anger and intense emotions. Linked to spastic colon, liver/gall bladder trouble, and muscular spasticity. Eases emotional pain, bringing laughter and enjoyment of life.

PINK ROSE For those with a 'fat' complex, always trying the latest diet, rejecting themselves. Also for those who are genuinely overweight or plagued by cellulite. Promotes a better self-image and a perspective that acknowledges and focuses on what can be changed.

POPPY For demanding, selfish people who can be jealous and covet other's belongings. Also for mucoid colitis, constipation and tuberculosis. Cultivates generosity and service to others.

PRIMROSE For those rejecting love as not being good enough, having a romantic and idealistic view of what 'love' should be. Physically manifests as diabetes, hypoglycaemia. Cultivates an appreciation of relationships and an acceptance of love.

RANUNCULUS For mental instability, imbalance in the brain expressed as schizophrenia, violence, rage, psychosis. Sufferers may have been abused in childhood and/or deprived of tender loving care by their mother. Also for premature birth, epilepsy, poor muscle tone and immature nervous system. Restores a balance of energy to the pleasure centres of the brain.

RED CARNATION For those with an inferiority complex, feeling unworthy and lonely, unable to accept success. Prone to lymphatic congestion, swollen glands, skin afflictions, hair loss and baldness. Enhances self-image and feelings of worthiness.

RED ROSE For gloominess and occasional depression. Replaces negative thoughts with enthusiasm and joy.

ROSE OF SHARON For those who are idealistic, straightforward, honest, highly creative and successful but sometimes feel burdened by responsibilities and want to escape from reality. Indicated for heart action – angina pectoris. Attracts just rewards for creativity.

SALVIA For self-dislike and feeling ugly. Brings constructive changes to one's self-image. Improves acne, warts, moles, birthmarks and other blemishes, and skin diseases.

SHRIMP For those who are dissatisfied with themselves, disliking and feeling lumbered with their lifestyle, keenly aware of others' achievements and assets. This attitude upsets the immune system's ability to handle everyday stress. Also for combating the ageing process. Speeds the process of change and allows creative ideas to flow.

STOCK For tense, nervous, hyperactive types – dependent on nicotine and other chemicals – susceptible to physical exhaustion and mood swings because they are unable to pace themselves. Slows down and balances out energy, enabling completion of projects.

SUNFLOWER For those feeling separated from the universal spirit, rejected and left to fend for themselves – persecuted, fearing death, feeling suicidal. Brings a sense of responsibility for actions. Integrates the personality and soul/spirit.

TIGER'S JAW CACTUS For those who like sitting and watching others do the work. Essentially immobilized by fear of failure to the point of apathy and laziness. May be spoiled and inconsiderate or a 'non-participant' (out of hypochondria). Brings the motivation to be confident and productive.

VANILLA For those overwhelmed by negative energy from others and themselves, feeling tired, depressed and irritated for no apparent reason, needing to withdraw from a situation or individual. Also for neurological overload or psychic attack. Offers protection against such influences, helping you stay clear and in control of your individual environment without unnecessary interference.

VERBENA For inner turmoil, frustration, impulsive action. Induces a meditative feeling of inner peace. Allows mind and body to relax and regenerate.

WANDERING JEW For those who are easily discouraged, lacking discipline, giving up easily. Prone to inflammation or neuritis/shingles. Helps us to achieve greater confidence and self-discipline so projects can be completed; to learning patience and tolerance.

WHITE CARNATION For those who are stubborn and headstrong, resulting in constant anxiety, tension and mood swings. Adrenal hormone upsets (the fight-or-flight syndrome). Eases fear of failure, balances desire and releases anxiety. Brings contentment.

WHITE HYACINTH For shock and trauma, especially that of birth which is linked with feelings of uncertainty and insecurity. Nervous exhaustion. Releases the shock of emotional and physical trauma (e.g. accidents, operations and violence). Enhances sense of self-reliance.

WHITE PETUNIA For those who have difficulty making decisions and acting on them, unable to synchronize thoughts, concentration and body movements. For dyslexia, stuttering – and also past negative programming. Aids co-ordination and the synergy of right and left brain function.

WHITE ROSE For those attracting negativity from others, feeling undefined fears. For 'psychic attack', and also loss of memory. Offers protection from negative thought-forms; cultivates self-confidence and ability to feel comfortable with anyone.

WISTERIA For those who are unaware of loving feelings, not feeling love at all. Opens us up to receive and give unconditional love. A heart tonic for enjoying everyone.

ZINNIA For those feeling unloved, hurt and angry, critical of themselves and others, bitter at being deprived of nurturing attention. Often affected by arthritic or rheumatic pain. Heavy metal toxicity. Encourages self-nurturing, releases bitterness and cultivates generosity.

NATIVE TEXANS

ASTER Promotes strength within and gentleness without. Increases powers of concentration and encouragement to promote loyalty and honesty in others. Stimulates the immune system to cleanse the internal environment of toxins in cases of disease.

CARROT Enhances initiative for developing healthy disciplines and organizing priorities so that ambitions are realized through natural rhythm and cycles. Improves the properties of mucus in respiration and reproductivity, enhancing fertility.

CHRISTMAS CACTUS Lends psychological support to help us focus on what is right for ourselves and others. Reinforces strengths and helps healing of others from the heart. Supports genetic strengths and natural talents to enhance well-being. Compensates for inherent character weaknesses.

COLUMBINE Enhances ability to think and act independently, dropping role models imposed by others. Helps an infant to become independent of its mother's immune system, increasing antibody efficiency and destruction of bacteria.

DILL Releases fear of abandonment and death. Clears self-alienation and denial of feelings. Allows effective thinking and channelling of our 'self'.

ECHINACEA Purifies thoughts, clarifies visions, refines judgement and understanding. Enhances resistance to viral toxicity.

GAILLARDIA Enhances determination to succeed by overcoming obstacles. Lightens the personality through the joy of overcoming. Boosts immune system, enhancing resistance to viruses and toxicity.

INDIA HAWTHORN Works with group karma, dispels confusion, accents impersonal love by expressing this through deed and example. Loving all as one.

KNOTTED MARJORAM Enhances clarity of thought to work out details when change is needed. For avoiding premature action, aiding a calculated transformation. Enhances immune system's defence mechanisms.

KOLANCHOE Helps correct ingrained illusion of opposites, such as good and bad consciousness, creating dualism, polarity in personality and separation. Mends this fragmentation so we can see our blind spots.

MEADOW SAGE Aids expression of strong emotions such as anger without transgressing or being vindictive. Allow us to express emotions and feelings without being controlled by them.

MEXICAN OREGANO Enhances ability to understand quickly and respond to new situations correctly, teaching by example and drawing to one experiences that develop character. Helps lubricate and cleanse the skin.

ROSE CAMPION Strengthens the body's natural defences when there is a congenital weakness which is karmic. Develops character by uprooting old ingrained patterns that prevent movement forward. Creates liberation in the subconscious.

SILVER LACE Aids contemplation and learning from set-backs, seeing them as a potential for growth rather than failures. Help us to ride the waves and know when to advance or to retreat. Aids synthesis of interferon, the body's antiviral agent.

SNAPDRAGON Increases perception and discernment. Helps us to recognize what brings us into alignment with others and define guidelines so that we can clarify and refine plans with reasonable expectations. Enhances internal and external judgement, raising consciousness of the immune system.

ANTIQUE ROSE COLLECTION

ALFREDO DE DEMAS Assists command over body and mind to affect constructive habits. Tunes the mind with the environment. Affords clarity of perception and grounding for those who are 'air-headed'.

FORTUNIANA Aids realization and penetration of universal truths. Leadership qualities emerge, inspiring co-operation in others by integrating the universal soul's desires with personal desires. Enhances intuition or sixth sense.

LADY EUBANKSIA Expands inner awareness. Brings integration of mind, body and spirit – the expression of all talents in a new and unique way. A previous reclusive person will realize goals through others, emerging as a teacher of wisdom and understanding.

OLD BLUSH Enhances stamina, catalyzing inner strength and the ability to keep going. Allows creativity to be expressed and adapted to every aspect of life and health, so that we accomplish more in life than seemed possible. Strengthens will-power to integrate motor pathways and neural systems to initiate muscular contraction.

VIRIDIFLORA Helps those who are extra-sensitive to their environment by maintaining alignment of their personal power centres. Enhances grounding and personal power, feeling centred and integrated by clarity of purpose.

MASTER REMEDIES

BLUEBONNET For those awakened by the call of their own destiny, the quest for one's true identity revealing great powers within. Increased inner awareness creates important changes (e.g. career, relationships and health) that foster our service to humanity.

GARDENIA Integration of personal life with future goals. Encourages long-range planning; awakens teaching, writing and speaking talents so concepts can be translated into reality. Dreams come true. Nourishes creativity, inspiration and achievement, encompassing home and family as well as the environment and career.

INDIAN PAINTBRUSH Brings the source of spirit and light into daily life, so that every challenge is met with a consciousness of success. Confers wisdom and a positive attitude, transforming and illuminating health, career and relationships. Makes every day a miracle.

YELLOW ROSE For the reformer who has chosen the life of service, who desires to serve society unselfishly. Helps us to be attuned to the times and environment, so that our good works benefit and improve the established order and are an inspiration to others. 'Love isn't love until you give it away.'

✤ PERELANDRA ROSE AND ✤ GARDEN ESSENCES

Back in 1976 Machaelle Small Wright established the Perelandra Garden, a nature research centre, with a view to researching and discovering the principles and dynamics of co-creation between man and nature. Tucked away in 22 acres of woodland at the foothills of the Blue Ridge Mountains of Virginia, she has succeeded in creating a garden environment which is integrally balanced with nature in such a way that every living thing enhances the life and health of everything else. Plants growing here flourish without the use of organic or inorganic pesticides, nor does Machaelle remove insects by hand. The state of balance provides a niche for the insects who, given their proper place, do not act in a destructive manner. The garden has now reached a level where all its inhabitants do truly enhance the life and health of one another.

Like many, Machaelle feels there is an intelligence in nature which serves to keep everything in balance. She communicates directly with the nature spirits, devas and the nature intelligences (the intelligent levels of consciousness within nature) in order to obtain specific information on how to create a balanced environment. It is said that the deva of each plant type holds the architectural blueprints of that plant.

The Perelandra Rose and Garden essences grew from this co-creative relationship and are one result of the work being done in this research centre. The essences benefit additionally by being made from the flowers of vegetables, herbs and other plants growing in this unique garden.

The first eight Rose essences (Set 1) were developed in 1984. Made from the roses in the Perelandra garden, these essences function with one another to support and balance an individual's physical body and soul as he proceeds in *day to day evolutionary process*. As we move forward in daily process, there are mechanisms within us which are set in motion to facilitate our periods of growth. The Perelandra Rose essences help stabilize and balance us and our process mechanisms.

The next set of 18 Garden essences is made from flower petals of vegetables, herbs and flowers grown in the Perelandra garden. Their balancing and restorative patterns address physical, emotional, mental and spiritual *issues* that we face in today's world.

The Perelandra Rose essences Set 2 was developed in 1992. The eight essences are made from roses growing in the Perelandra garden and address the specific functions within the body that are activated and/or impacted during a *deep expansion experience*. Here, one is not simply processing ordinary, everyday occurrences. Rather, one is faced with an experience that is new and challenging to the present balance and functioning of the body. When faced with this kind of expansion, the body is required to function in ways that are new, and with patterns and rhythms yet to be experienced. The Rose Essences II address this expansion phenomenon by fine-tuning, balancing and stabilizing the specific steps of the process one must go through to expand.

The Perelandra essences are one meaningful way the extraordinary benefits derived from this special balanced, natural environment can be shared with mankind.

GARDEN ESSENCES

BROCCOLI For the power balance which must be maintained when one perceives himself to be under siege from outside. Stabilizes the body/soul unit so the person won't close down, detach and scatter.

CAULIFLOWER Stabilizes and balances the child during the birth process. Stabilizes the body/soul balance in the adult.

CELERY Restores balance in the immune system when it is being overworked or stressed and during long-term viral or bacterial infections.

CHIVES Re-establishes the power one has when the internal male/female dynamics are balanced and the person is functioning in a state of awareness within this balance.

COMFREY Repairs higher vibrational soul damage that occurred in the present or a past lifetime.

CORN Stabilization during universal spiritual expansion. Assists transition of experience into useful, pertinent understanding and action.

CUCUMBER Re-balancing during depression. Vital reattachment to life.

DILL Assists the individual in reclaiming power balance one has released to others. Releases victimization.

NASTURTIUM Restores vital physical life energy during times of intense mental level focus.

OKRA Returns ability to see the positive in one's life and environment.

SALVIA Restores emotional stability during times of extreme stress.

SNAP PEA Re-balances child or adult after a nightmare. Assists in ability to translate daily experience into a positive, understandable process.

SUMMER SQUASH Restores courage to the person who experiences fear and resistance when faced with daily routine. Releases shyness and phobia issues.

SWEET BELL PEPPER Restores inner peace, clarity and calm when faced with stressful times. Stabilizes body/soul balance during times of stress.

TOMATO Cleansing. Assists the body in shattering and throwing off that which is causing infection or disease.

YELLOW YARROW Supplies emotional protection during vulnerable times. Its support softens resistance and assists the integration process.

ZINNIA Reconnects one to the child within. Restores playfulness, laughter, joy and a sense of healthy priorities.

ZUCCHINI Helps restore physical strength during convalescence.

THE ROSE ESSENCES I

GRÜSS AN AACHEN Stability. Balances and stabilizes the body/soul unit on all physical/ emotional/mental/spiritual (p.e.m.s.) levels as it moves forward in its evolutionary process.

PEACE Courage. Opens the individual to the inner dynamic of courage, which is aligned to universal courage.

ECLIPSE Acceptance and insight. Enhances the individual's appreciation of his own inner knowing. Supports the mechanism which allows the body to receive the soul's input and insight.

ORANGE RUFFLES Receptivity. Stabilizes the individual during the expansion of his sensory system.

AMBASSADOR Pattern. Aids the individual in seeing the relationship of the part to the whole, in perceiving his pattern and purpose.

NYMPHENBURG Strength. Supports and holds the strength created by the balance of the body/ soul fusion, and facilitates the individual's ability to regain that balance.

WHITE LIGHTNIN' Synchronized movement. Stabilizes the inner timing of all p.e.m.s. levels moving in concert and enhances body/soul fusion.

ROYAL HIGHNESS Final stabilization. The 'mop-up' essence which helps to insulate, protect and stabilize the individual and to stabilize the shift during its final stages, while vulnerable.

THE ROSE ESSENCES II

BLAZE IMPROVED CLIMBING ROSE Softens and relaxes first the central nervous system, then the body as a whole, thus allowing the input from an expansion experience to be appropriately sorted, shifted and integrated within the body.

MAYBELLE STEARNS Stabilizes and supports the sacrum during an expansion experience.

MR. LINCOLN Balances and stabilizes the cerebrospinal fluid pulse while it alters its rhythm and patterning to accommodate the expansion.

SONIA Stabilizes and supports the cerebrospinal fluid pulse *after* it has completed its shift to accommodate the expansion.

CHICAGO PEACE Stabilizes movement of and interaction among the cranial bones, cerebrospinal fluid and sacrum during an expansion experience.

BETTY PRIOR Stabilizes and balances the delicate rhythm of expansion and contraction of the cranial bones during the expansion.

TIFFANY Stabilizes the cranials as they shift their alignment appropriately to accommodate the input and impulses of expansion.

OREGOLD Stabilizes and balances the cranials, central nervous system, cerebrospinal fluid and sacrum after an expansion process is complete.

This material is reproduced by kind permission of Machaelle Small Wright, *Perelandra Guide to Rose and Garden Essences*, © 1992, and Perelandra 1995–6 catalogue, © 1995, Perelandra Ltd.

❋ PACIFIC ESSENCES ❋

These are the first Canadian essences and are made by Sabina Pettitt from the plants and marine life of the Pacific Northwest. Sabina learned about flower essences through her healing work with Dr John LePlante, a naturopath and chiropractor, in the early 1970s.

On moving to Vancouver Island, in the Canadian province of British Columbia, Sabina was excited to discover new kinds of plants, and began making some of them into vibrational medicines. The Arbutus trees of the west coast of Canada were among the first to catch her attention. The Arbutus essence acts as a spiritual tonic; one of the qualities it promotes is wisdom.

In 1983 Sabina formed Pacific Essences with Fiona Macleod and together they proceeded to research the plant energies that attracted them. By 1985 they had researched 24 Wildflower remedies and 13 Spring Flowers.

One day when walking along a sandy beach Sabina came across a Sand Dollar (a type of sea urchin). Sabina knew instinctively that this Sand Dollar had to be made into a remedy to treat a friend with a rare form of skin cancer. To capture its essence she placed the Sand Dollar in a glass of seawater and left it under a pyramid in the sun. This incident marked the beginning of her work with essences from the ocean, from which a whole new realm of energetic medicine began to unfold.

Sabina pioneered the first set of 12 sea essences which introduces us to a range of entirely new frequencies in the world of vibrational medicine. They are about transformations in consciousness and are indicated for major breakthroughs, for they help us to contact the basic rhythms of the universe when we are going through change. They are best taken individually, as each one is very precise and powerful. Being quick-acting, they usually have quite noticeable results.

Sabina's sea essences differ from her flower remedies in that they come from salt water, which is very similar in composition to our own blood plasma and seems to have a special affinity for the body. In Chinese medicine the water element is related to reproduction, growth and maturation. At the level of the spirit it is linked to chi or psychic strength, which leads us through obstacles to growth. It is also the symbol for the unconscious.

Sabina proposes that, by their very nature, sea essences reveal the unconscious and strengthen consciousness in order to move forward towards a unique unfolding. Each of her essences (Wildflower, Spring Flower or Sea Essence) is also linked to particular chakras and meridians.

NATIVE WILDFLOWERS – KIT 1

BLUEBELL For giving up constraints, releasing old programmes, opening the channels of communication, engaging in what is fulfilling. Helpful for emotionally-caused speech disorders, autism. Combats shyness. Boosts low energy, combats fatigue, alleviates fear, strengthens the will and ability to breathe during panic or anxiety attacks. Chakra – throat. Meridians – lung and kidney.

BLUE CAMAS For acceptance and objectivity. Balances the intuitive and rational, unifies the left and right brain. For the creative person who is impractical, and the down-to-earth person unable to access his or her intuition. Also for dyslexia, learning disabilities, inability to learn from experience. Releases stored memory from past lives. Chakras – solar plexus and throat. Meridians – kidney and bladder.

BLUE LUPIN For clear and precise thinking. Links the pineal gland (organ of spiritual perception) with the pituitary gland (organ of metabolic control and balance). Also for toxin-related headaches and digestive disorders. Eliminates confusion about who we are. Alleviates depression, frustration and despair. Focuses attention and simplifies issues. Chakra – base/root. Meridian – liver.

EASTER LILY Truth, purity, integrity. Helps to integrate different aspects of our personalities, allowing open and honest self-expression. For by-passing acquired personas of illusion, duplicity and dishonesty. Also effective for pre-menstrual syndrome and gynaecological imbalances. Chakras – heart and third eye and crown. Meridians – kidney and bladder.

FIREWEED For realizing the abundance of love, both within and without. For emotional experiences recorded in the heart. Eases a broken heart, clears emotional wounds, coldness and the inability to feel. For embracing new relationships without residue from past ones. Improves circulation, softens muscle fascia in chest and upper back. Chakra – heart. Meridian – heart.

GOATSBEARD For meditation, creative visualization. To visualize oneself in a deep state of relaxation, being calm and relaxed in stressful situations. Resolving tension by creating inner alignment before action. Activates thymus to deal with stress. Strengthens immune system, white blood cell production. Chakra – third eye. Meridians – small intestine and spleen.

HARVEST LILY Community, relationships, social interaction. Encourages expansion and awakening. Supports group energy and the ability to see another's point of view. For problems linked to reproduction, elimination, digestion, absorption, respiration and heart. Chakras – solar plexus and crown. Meridians – triple warmer and heart protector.

HOOKER'S ONION For freedom, inspiration, spontaneity. Replaces overwhelmed, stuck and heavy feelings with being refreshed and light-hearted. Nurtures creativity. Remedy for the spirit. Potential for releasing birth traumas and resolving the emotional attachment between mother and child. Chakras – all. Meridians – all 12.

ORANGE HONEYSUCKLE Inner direction, expression and identity. For crisis of personal identity and related physical tension. Releases creative blocks, diffuses anger and frustration. Evokes peaceful creativity. Useful for the turmoil of the teenage years. Also a powerful tonic for digestive disorders. Chakras – hara or sacral and solar plexus. Meridian – triple heater or warmer.

PLANTAIN For releasing mental blocks and drawing off negativity. Purifies and cleanses the effects of poisonous thoughts, attitudes and resentment. Also for blood and liver disorders; any physical toxicity resulting from emotional or mental poisons, such as migraines and indigestion. Chakras – hara or sacral and crown. Meridians – liver and gall bladder.

SALAL For grudges or resentment. Releases power to forgive yourself and others; to let go. Clears stress and allows you the freedom and joy to experience the embodiment of the spirit in mysterious ways. Chakra – heart. Meridians – heart and small intestine.

SNOWBERRY For accepting life as it is at the moment, dissolving resistance to what is – even when it is painful. Also helpful for chronic fatigue and seasonal affected disorder. Chakras – crown and heart. Meridians – kidney and bladder.

NATIVE WILDFLOWERS – KIT 2

ARBUTUS Spiritual tonic – enhances qualities of depth and integrity. For homesickness, abandonment. For hanging on tightly while letting go lightly. Also benefits the lungs when their energy is depleted by sadness. Chakra – crown. Meridians – lung and liver.

CANDYSTICK Physical tonic – releases pelvic tension and promotes pelvic alignment. Releases blocked energy surrounding the experiences of abortion, miscarriage, birth, sexuality. Transforms self-anger and frustration to honour of self despite trauma. Survival and free will. Also for injuries to the sacrum and pelvic girdle, any insult to the reproductive system. Chakras – hara or sacral and throat. Meridians – kidney and bladder.

CHICKWEED For acknowledging and experiencing timelessness, being fully present and able to respond. Allows free and easy expression. Works on gall bladder channel to release tension and give up control. Useful for losing excess weight that is caused in part by old emotional baggage. Good for health practitioners. Chakras – throat and base or root. Meridian – gall bladder.

DEATH CAMUS Spiritual rebirth: Awareness of spiritual connection with all life, for new beginnings and change. Alleviates stress and worry in times of transition. Helpful for new jobs, relationships, adventure. Assists self-cleansing efforts such as fasting, examining beliefs. Chakras – hara or sacral and heart. Meridians – lung and kidney.

GRASS WIDOW Releases old beliefs and limited patterns, and the fear of being judged by others. Challenges mental structures and beliefs (linked to family, work, religion) that are not working for us. For fear of letting go. Also helpful for digestive problems and food intolerance. Chakra – heart. Meridians – stomach and large intestine.

NOOTKA ROSE For expressing love, laughter and joy. Kindles enthusiasm. Reminds us that the life of the soul does not begin with birth or end with death. Excellent for spiritual crisis, abuse, abandonment, psychic, emotional or physical assault. Re-integrates the psyche after assault, heals fragmentation after years of self-abuse – such as with drugs, alcohol. Chakras – all. Meridians – all 12.

OX-EYE DAISY For vision and the visionary. Brings a greater perspective when we cannot see the woods for the trees. Dissolves the blockage of fear which prevents clear sight. Develops better vision. Benefits the eyes and ears. Chakra – third eye. Meridians – heart protector and kidney.

PIPSISSEWA For making decisions. Clears ambivalence and indecisiveness. Releases worry and confusion around choices in life. Benefits the area of the brain involved in choice. Chakras – solar plexus and throat. Meridians – spleen, liver and kidney.

POISON HEMLOCK For letting go, moving through transition periods without getting stuck and holding on to old structures and beliefs. Dissolves emotional, mental, physical paralysis arising from periods of major change. Releases rigid feelings, ingrained thought-patterns, no longer relevant unconscious thoughts. Also beneficial for constipation, fluid retention, weight problems, paralysis of the physical structure or nervous system, stalled labour during the birthing process. Chakra – crown. Meridian – gall bladder.

SALMONBERRY A physical tonic – for spinal alignment and structural balancing. Works on bone muscles, fascia. Helps chronic misalignments of physical structure due to injury. Chakra – third eye. Meridian – bladder.

TWIN FLOWER Acceptance and compassion. Clears judgement and a critical attitude towards everything. Teaches discernment to make choices without criticizing others. Fosters optimism and humility. Chakras – base and heart. Meridians – liver and gall bladder.

VANILLA LEAF For affirmation and acceptance of oneself. Replaces self-loathing with self-esteem. A grounding remedy of exuberance, joy, acceptance. For skin disorders and any problem rooted in self-denigration and lack of self-love. Chakras – third eye and crown. Meridians – lung and large intestine.

SPRING FLOWERS

CAMELLIA A catalyst for opening up to new attitudes which reflect one's true inner nature. Replaces guilt and shame with openness and flexibility. Stimulates expansion beyond self-inflicted limitations, and expression of our uniqueness and inner power. Releases cell memory of earlier experiences in this life. Accesses self-trust and creates shifts in attitude. Chakra – solar plexus. Meridian – large intestine.

FORSYTHIA Catalyst for change. Provides motivation for transforming old useless thought- and behaviour-patterns which may be self-destructive (such as addictive habits: mental, emotional and physical addiction, especially to alcohol, drugs and tobacco). Liberates dysfunctional relationships. Detoxifies the liver. Chakra – crown. Meridian – gall bladder.

GRAPE HYACINTH For times of external shock, despair and stress. Allows one to step back from the situation while harnessing inner resources to meet the challenge. Replaces shock and trauma with balance. Dissolves hopelessness, despair and depression. Eases stress felt in the stomach and aids breathing in times of stress. Also for bumps, bruises, accident shocks and all forms of trauma. Chakra – third eye. Meridians – stomach and lung.

LILY OF THE VALLEY For freedom of choice by discovering the simplest form of behaviour. Replaces sophistication and over-control with innocence. An emotional tonic that helps us to see through the eyes of a child. Used in Europe as a cardiac tonic. Brings inner radiance and vitality. Chakra – throat. Meridian – heart.

NARCISSUS For identifying and resolving conflicts by going to the centre of the problem or fear. Slays internal dragons, calms butterflies in the stomach, alleviates worry. Clears obsessive thinking, connects us to the impulse for survival, assists in feeling grounded. Also promotes digestion and eases digestive disorders (such as excess stomach acid, ulcers, gas). Chakras – base/root and hara/sacral. Meridian – stomach.

PERIWINKLE Helps us to be responsible for our own depression and thereby dispel it. Lifts the dark cloud of depression, moves us to a place of inner knowing. Calms the mind and clears the memory. Also for hypertension, haemorrhaging, nervous disorders especially anxiety and seasonal affective disorders. Chakras – hara/sacral and crown. Meridian – heart.

POLYANTHUS Dissolves blocks to abundance and transforms attitudes of inadequacy into those of worthiness and willingness to receive. Increases sense of self-worth. Also benefits the respiratory and elimination systems. Chakra – base. Meridians – large intestine and lung.

PURPLE CROCUS Enhances ability to tune in to all aspects of pain and grief in order to release the tension and restriction associated with these feelings. For embracing issues; beneficial for those who turn their blocked energy against themselves after grief, causing life-threatening disease. Helps tension in the upper back and shoulders, releases the heaviness related to loss and grief. Also assists the lungs. Chakra – throat. Meridian – lung.

PURPLE MAGNOLIA Promotes intimacy and non-separateness, enhances all the senses. Replaces withdrawal, coldness and frigidity with open intimacy. Elevates sexuality to its fullest potential for intimacy and non-separateness. Benefits the senses of smell, touch and feeling. Also a remedy for the spirit. Chakras – solar plexus and crown. Meridian – heart protector (circulation/sex).

SNOWDROP For letting go, having fun and lightening up. Combines enthusiasm and joyful exploration of life. Embodies qualities of personal power and leadership. Dissolves energy blocks and personal holding patterns that prevent the free flow of energy or qi. Strengthens the will to dissolve paralysing fear. Physically good for paralysis problems – arthritis, multiple sclerosis, polio myelitis, cerebral palsy. Chakras – base, solar plexus and crown. Meridians – kidney and bladder.

VIBURNUM Strengthens our connection with the subconscious and our psychic abilities. Excellent aid to channelling, meditating or centring. To hear and trust the voice within. Fosters clarity of sight. Affects the ears and ability to listen. Helps relax the nervous system. Chakra – third eye. Meridians – spleen and triple warmer.

WEIGELA For integrating experiences on the physical and emotional planes. For realizing that others are our teachers and mirrors who reflect our own negative and positive energy patterns. Fosters trust. Also for accidents and unexpected physical/emotional traumas. Chakras – throat and third eye. Meridians – liver and gall bladder.

WINDFLOWER A spiritual tonic providing grounding and inner security. Provides the security necessary to express our spiritual being, allowing the soul to dance. Also for stomach disorders, both physical and emotional – for nourishment on all levels. Chakras – throat and heart. Meridian – stomach.

SEA ESSENCES

ANEMONE For acceptance of ourselves and others, by helping us to take responsibility for our own reality, allowing us to be organized by the universe. Aligns the mental body with higher soul purpose: Empowerment versus victim mentality. Releases karmic blockage in the solar plexus. Also for physical pain, allowing movement through pain rather than resistance to it. Helps eye problems. Also for over-controlling emotionally and mentally; for those prone to tension, muscle spasms and injuries. Chakra – solar plexus. Meridian – liver.

BARNACLE For attuning with the feminine aspect of the self in order to develop complete trust. Embodies wisdom, nurturing, fertility and abundance. Also for the female reproductive system, especially cysts and fibroids. Regulates hormone production and release. A powerful birthing remedy. Chakra – heart. Meridian – small intestine.

BROWN KELP For shifts in perception leading to clarity. For those who get in their own way because of fear and confusion. Balances energy between the base/root and crown chakra. Also dissolves back tension, helps bladder infections and ear problems – especially fluid imbalance of the middle, inner ear. Chakras – base/root and crown. Meridian – bladder.

JELLY FISH A birthing and rebirthing essence. Dissolves resistance that causes pain, helping us to be fluid and flexible rather than rigid and stuck. Spiritually connects us to the rhythms of our own being. Helps self-expression and depression. Also works against arterial plaque and hardening of arteries. Dissolves bitterness and hardness on the mental and emotional level before physical manifestation of disease occurs. Chakra – throat. Meridians – heart and heart protector.

MOON SNAIL To cleanse the mind and let in light. Eliminates physical toxins which cloud the mind. Helps cultivate innocent wonderment instead of rigid thought structures. A helpful tool for meditation and inner journeys. For mapping unconscious territory in order to harness and explore creative expression. Chakra – hara/sacral. Meridian – triple warmer.

MUSSEL For releasing the burden of anger, enabling one to stand up straight. Transforming anger, it allows creativity and inner radiance to shine through. Excellent for a 'victim consciousness' that prevents our alignment with inner power and strength. Resolves irritability, frustration and anger. Also relaxes neck and shoulder tension and eases headaches and dizziness. Helpful for whiplash; promotes the flow of bile and aids digestion. Chakra – hara/sacral. Meridian – gall bladder.

PINK SEAWEED A grounding remedy for the patience needed before new beginnings, to harmonize thought before action. Helps us to move out of our 'comfort zone' into the new and challenging. Softens and allows change to occur with grace. Helpful when beginning new jobs, schools, relationships and experiences. Physically strengthens the bones and teeth; aids constipation. Chakras – hara and solar plexus. Meridian – heart protector.

SAND DOLLAR For 'coming to your senses', awakening to reality versus illusion. For positive thinking that helps us to overcome the underlying cause of disease in the physical body. Effective for bronchitis, asthma, throat problems and self-expression. Chakra – throat. Meridian – lung.

SEA PALM For breakthroughs in consciousness. For those who hurry for no reason, who are busy, preoccupied and controlling but not really allowing themselves just to be. For activity which is a hindrance to success and

meaningful relationships. For those who crave nurturing and emotional/physical nourishment. Also helps digestive problems and eating disorders. Chakra – heart. Meridians – stomach.

STARFISH A grief remedy: For willingly giving up the old and allowing the experience of being empty. For appreciating our own unique soul path. Helps us to remember that 'to everything there is a season and a time for every purpose under heaven.' Stimulates a deep spiritual connection with those we love. Chakra – crown. Meridian – large intestine.

SURFGRASS For courage, strength and power rooted in stability and flexibility. Encourages integration of opposites by embracing paradox. Brings us the courage to be. For achieving goals that reflect our life's purpose, not our ego's desires. Alleviates fear and integrates courage. Strengthens will and gives a second wind. Also benefits kidney disease, infections, calcifications, inflammations. Balances the adrenal glands, enabling adrenaline to be used in a life-supporting way: stress without distress. Chakra – heart. Meridian – kidney.

URCHIN For safety and psychic protection. For charting unknown territory, such as past-life regressions. A spiritual essence that expands the mind to access stored memories from early childhood or a previous life. Also for the effects of childhood abuse which have created self-abuse patterns (e.g. alcoholism, eating disorders, suicidal tendencies). Helps to dispel panic attacks, respiratory problems that arise from feeling unsafe. Chakras – crown and solar plexus. Meridian – spleen.

❋ GEM REMEDIES ❋

Gem essences are made in the same way as flower essences. They have similar emotional/psychological benefits but also act at the physical level like homoeopathic remedies. They play a supportive role when used in combination with flower essences. (Available from the Flower and Gem Remedy Association [Gem], Pegasus [Peg], AK [Andreas Korte] and Ask [Alaskan Flower and Environmental Essences].)

AMETHYST (Gem) Soul stone. Excellent for the build-up of stress or overwhelming emotional states that lead to tension-type migraine headaches, easing mental anxieties that cause the physical symptoms. Balances the metabolism and the endocrine and immune systems. Enhances the pineal and pituitary glands. Cleanses the blood and aids blood sugar problems such as diabetes and hypoglycaemia. Also initiates self-esteem and is useful for mental disorders and brain imbalances (such as autism, dyslexia and epilepsy).

AURIC PROTECTION (Gem) Strengthens the aura. Ideal for therapists/practitioners who feel drained after seeing a number of clients. Also protects anyone who is sensitive to other people's vibrations, such as in the workplace or crowded city environments.

AZURITE (Gem) A catalyst for releasing past programmed belief systems, enabling us to shed beliefs that are no longer appropriate or useful. For negative thought-patterns, which can lead to bone and joint problems, especially arthritis, inflammation of the joints and so on. Expands consciousness, drawing in light and truth to cleanse the mind and soul, integrating the spiritual and physical. Enhances the body's ability to absorb copper, zinc, magnesium and calcium.

CRYSTAL FIRST AID REMEDY (Gem) Restores balance after a shock to the body, either on the emotional/psychological/spiritual or physical levels.

ETTRINGITE (Peg) Self-empowerment. For greater awareness of the flow of energy into people. May bring a greater sense of the combination of love, power, strength, will, purpose and spiritual guidance.

FUCHSITE (Peg) Purpose. For deeper insight into the way our evolution has been affected by our own thoughts. Brings alignment and harmony to our life purpose and a clear image of ourselves in the future. Helps us to perceive the future and act on it. Assists those engaged in time travel.

GOLD (Gem) A major healer which balances the heart chakra and aids in the absorption and assimilation of gold as well as all vitamins and minerals. Strengthens the nervous and muscular systems, improves circulation, balances right and left hemispheres of the brain. Aids regeneration of the body as a whole and attracts positive energy to the aura.

HERKIMER DIAMOND (Gem) Realigns the chakra system. Reduces and alleviates stress, draws off and eliminates toxins from the body, cleanses the subtle bodies. For pre-cancerous conditions; for people who are resistant to connecting to the physical plane, it allows the soul's force to come through. Good for couples wanting a child.

IUG KENYA ENERGETIC PROTECTIVE SHIELD Made from a meteorite which fell to the earth in Kenya, this throws a protective shield around the body's entire energy system. For neutralizing the negative effect of geopathic stress and manmade fields of power lines, radiation, radar, radio and television as well as other electronic and electrical instruments. There are three potencies from which to choose.

LAPIS LAZULI (Gem) A mental healer and cleanser, soul purifier and spiritual rejuvenator. By developing stability and power of the mind, the soul's force can function smoothly. Heals the memory of emotional wounds, brings strength and vitality, mental clarity and enhances psychic abilities. Eases anxiety and tension in the throat chakra and soothes related problems such as sore throat and tonsillitis. Stimulates expression on personal level for shy, retiring types. Also a powerful cleanser of toxicity in the lymphatic system. Invigorates the pituitary, thymus and thyroid glands, the spleen and the lungs.

MOONSTONE (Gem) Soothes, balances and heals emotions. For stress affecting the solar plexus, stomach, abdomen, spleen, pancreas and intestinal tract. Stimulates digestive enzymes for better digestion and absorption of food. Eases ulcerous conditions. Cleanses the lymphatic system, aids female problems and helps the birth process. Eases anxiety and stress, especially associated with mothering.

MOSS AGATE (Gem) Grounding, strengthening mind and body. Eases depression, develops confidence and security, allows spirituality to be grounded and practical. Beneficial effect on the lymphatic system, spleen, liver, circulation and intestinal tract. Helps treat water retention, hyperglycaemic, anorexia and allergies.

OKENITE (Peg) Change. For better affinity in working with and integrating change. Works with movement, air travel. Balances and strengthens the astral body. Furthers understanding of the Earth's etheric body.

ROSE QUARTZ (Gem) A powerful restorer of balance and healer of the emotions. Focuses on the heart. Heals internal wounds held in the heart, especially those stemming from childhood due to a lack of fulfilment of basic emotional needs. Restores the self-love needed for a positive self-image, dispels feelings of unworthiness that lead to loneliness and low self-esteem. Heals the inner child. Helps ease anger and tension with father figures. Dissolves trauma and reprogrammes the heart to learn to nurture, increasing self-confidence and creativity. Good for circulation, heart, kidney, liver and lungs. Enhances fertility.

SILVER (Gem) Stimulates mental functions, improves circulation of energy to the brain, enhances the pituitary and pineal glands. Indicated for left and right brain imbalance, visual and co-ordination problems, epilepsy, autism, speech difficulties, dyslexia. Relieves stress, works with the feminine principles and emotional balance.

SUNSTONE (Peg) Inner strength. For calling on the regenerative powers of the sun. Enhances understanding of the patterns of past lives. Helps in overcoming obstacles. Increases communion and understanding of the energies of the sun.

TURQUOISE (Gem) Strengthens the entire body as well as realigning the whole subtle anatomy. Increases circulation and absorption of nutrients. Revitalizes the nervous system. Useful in treating anorexia nervosa. Used by Native Americans for protection and balance.

VANADINITE (Peg) A transparent shield. Helps to safeguard or protect, creating a stronger awareness of inner influences. A true shield is one which allows energies to pass through. Aids in the understanding of those fears, struggles and difficulties we may be trying to shield in the first place.

These Pegasus Gems are an example of the many Gem Elixirs (several hundred) and other Vibrational Remedies to be described and included in a forthcoming book by Fred Rubenfeld and Michael Smulkis (1995).

PART THREE

FIVE

AILMENT CHART

ESSENCE KEY

- **Africa and the Amazon**
  Andreas Korte Essences (AK)

- **Australia and New Zealand**

  Australia:
  Bush Flower Essences (Aus B)
  Living Flower Essences (Aus L)

  New Zealand:
  New Perception Flower Essences (NZ)

- **Europe**

  Britain:
  Bach Flower Remedies (B)
  Bailey Essences (Ba)
  Findhorn Flower Essences (F)
  Green Man Tree Essences (GM)
  Harebell Remedies (Hb)

  France:
  Deva Flower Elixirs (Dv)

- **India**
  Himalayan Aditi Flower Essences (Him A)
  Himalayan Flower Enhancers (Him E)
  Himalayan Indian Tree and Flower Essences
    (Him I)

- **USA and Canada**

  USA:
  Alaskan:
  Alaskan Flower and Environmental
    Essences (Ask)
  Arizona:
  Desert Alchemy Flower Essences (DAl)
  California:
  FES and Californian Research Essences
    (Cal)
  Flower Essence Society (Fes)
  Master's Flower Essences (Ma)/Yoga Flower
    remedies
  Colorado:
  Pegasus Essences (Peg)
  Hawaiian:
  Hawaiian Tropical Flower Essences (Haii)
  Texas:
  Petite Fleur Essences (PF)
  Virginia:
  Perelandra Virginian Rose and Garden
    Essences (PVi)

  Canada:
  Pacific Essences (Pac)

- **Gem Essences: Flower and Gem Remedy
  Association (Gem)**

✻ PHYSICAL ✻

ABUSE Cotton Grass, Tundra Twyblade (Ask); Luffa (Cal)

ACCIDENTS Rose Bay Willow Herb (Ask); Mountain Devil (Aus B); Rock Rose, Star of Bethlehem (B); Arnica (Dv); Dogwood, Love Lies Bleeding (Fes); Ulua (Haii); Pear (Ma); Grape Hyacinth, Weigela (Pac)

ACHES – GENERAL Dandelion (Fes); Mussel (Pac))

ACIDITY (EXCESSIVE) Chamomile (Cal); Curry Leaf (Him A); Narcissus (Pac)
See also **Digestive problems**

ACNE Spinifex (Aus B); Luffa (Cal); Salvia (PF)
See also **Skin problems**

ADDICTIONS (SYMPTOMS) Bush Iris (Aus B); Rose Damacea, Skullcap (Cal); Morning Glory (Cal, Fes, Him A, Him E); Hedgehog Cactus (DAl); Fairy Lantern, Five Flower Formulae, Mallow, Nicotiana (Fes); Pua Kenikeni (Haii); Peacock Flower (Him I); Nootka Rose, Forsythia (Pac)

ADDICTIONS (WITHDRAWAL) Morning Glory (AK); Rose Damacea, Skullcap (Cal); Harmonizing Addictive Patterning (DAl); Angelica, Nicotiana (Fes); Pua-kenikeni (Haii); Anti-Addiction Remedy (Him A); Forsythia (Pac); Purple Nightshade (Peg)
See also **Caffeine problems**

ADRENALS Chamomile (Cal, Fes); Rose Quartz (Gem); White Carnation (PF)

AGEING Almond Tree (AK); Mulla Mulla (Aus B); Almond (Dv); Mallow (Dv, Hb); California

Wild Rose, Hibiscus, St John's Wort, Star Tulip (Fes); Ukshi (Him A); Shrimp (PF)

ALLERGIES Apricot, Green Rose (Cal); Yarrow Special Formula (Fes); Moss Agate (Gem); Wood Apple Tree (Him I); Grass Widow (Pac); Lantana (PF)

ANAEMIA Kapok Bush (Aus B); Paw Paw (Cal); Rose Quartz (Gem); Dianthus (PF)

ANOREXIA NERVOSA Five Corners (Aus B); Banana, Paw Paw (Cal); Black-eyed Susan, Fairy Lantern, Manzanita, Pretty Face (Fes); Moss Agate, Turquoise (Gem); Sea Palm, Sea Urchin (Pac)

APPETITE DISORDERS Moonstone, Moss Agate, Turquoise (Gem); Urchin (Pac)

ARTHRITIS Mountain Devil (Aus B); Azurite, Gold (Gem); Ohai-ali'i (Haii); Snowdrop (Pac); Zinnia (PF)

ASSIMILATION (OF NUTRIENTS) Paw Paw (Aus B); Cedar, Jasmine (Cal); Self Heal (Dv, Hb); Star Jasmine (Hb); Azurite, Gold, Moonstone, Turquoise (Gem); Blackthorn (GM); Magnolia (PF)

ASTHMA Tall Mulla Mulla (Aus B); Green Rose, Hyssop, Lungwort (Cal); Eucalyptus (Cal, Fes); Sand Dollar (Pac); Babies Breath (PF)

BACK PROBLEMS Amazon River (AK); Centuary, Vine (B); Lilac (Dv, GM); Red Oak (GM); Ohai-ali'i (Haii); Brown Kelp (Pac); Indian Pipe (Peg); Chicago Peace, Maybelle Stearns (PVi))

✻

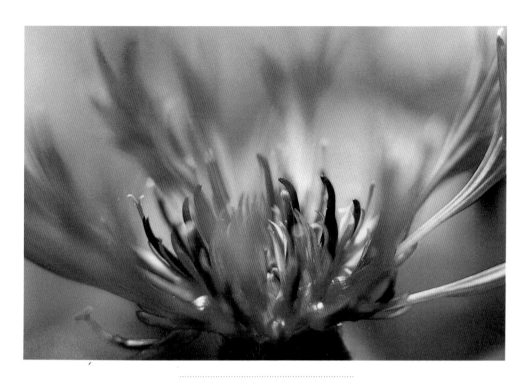

Corn Flower

CAROL BRUCE

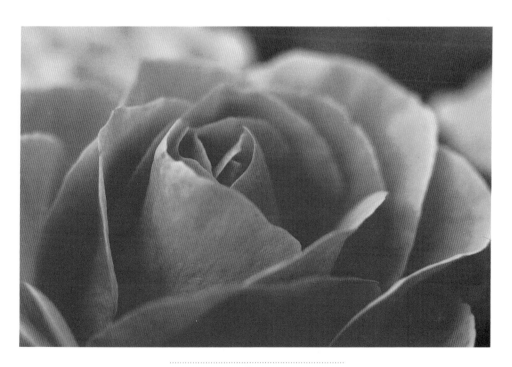

Rose

CAROL BRUCE

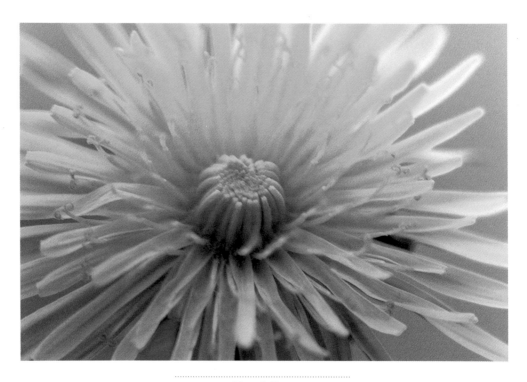

Dandelion
CAROL BRUCE

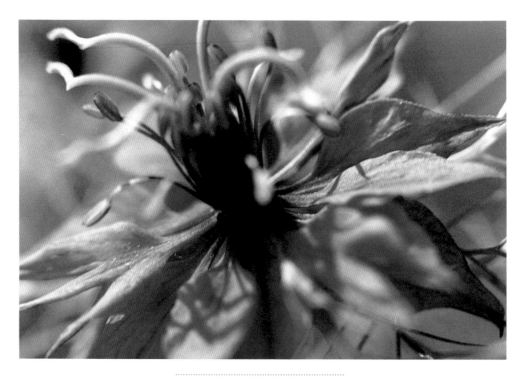

Love in a Mist
CAROL BRUCE

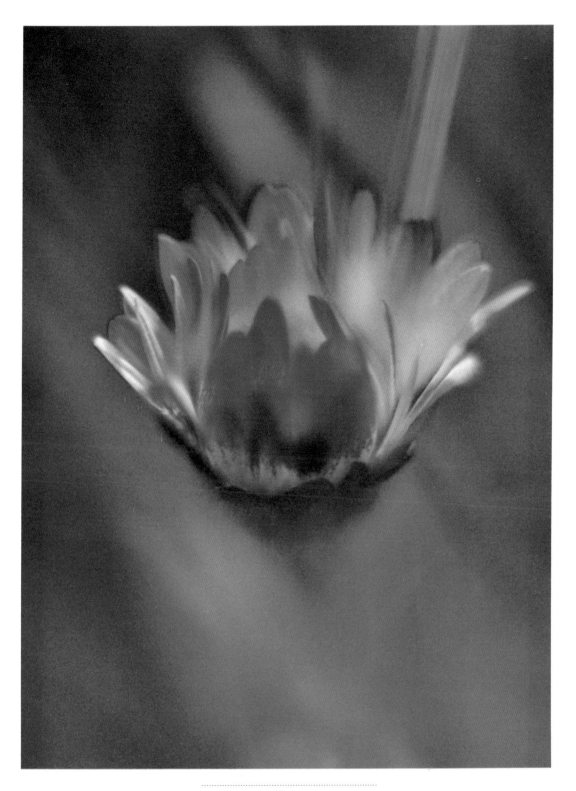

Daisy

CAROL BRUCE

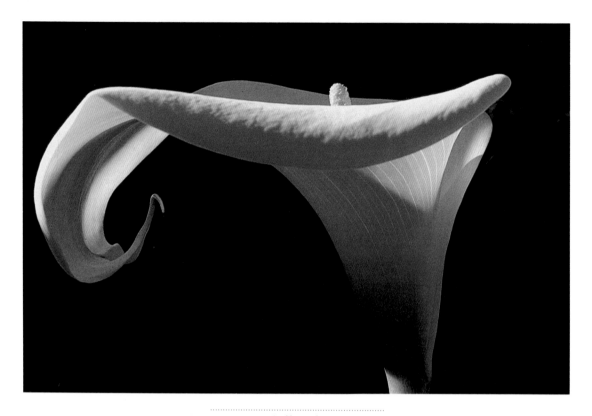

Calla Lily

HELMUT MAIER

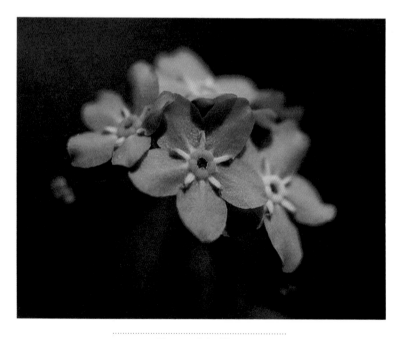

Forget Me Not

HELMUT MAIER

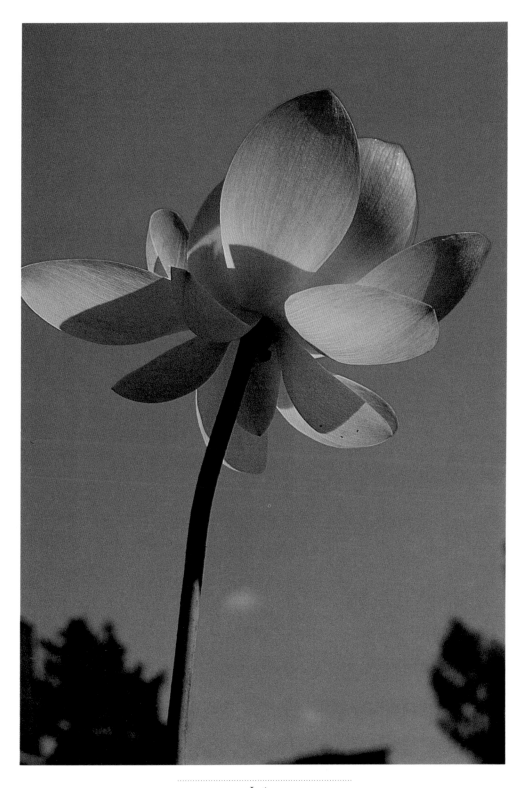

Lotus

HELMUT MAIER

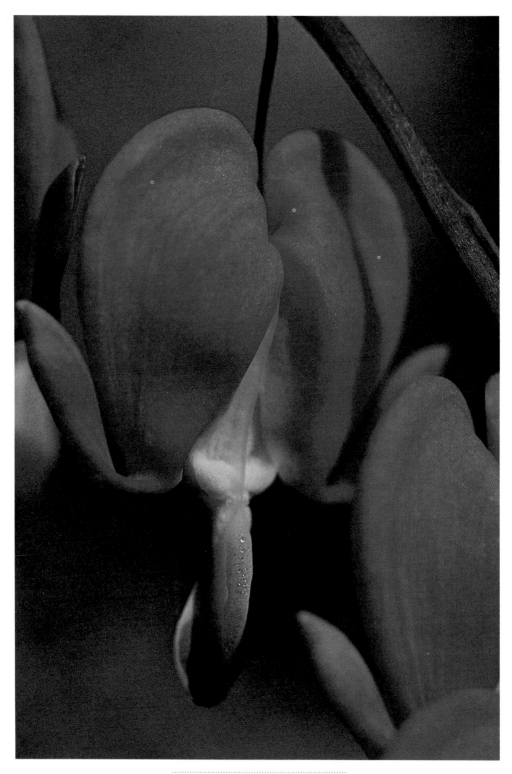

Bleeding Heart

HELMUT MAIER

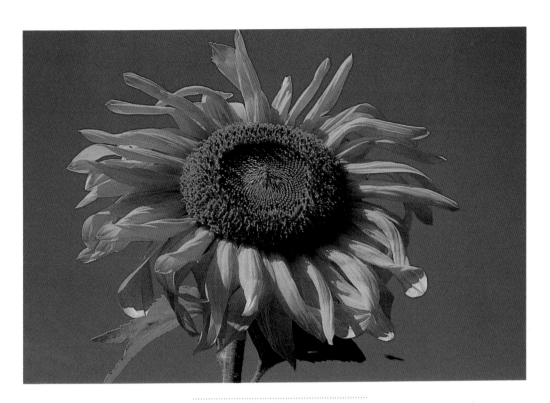

Sunflower
HELMUT MAIER

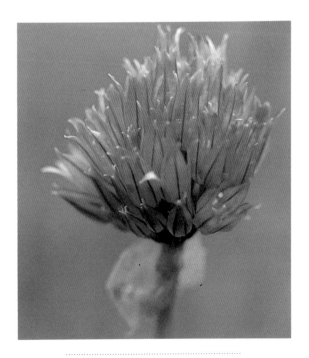

Wild Garlic
HELMUT MAIER

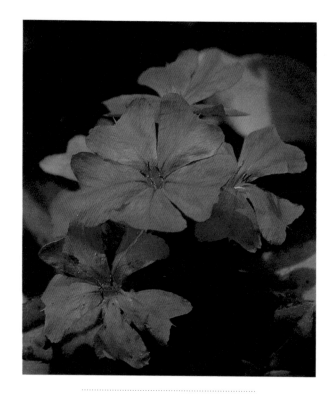

Cerato
HELMUT MAIER

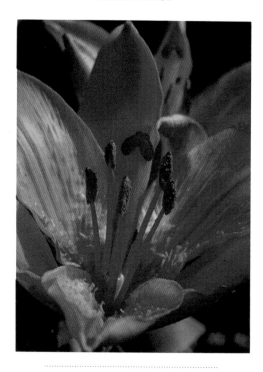

Fire Lily
HELMUT MAIER

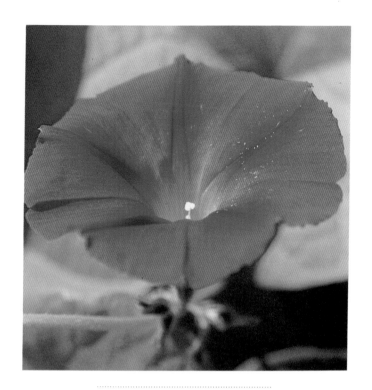

Morning Glory
REGINA HORNBERGER

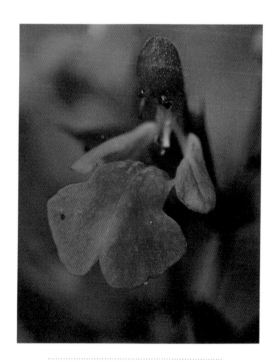

Self Heal
HELMUT MAIER

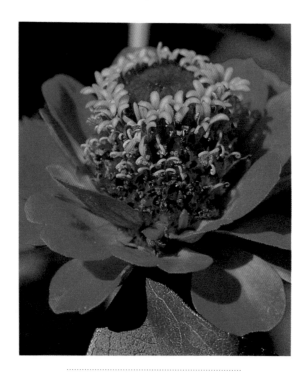

Zinnia

REGINA HORNBERGER

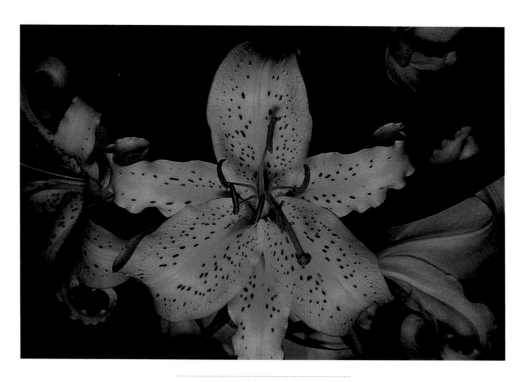

Golden Lily

ELIZABETH MACINTOSH

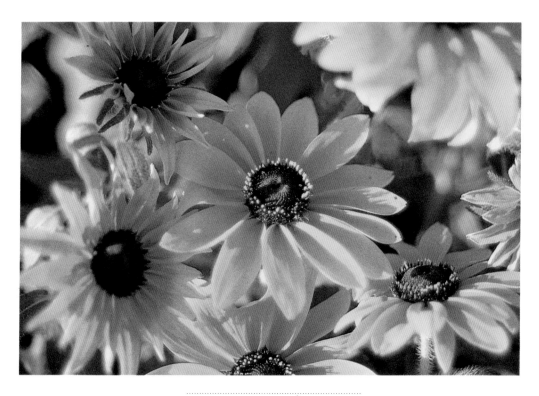

Black Eyed Susan
DEVA

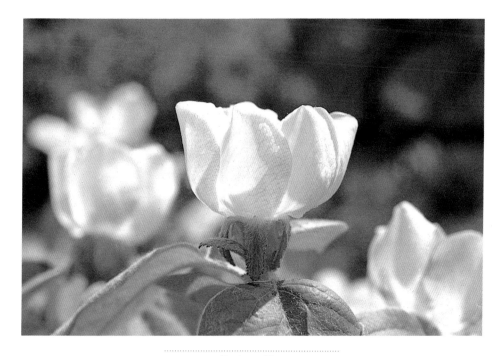

Quince Tree
DEVA

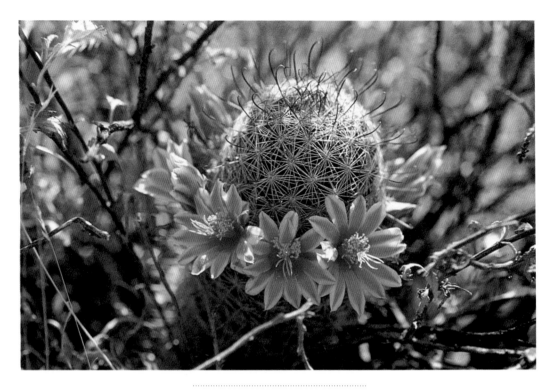

Fish Hook Cactus
DESERT ALCHEMY

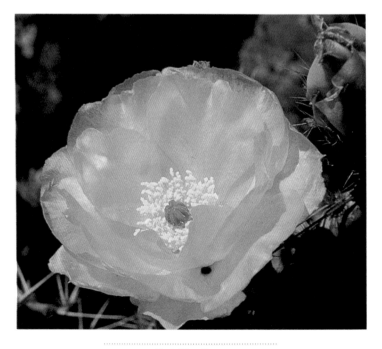

Prickly Pear
DESERT ALCHEMY

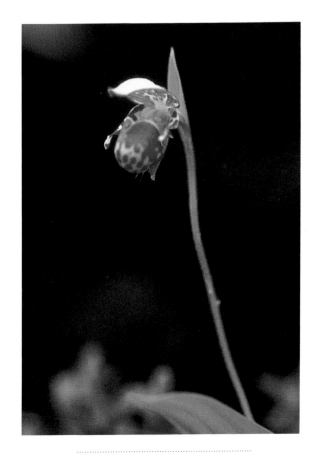

Lady's Slipper
ALASKAN

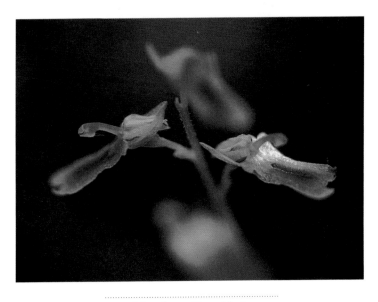

Northern Twayblade
ALASKAN

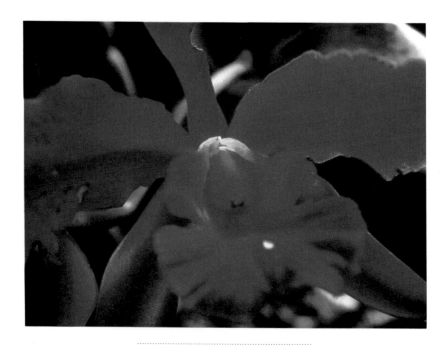

Heart Orchid
AMAZONIAN

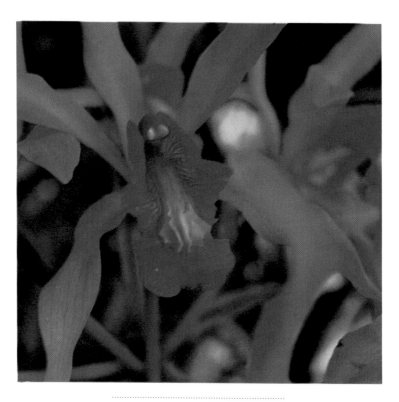

Higher Self Orchid
AMAZONIAN

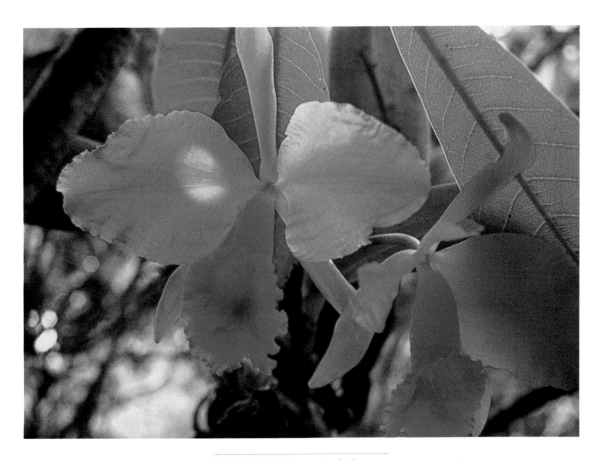

Inspiration Orchid
AMAZONIAN

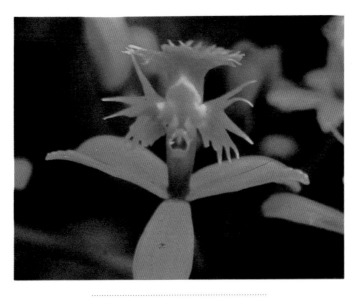

Angel Orchid
AMAZONIAN

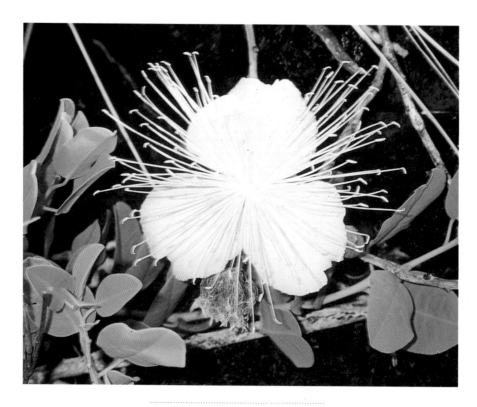

Poa Poa
HAWAIIAN ALOHA

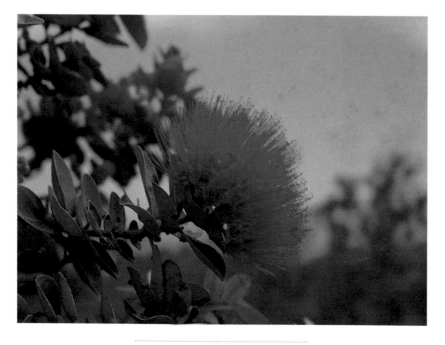

Lehua
HAWAIIAN ALOHA

BACTERIAL INFECTIONS Pansy (Cal); Wild Garlic (Dv); Brown Kelp (Pac)

BLOOD DISORDERS Avocado, Nettle (Cal); Amethyst (Gem); Blackthorn (GM); Hawaiian Tree (Haii); Periwinkle, Plantain (Pac); Basil (PF)

BLOOD-PRESSURE – HIGH Vine (B); Morning Glory (Cal.); Periwinkle (Pac)

BLOOD-PRESSURE – LOW Kapok Bush (AusB); Penta (PF)

BLOOD SUGAR (BALANCE) Apricot, Banana, Jasmine, Sugar Beet (Cal); Iris (Fes); Amethyst, Moss Agate (Gem); Moss Rose, Primrose (PF)

BOILS/ABSCESSES Avocado, Luffa, Nettle, Saguaro (Cal)

BONES (HEALING) Azurite (Gem); Red Oak (GM); Pink Seaweed, Salmonberry (Pac); Jasmine (PF)

BREATHING TROUBLES Eucalyptus, Lungwort (Cal); Rhododendron (Dv); Yerba Santa (Fes); Polyanthus, Sand Dollar (Pac)

BRONCHIAL CONDITIONS Eucalyptus, Hyssop, Lungwort (Cal); California Pitcher Plant (Fes); Drum Stick (Him A); Polyanthus, Sand Dollar (Pac); Babies Breath (PF)

BULIMIA Paw Paw (Cal); Black-eyed Susan, Manzanita (Fes); Moonstone, Turquoise (Gem); Sea Palm, Urchin (Pac)

BURNS Mulla Mulla (Aus B); Aloe Vera (Fes); Anemone (PF)

CAFFEINE PROBLEMS Coffee (Cal, Haii); Skullcap (Cal); Purple Nightshade (Peg)

CANCER Koenign Van Daenmark, Peach (Cal); Herkimer Diamond (Gem); Nani ahiahi (Haii); Lilac (PF)

CATARRH Eucalyptus, Jasmine (Cal); Yerba Santa (Fes); Polyanthus (Pac)

CELLULITE Pink Rose (PF)

CHILDBIRTH Balsan Poplar, Green Bells of Iceland, Grove Sandwort, Hairy Butterworth, Shooting Star, Sticky Geranium (Ask); Star of Bethlehem (B); Watermelon (Cal); Pomegranate (Fes); Moonstone (Gem); Noni (Haii); Pear (Ma); Barnacle, Hookers Onion, Jelly Fish (Pac); Cauliflower (PVi)

CHILDBIRTH – PREMATURE Poison Hemlock (Pac); Ranunculus (PF)

CIRCULATION PROBLEMS Queen Anne's Lace (Fes); Gold, Moss Agate, Rose Quartz (Gem); Blackthorn (GM); Yellow Ginger (Haii); Fireweed (Pac); Morning Glory (PF)

CLEANSING Sage (AK, Cal); Morning Glory (Cal); Ragged Robin (F); Lungwort, Primrose, Yarrow in Seawater (Hb); Wood Apple Tree (Him I); Moonsnail (Pac); Dutchman Breeches, Shamp Onion, Sourgrass (Peg)

COLIC Sage (Cal); Chamomile (Cal, Fes)

COLON SPASM Cedar, Green Rose (Cal); Moonstone (Gem); Barnacle (Pac); Bamboo (PF)

COMMON COLD Eucalyptus, Jasmine, Pansy (Cal); Yerba Santa (Fes)

CONSTIPATION Cedar (Cal); Moonstone (Gem); Caster Oil Plant (Him I); Barnacle, Pink Seaweed, Poison Hemlock (Pac); Poppy (PF)

CONVALESCENCE/RECUPERATION Golden Waitsa (Aus L); Hornbeam (B); Elder (F); Self Heal (Dv, Fes); Lotus, Peacock Flower (Him A)

CRAMPS (MUSCLE) Impatiens (B); Anemone (Pac)

CYSTITIS Pansy (Cal); Surfgrass (Pac)

CYSTS (ON OVARIES)/FIBROIDS Pomegranate (Fes); Barnacle (Pac)

DETOXIFICATION Arnica (AK); Avocado, Coffee, Morning Glory, Skullcap, Spruce (Cal); Herkimer Diamond (Gem); Apple, Laburnum (GM); Noni, Yellow Ginger (Haii); Primrose (Hb); Blue Lupin, Moonsnail (Pac); Coralroot-spotted, Pine Drops, Sourgrass (Peg)

DIARRHOEA Black-eyed Susan (Aus B); Cedar (Cal); Moss Agate (Gem); Barnacle (Pac)

DIGESTIVE PROBLEMS Crowea (Aus B); Cedar, Chamomile, Sage (Cal); California Pitcher Plant (Fes); Jujube Tree (Him I); Orange Honeysuckle (Pac); Red Spider Lily (Peg); Moss Rose (PF)

DIZZINESS/FAINTNESS Aspen, Clematis (B); Sober Up (Him E); Mussel (Pac)

DRUG TOXINS (DISCHARGING) Arnica (AK); Bottlebrush, Skullcap, Spruce (Cal); Morning Glory (Fes, Cal); Apple (GM); Peacock Flower (Him I)

DYSLEXIA Bush Fuchsia (Aus B); Amethyst, Silver (Gem); Blue Camas (Pac); White Petunia (PF)

EAR PROBLEMS Star Tulip (Fes); Brown Kelp, Ox-eye Daisy, Viburnum (Pac);

ECZEMA Billy Goat Plum, Spinifex (Aus B); Luffa (Cal); Wood Apple Tree (Him I); Vanilla Leaf (Pac)

ELIMINATION Avocado, Cedar, Chamomile (Cal); Moss Agate (Gem); Star Jasmine (Hb); Narcissus, Polyanthus (Pac)
    See also **Digestive problems**

ENDOCRINE SYSTEM Koenign Van Daenmark (Cal); Lotus (Fes); Amethyst (Gem)

ENERGY Macrocarpa, Old Man Banksia (Aus B); Leafless Orchid (Aus L); Firethorn (Ba); Cherry, Sugar Beet (Cal); California Pitcher Plant (Fes); Bay (GM); Ohi'a-ai (Haii); Flowering Currant, Nasturtium (Hb); Longevity, Vital Spark (Him E); Cherry, Corn (Ma); Bluebell, Goatsbeard (Pac); Cape Honeysuckle (Peg); Tonic – Nasturtium (PVi)

ENVIRONMENTAL CLEANSING Delph, Ti (AK); Grass of Parnassus, Sweetgrass, Yarrow (Ask); Kamani, T-Leaf Flower (Haii); Environmental Protector, Office Flower (Him A)

EPSTEIN BARR VIRUS (ME) K9 (AK); Koenign Van Daenmark, Pansy (Cal)

EXHAUSTION Aloe Vera (AK); Macrocarpa (Aus B); Elm, Vervain (B); Staghorn Cholla Cactus, Whitehorn, Woven Spine Pineapple (DAl)

EYE PROBLEMS Alder (Ask); Queen Anne's Lace, Star Tulip (Fes); Cotton (Haii); Nasturtium, Speedwell (Hb); Anemone, Ox-eye Daisy (Pac)
    See also **Sight (enhancing)**

FATIGUE California Wild Rose, Indian Paintbrush, Lavender, Yerba Santa (Fes);

English Elm (GM); Hornbeam, Lungwort (Hb); Snowberry (Pac); Pine, Stock (PF)

FERTILITY (PROBLEMS) She Oak (Aus B); Fig, Gooseberry, Watermelon (Cal); Pomegranate (Fes); Rose Quartz (Gem); Noni (Haii); Blackberry, Lady's Mantle, Rose-red (Hb); Barnacle (Pac)

FEVERS Onion (PF)
See also **Common cold**

FLUID RETENTION She Oak (Aus B); California Pitcher Plant (Fes); Moss Agate (Gem); Water Poppy (Haii); Indian Almond (Him I); Poison Hemlock (Pac); Bachelor Button, Japanese Magnolia (PF)

FRIGIDITY Canary Island Bellflower, Pumpkin (AK); Wisteria (Aus B); Lehur (Haii); Cannon Ball Tree (Him A); Ixora (Him A, Him I); Barnacle (Pac); Marigold (PF)

GALL STONES Mussel (Pac); Garden Mum (PF)

GLANDULAR FEVER K9 (AK); Koenign van Daenmark, Pansy (Cal)

HAIR LOSS/BALDNESS Cedar (Cal); Red Carnation (PF)

HAYFEVER K9 (AK); Eucalyptus, Green Rose (Cal); Wood Apple Tree (Him I)

HEADACHES Black-eyed Susan (Aus B); Aspen, Vervain, White Chestnut (B); Apricot, Clove, Feverfew, Green Rose (Cal); Ameythst (Gem); Meadowsweet (Hb); Clarity (Him E); Blue Lupin, Mussel, Plantain (Pac); Japanese Mongolia (PF)

HEALING (SELF) Coordination Orchid (AK); Self Heal (AK, Dv, Fes, Hb); Bog Rosemary (Ask); Spinifex (Aus B); Star of Bethlehem (B); Aloe (DAl); Star Tulip (Fes); Rose Quartz (Gem); Gean/Wild Cherry, Norway Maple (GM); Creeping Thistle, Milkmaid (Peg); African Violet (PF)

HEART PROBLEMS Foxglove (Ask, Hb); Gold, Rose Quartz (Gem); Borage, Rosemary (Hb); Jelly Fish (Pac); Rose of Sharon (PF)

HORMONE IMBALANCE – FEMALE She Oak (Aus B); Evening Primrose, Watermelon (Cal); Mala Mujer (DAl); Pomegranate (Fes); Barnacle (Pac); Marigold (PF)

HORMONE IMBALANCE – MALE Evening Primrose, Watermelon (Cal); Marigold (PF)

HYPERACTIVITY Chamomile (Dv); Nasturtium (Fes); Stock (PF)

IMMUNE SYSTEM (BOOSTING) K9 (AK); Wild Garlic (AK, Dv); Macrocarpa (Aus B); Khat, Koenign Van Daenmark (Cal); Gorse (F); Echinacea, Garlic, Lavender, Love Lies Bleeding, Morning Glory (Fes); Amethyst (Gem); Ivy, Yew (GM); Hawaiian Tree, Ohi'a-ai (Haii); Hawthorn, Pansy (Hb); Immunity Booster (Him A); Rata Berries White (NZ); Celery (PVi)

IMPOTENCY Banana, Swiss Cheese Plant (AK); Larch (B); Queen of the Night (DAl); Ixora (Him A, Him I); Marigold (PF)

INCONTINENCE Cedar (Cal); St John's Wort (Fes); Surfgrass (Pac)

INDIGESTION (DYSPEPSIA) Sage (Cal); Chamomile (Fes, PF); Moonstone (Gem); Sea Palm (Pac); Ligustrum (PF)

INFLAMMATIONS Apricot, Eucalyptus, Saguaro (Cal); Surfgrass (Pac)

INFLUENZA Eucalyptus, Jasmine, Pansy (Cal); Lily (PF)

INJURIES Cotton Grass (Ask); Love Lies Bleeding (Fes)

INSOMNIA Valerian (AK, Cal, Dv, NZ); Boronia (Aus B); Hops Bush (Aus L); White Chestnut (B); Licorice, Ylang Ylang (Cal); Chamomile (Cal, Dv, Fes); Black-eyed Susan, Dill, Lavender, Mugwort, St John's Wort (Fes); Yellow Ginger (Haii)

ITCHING Luffa (Cal); Vanilla Leaf (Pac)

JET LAG Dill (AK); Banksia Robur (Aus B); Ylang Ylang (Cal)

KIDNEY PROBLEMS Chamomile (Cal); Rose Quartz (Gem); Surfgrass (Pac); Red Spider Lily (Peg); Begonia (PF)

LARYNGITIS Lungwort (Cal); Lapis Lazuli (Gem); Snapdragon (Hb); Sand Dollar (Pac)

LIVER DISORDERS Moss Agate, Rose Quartz (Gem); Speedwell (Hb); Forsythia, Plantain (Pac); Ligustrum (PF)

LONG-TERM ILLNESS Peacock Flower (Him A); Coralroot-spotted (Peg)

LUNG IMBALANCE Hyssop, Jasmine, Lungwort (Cal); Eucalyptus (Cal, Fes); Yerba Santa (Fes); Lapis Lazuli (Gem); Flowering Currant (Hb); Arbutus (Pac)

LYMPHATIC SYSTEM Apricot, Avocado, Saguaro (Cal); Lapis Lazuli, Moss Agate, Moonstone (Gem); Caster Oil Plant (Him I); Red Carnation (PF)

MENOPAUSE She Oak (Aus B); Evening Primrose, Gooseberry (Cal); Alpine Lily, Borage, Easter Lily, Fuchsia, Hibiscus, Mariposa Lily, Pomegranate, Rosemary, Tiger Lily (Fes); Orange Honeysuckle (Pac)

MENSTRUATION – ABSENCE OF She Oak (Aus B); Evening Primrose (Cal); Fairy Lantern, Mugwort, Pomegranate (Fes); Moonstone (Gem)

MENSTRUATION – IRREGULAR Evening Primrose (Cal); Fairy Lantern, Mugwort, Pomegranate (Fes)

MENSTRUATION – PAINS Feverfew (Cal); Black Cohosh, Love Lies Bleeding, Pomegranate (Fes)

MERIDIAN BALANCE Northern Lady's Slipper (Ask); Silver Maple (GM)

METABOLISM (RE-BALANCING) Nasturtium, Peppermint, Rosemary, Snapdragon (Fes); Caster Oil Plant (Him I)

MIASMS Lotus essence (AK, Dv, Fes, Haii)

– HEAVY METALS Hyssop (Cal); Bloodroot, Daffodil (Peg)

– PETROCHEMICAL Apricot, Coffee (Cal); Garlic (Fes); Almond (Peg)

– PSORA Dandelion, Fig, Grapefruit, Lemon (Cal); Eucalyptus, Garlic (Fes); Camphor (Peg)

– RADIATION Lemon (Cal); Garlic (Fes); Bloodroot (Peg)

– SYPHILITIC Banana, Bottlebrush, Chamomile (German), Comfrey, Jasmine (Cal); California Poppy, Chaparral, Iris-Blue Flag (Fes); Bells of Ireland, Celandine, Four-leaf Clover (Peg)

– SYCOSIS Dandelion, Lilac (Fes)

– TUBERCULOSIS Eucalyptus, Green Rose (Cal); Blackberry (Fes); Cotton, Hops, Live Forever, Red Clover (Peg)

MIGRAINE Feverfew, Green Rose (Cal); Amethyst (Gem); Plantain (Pac); Narcissus (PF)

MORNING LETHARGY Banksia Robur (Aus B); Hornbeam (B); Morning Glory (Cal, Him E, Fes); Rosemary, Tansy (Fes); Night Queen (Him I)

MOSQUITO BITES Mountain Devil (Aus B); Garlic (Fes)

MUCOUS COLITIS Cedar, Green Rose (Cal); California Pitcher Plant (Fes); Moss Agate (Gem); Poppy (PF)

MULTIPLE SCLEROSIS Comfrey (Cal); Dandelion (Dv); Gold (Gem); Snowdrop (Pac)

MUSCULAR DISORDERS Dandelion (AK, Ask, Dv, Fes, Hb); Vervain (B); Comfrey (Cal); Gold (Gem); Anemone, Salmonberry (Pac); Pink Geranium (PF)

NASAL CONGESTION Eucalyptus, Jasmine (Cal); California Pitcher Plant, Yerba Santa (Fes); Peepal Tree (Him I)

NAUSEA Sage (Cal); Jujube Tree (Him I); Windflower (Pac)

NECK AND BACK STIFFNESS Dandelion (Dv, Fes, NZ); Iris (Fes); Pau Pilo (Haii); Meadowsweet (Hb); Mussel (Pac)

NERVOUSNESS Almond, Banana (Ma); Aspen (B); Coffee, Comfrey (Cal); Chamomile (Cal, Dv, Fes); Whitehorn (DAl); Wild Garlic (Dv); Hau (Haii)

NERVOUS SYSTEM (TONIC) Angelica (Cal); Comfrey (Cal, DV); Morning Glory (Cal, Dv, Fes, Him E); Fairy Duster (DAl); Arnica (Fes); Gold (Gem); Pear (GM); Hau (Haii); Commelina, Peacock Flower (Him I); Viburnum (Pac); Blaze Improve, Oregold (PVi)

NERVOUS EXHAUSTION Buffalo Gourd, Fairy Duster (DAl); Lady's Slipper (Fes); Alder (GM)

OBESITY Evening Primrose, Golden Rod, Hound's Tongue, Nicotiana, Pink Monkeyflower, Tansy (Fes); Poison Hemlock (Pac); Pink Rose (PF)

PAIN (RELIEF) Cotton Grass (Ask); Dog of the Wild Forces (Aus B); Illyarrie, Menzies Banksia (Aus L); Valerian (Cal); Love Lies Bleeding (Fes); Gean/Wild Cherry (GM); Foxglove (Hb); Day-blooming Jessamine (Him A); Commelina (Him I); Anemone (Pac); Bourgainvillea (PF)

PARALYSIS Scottish Primrose (F); Azurite (Gem); Poison Hemlock, Snowdrop (Pac)

PARASITES Garlic (Fes); Amaryllis (PF)

PELVIC INFLAMMATORY DISEASE (PID) Billy Goat Plum, Spinifex (Aus B); Pomegranate (Fes); Snowdrop (Hb)

PHYSICAL STRENGTH/GROWTH Milky Nipple Cactus (DAl); Zucchini (PVi)

PRE-MENSTRUAL SYNDROME Peach-flow-ered Tea Tree, She Oak (Aus B); Evening Primrose, Feverfew (Cal); Immortal, Mala Mujer, Tar Bush (DAl); Pomegranate (Fes); Indian Almond (Him I)

PREGNANCY PROBLEMS (E.G. MORNING SICKNESS) Pumpkin (AK); Papaya (Cal); Watermelon (Cal, Dv); Chamomile (Cal); Forget-me-not, Zucchini (Dv); California Wild Rose, Calla Lily, Evening Primrose, Mugwort, Pomegranate (Fes); Noni (Haii); Rosebud-white (Hb)

PROTECTION FROM – POLLUTION Spider-wort (Cal); White Yarrow (Dv)

PROTECTION FROM – RADIATION Spider-wort (Cal); White Yarrow (Dv); Yarrow in sea-water (Hb)

PSORIASIS Billy Goat Plum, Spinifex (Aus B); Angelica, Luffa (Cal); Aloe Vera (Fes); Vanilla Leaf (Pac)

PSYCHOSOMATIC ILLNESS Strawberry Cactus (DAl); Canyon Dudleya, Fuchsia, Purple Monkeyflower, Yerba Santa (Fes); Wood Apple Tree (Him I)

PUBERTY Bottlebrush (Aus B); Walnut (B); Fairy Lantern, Sagebrush, Saguaro, Sticky Monkeyflower (Fes); Mallow, Rosebud-red (Hb); Orange Honeysuckle (Pac)

RADIATION PROBLEMS Mulla Mulla (Aus B); Spiderwort (Cal)

REPRODUCTIVE PROBLEMS – FEMALE She Oak (Aus B); Watermelon (Cal); Alpine Lily, Pomegranate (Fes); Candysticks (Pac); Red Spider Lily (Peg)

REPRODUCTIVE PROBLEMS – MALE Water-melon (Cal); Pomegranate (Fes); Red Spider Lily (Peg)

RESPIRATORY SYSTEM Eucalyptus, Lungwort (Cal); Grape Hyacinth (Pac); Babies Breath (PF)

SCAR TISSUE Aloe Vera (Fes); Anemone (PF)

SEXUAL DISEASES (CHLAMYDIA, HERPES) K9 (AK); Billy Goat Plum (Aus B); Pansy (Cal); Pomegranate (Fes)

SHOCK Arnica (AK, Fes); Cotton Grass, Fireweed (Ask); Emergency Essence, Fringed Violet (Aus B); Rescue Remedy (B); Self Heal (Fes); Privet (GM); Ulua (Haii); First Aid Remedy (Him A); Grape Hyacinth (Pac); White Hyacinth (PF)

SIGHT (ENHANCING) Queen Anns Lace (Fes); Silver (Gem); Cotton (Haii); Anemone, Ox-eye Daisy (Pac)

SINUSITIS Jasmine (Cal); Eucalyptus (Cal, Fes)

SKIN PROBLEMS Billy Goat Plum (Aus B); Angelica, Luffa (Cal); Office Flower (Him A); Gilia Scarlet, Red Spider Lily (Peg); Lily (PF)

SKIN LESIONS Angelica, Luffa (Cal); Anemone (PF)

SMOKING (EFFECTS OF) Morning Glory (AK, Cal, Fes, Him E); Bo Tree, Hyssop, Tobacco (Cal); Nicotiana (Fes); Drum Stick (Him A)

SPEECH PROBLEMS Mimulus (B); Petunia, Snapdragon (Hb); Parrot (Him A); Bluebells, White Petunia (PF)

SPLEEN Lapis Lazuli, Moonstone, Moss Agate (Gem); Goatsbeard (Pac)

SPINAL PROBLEMS Lilac (Dv); Azurite (Gem); Ohai-ali'i (Haii); Sunflower (Hb); Salmonberry (Pac); Indian Pipe (Peg); Mushroom, Orchid (PF)

STRESS Valerian (AK, Cal); Black-eyed Susan (Aus B); Peanut, Ylang Ylang (Cal); Corn (Fes); Sweet Pea (Fes); Silver (Gem); Laburnum (GM); Ma'o (Haii); Urban Stress Remedy (Him A); Spinach (Ma); Goatsbeard (Pac)

SUNBURN Mulla Mulla (Aus B)

SWELLING Apricot (Cal); Caster Oil Plant (Him I); Red Carnation (PF)

TEETH-GRINDING Black-eyed Susan (Aus B); Morning Glory (Cal, Fes)

TEETHING (BABIES) Pink Seaweed (Pac)

TENSION Dandelion (AK, Cal, Dv, Fes, Hb); Purple Flag Flower, Rose Cone Flower (Aus L); Beech, Impatiens, Vervain, Water Violet (B); Comfrey (Cal); Comfrey, Forget-me-not, Passion Flower, Spruce (Dv); Chamomile (Cal, Dv, Fes, Hb); Lavender (Fes); Cherry Plum, Lilac (GM)

THROAT (SORE) Lungwort, Pansy (Cal); Lapis Lazuli (Gem); Pennyroyal (NZ); Blue Camas, Sand dollar (Pac)

TIREDNESS Leafless Orchid (Aus L); Aspen, Hornbeam, Pine (B); Tansy (Fes)

TONSILITIS Jasmine, Lungwort (Cal); Lapis Lazuli (Gem); Sand dollar (Pac)

TOXICITY/TOXAEMIA Bottlebrush, Skullcap, Spruce (Cal); Coffee (Cal, Haii); Ragged Robbin (F); Chaparral (Fes); Blue Lupin (Pac); Coralroot spotted (Peg); Crossandra, Pansy (PF)

TRAVEL SICKNESS Dill (AK); Ylang Ylang (Cal); Jujube Tree (Him I)

ULCERS Cedar, Green Rose (Cal); Moonstone (Gem); Peppermint (PF)

VIRAL INFECTIONS K9 (AK); Koenign Van Daenmark, Sugar beet (Cal); Pansy (Cal, Hb); Wild Garlic (Dv, Fes); Echinacea, Onion (PF)

VITALITY Alpine Mint Bush, Crowea, Macrocarpa, Wild Bush Potato (Aus B); Leafless Orchid, Pink Fountain Triggerplant (Aus L); Almond, Morning Glory (Dv); Nasturtium (Dv, Hb, Fes); Gorse, Sycamore (F); Tansy (Fes); Blackberry (Hb); Apple (Ma)

WARTS Pansy (Cal); Salvia (PF)

WEIGHT CONTROL Hound's Tongue, Yerba Santa (Fes); Moonstone (Gem); Mango, Naio, Pua-Pilo (Haii); Chickweed, Poison Hemlock (Pac); Dayflower (Peg)

❋ PSYCHOLOGICAL ❋
(MENTAL AND EMOTIONAL)

ABANDONMENT Arbutus, Nootka Rose, Sea Palm (Pac); Mesquite, Milky Nipple Cactus (DAl)

ABUSE (EMOTIONAL) White Fireweed (Ask); Black Cohosh, Black-eyed Susan, Bleeding Heart, Echinacea, Morning Glory, Purple Monkeyflower (Fes); Elder (Hb); Hibiscus, Rippy Hillox (Him I); Orange (Ma); Urchin (Pac)

ABUSE (SELF) Bisbee Beehive Cactus, Kleins Pencil Cholla Cacuts (DAl), Dogwood (Fes)

ACCIDENT, PRONE TO Jacaranda, Kangaroo Paw, Red Lily (Aus B); Impatiens (B); Ulua (Haii); Pill Bearing Spurge (Him A, Him I)

ADAPTABILITY Angel of Protection Orchid (AK); Bauhinia, Waratah (Aus B); Prickly Pear Cactus (DAl); Aloe Vera, Golden Yarrow (Fes); Healer (Him E)

ADDICTIVE BEHAVIOUR Blue China Orchid (Aus L); Rose Damacea, Skullcap (Cal); Hedgehog Cactus, Tarbrush (DAl); Morning Glory (Cal, Dv, Fes); Nicotiana, Scarlet Monkeyflower (Fes); Tulip Tree (GM); Nau, Pua kenikeni (Haii); Drum Stick (Him A); Forsythia, Urchin (Pac); Monkeyflower Bush (Peg)

ADDICTION withdrawal symptoms – Morning Glory (AK, Cal); Rose Damacea, Skullcap, Spruce (Cal); Angelica, Sagebrush (Fes); Nirjara (Him E); Tomato (Ma); Nootka, Urchin (Pac); Purple Nightshade (Peg)

AGGRESSION Aggression Orchid (AK); Mountain Devil (Aus B); Buffalo Gourd, Mountain Mahogany (DAl); Martagon Lily, Scarlet Monkeyflower (Dv); Oregon Grape, Snapdragon, Tiger Lily (Fes); Elder, Italian Alder (GM); Red Silk Cotton Tree (Him I)

ALCOHOLISM Morning Glory (AK); Angelica, Avocado, Pennyroyal (Cal); Chrysanthemum, Mountain Pennyroyal (Fes); Kou (Haii); Sober Up (Him E); Nootka Rose, Urchin (Pac)

ANGER Blue Elf Viola (Ask); Mountain Devil (Aus B); Fuchsia Grevillea, Orange Spiked Peaflower (Aus L); Holly (B); Compass Barrel Cactus, Foothills Paloverde, Star Primrose (DAl); Fuchsia, Scarlet Monkeyflower (Dv, Fes); Willowherb (F); Snapdragon (Fes); Kukui, Ulua (Haii); Nettle (Hb); Wellbeing (Him E); Mussel (Pac); Orange Flame Flower Cactus (Peg)

ANOREXIA NERVOSA Paw Paw (Cal); Black-eyed Susan, Manzanita (Fes); Moss Agate, Turquoise (Gem)

ANXIETY Purple Flag Flower, Woolly Smoke-bush (Aus L); Red Chestnut (B); Banana (Cal); Hoptree, Strawberry Cactus (DAl); Wild Garlic (Dv); Scottish Primrose (F); Filagree (Fes); Alder (GM); Kukui, Plemomele Fragrans (Haii); Chamomile (Hb); Jujube Tree (Him I); Periwinkle (Pac)

APATHY Kapok Bush (Aus B); Gorse (F); Blackberry, California Wild Rose, Tansy (Fes); Tulip (Him A)

APPREHENSION Water Violet (Aus L); Aspen (B)

❋

ARGUMENTATIVENESS Dagger Hakea, Isopogon (Aus B); Banana (Ma)

ARROGANCE Larkspur (Fes); Cup of Gold
(Haii); Sunflower (NZ)

ATTACHMENT Cotton Grass, River Beauty,
Sweetgale (Ask)

AUTISM Bluebell, Sundew (Aus B); Amethyst,
Silver (Gem)

BALANCE (EMOTIONAL) Labrador Tree (Ask);
Dog Rose of the Wild Forces, Hops Bush (Aus
L); Scleranthus (B); Chamomile (Fes); Buffalo
Gourd, Fairy Duster, Fire Prickly Pear Cactus
(DAl); Water Poppy (Haii); Forget-me-not,
Lavender, Red Tulip (Hb)

BEREAVEMENT Forget-me-not (Fes); Radish
(Him A); Purple Crocus, Starfish (Pac)

BITTERNESS Dagger Hakea, Southern Cross
(Aus B); Holly (B); Willow (B, Fes); Drum Stick,
Pill Bearing Spurge, Slow Match, Ukshi (Him
A); Mugwort (Hb); Slow Match Tree (Him I);
Raspberry (Ma); Jelly Fish (Pac)

BLAME Green Rose (Aus L); Star Primrose,
Syrian Rue (DAl)

BONDING (DEVELOPING) Bottlebrush (Aus
B); Watermelon (Cal); Linden (Dv); Mariposa
Lily (Fes); Noni (Haii); Plumeria (Peg)

BRAIN (LEFT AND RIGHT IMBALANCE) Bush
Fuchsia (Aus B); Amethyst, Gold, Silver (Gem)

BROKEN HEARTED Bleeding Heart (AK, Fes);
Boronia (Aus B); Love Lies Bleeding (Fes);
Field Maple (GM); Heartsease (Hb); Indian
Mulberry (Him I)

BURN-OUT Macrocarpa (Aus B); Fairy Duster,
Whitehorn, Woven Spine Pineapple Cactus
(DAl); Gorse (F); Aloe Vera, Lavender (Fes);
Papaya (NZ); Purple Nightshade (Peg)

CALMING – EMOTIONS French Lavender,
Valerian, Wild Garlic (AK); Dog Rose of the
Wild Forces, Mint Bush (Aus B); Many-headed
dryandra, Yellow Flag Flower (Aus L); Licorice
(Cal); Fairy Duster, Indian Tobacco (DAl);
Nettles (Dv); Chamomile (Dv, Hb, Fes); Lettuce
(Dv, Ma); Daisy (F); Indian Pink (Fes);
Gean/Wild Cherry (GM); Bluebell, Lavender,
Marjoram, Red Clover (Hb); Lotus (Him A);
Comelina (Him I); Purple Nightshade (Peg)

CALMING – THE MIND White Chestnut (B);
Foxglove (Ba); Candy Barrel Cactus (DAl);
Petunia, Ragwort, Salpglossis (Hb); The
Pongam, Yellow Canna (Him I)

CARING Immortal, Mesquite (DAl); Poison
Oak, Sunflower (Fes); Lucombe Oak (GM)

CHILDBIRTH (ATTITUDE TOWARDS) Dolphin
(AK); Grove Sandwort (Ask); Watermelon (Cal,
Fes); Evening Primrose (Fes); Noni (Haii)
See also **Pregnancy**

CITY STRESS Corn (AK, Cal); Antiseptic Bush,
Pink Fairy Orchid (Aus L); Clove, Rose Beauty
Secret (Cal); Pink Yarrow, Sweet Corn (Dv);
Indian Pink, Nicotiana, Yarrow, Yarrow Special
Formula (Fes); Sweet Pea (Fes); Buddleja (Hb);
Office Flower, Torroyia Rorshi Plant, Urban
Stress Remedy (Him A)

CLARITY (OF MIND) Bladderworth, Bunch-
berry, Twinflower (Ask); Alder (Ask, GM);
Bush Fuchsia, Isopogon (Aus B); Pink Trumpet
Flower, White Eremophila (Aus L); White
Chestnut (B); Lemon (Cal); Candy Barrel
Cactus, Star Primrose (DAl); Dill, Fig Tree,

Peppermint (Dv); Daisy (Dv, Hb, NZ); Deerbrush, Madia, Mountain Pennyroyal (Fes); Box, Pittespora (GM); Kou, Nana-honua (Haii); Teekwood Tree (Him I); Apple (Ma)

CLAUSTROPHOBIA Fuchsia Gum, W. A. Christmas Tree (Aus L); Glastonbury Thorn (GM); Authenticity (Him E); Five Fingers (NZ)

COMMUNICATION Fishhook Cactus (DAl); Cosmos, Linden, Zinnia (Dv); Calendula (Dv, Fes); Broom (F); Scarlet Monkeyflower (Fes); Jade Vine, Ulei (Haii); Authenticity (Him E); Indian Mulberry, Parrot Tree (Him I); Gentian (Peg)

COMMITMENT Compass Barrel Cactus, Prickly Pear Cactus (DAl); Basil, Evening Primrose (Fes); Ragwort (NZ)

COMPLAINING Wild Violet, One Sided Bottle Brush (Aus L)

COMPULSIVENESS Boronia (Aus B); Filagree (Fes)

CONCENTRATION Scleranthus (B); Hairy Sedge (Ba); Broom (F); Madia, Peppermint (Fes); Teak Wood Flower (Him A); Neem, Teak Wood Tree, Yellow Canna (Him I)

CONFIDENCE (INCREASING) Tamarack (Ask); Dog Rose, Illawarra Flame Tree (Aus B); Snake Vine (Aus L); Larch (B); Cerato (B, Fes); Buffalo Gourd, Cardon, Ephedra, Hedgehog Cactus (DAl); Borage (Dv, Hb); Bell Heather (F); Mullein, Trumpet Vine (Fes); Catalpa, Cherry Plum (GM); Cymbidium (Hb); Pineapple (Ma)

CONFUSION White Chestnut (B); Foxglove, Honesty (Ba); Blackberry (Dv); Broom, Daisy (F); Dill (Fes); Box (GM); Teak Wood Flower (Him A)

CONTEMPT Cowslip Orchid (Aus L); Holly (B)

CONTENTMENT Christmas Tree (Aus L); Bluebell, Rose – wild (Hb)

CONTROL (LOSS OF) Cherry Plum, Rock Rose (B); Desert Marigold, Hop Tree, Sacred Datura, Star Primrose, Strawberry Cactus (DAl); Daisy (F); Self-heal (Hb); Sea Palm (Pac)

COPING (WITH PROBLEMS) Waratah (Aus B); Rose Cone Flower, Yellow Flag Flower (Aus L); Cow Parsnip, Immortal, Jojoba, Spineless Prickly Pear (DAl); Fig Tree (Dv); Milkweed (Fes); White Poplar (GM); Dandelion (Hb); Radish (Him A)

COURAGE Borage (AK, Dv, Hb); Monk's Hood, Prickly Wild Rose (Ask); Dog Rose, Green Spider Orchid, Grey Spider Flower, Waratah (Aus B); Menzies Banksia (Aus L); Mimulus (B); Sacred Datura, Saguaro (DAl); Thistle (F); Black Cohosh, Mountain Pride, Penstemon (Fes); Italian Alder, White Poplar GM); Wiliwili (Haii); Swallow Wort (Him A); Rangoon Creeper (Him I); Tomato (Ma); Surfgrass (Pac); Summer Squash (PVi)

CREATIVITY Blue Flag Iris, Inspiration Orchid (AK); Golden Corydalis, Sticky Geranium, Wild Iris (Ask); Turkey Bush (Aus B); Pink Impatiens (Aus L); Indian Root (DAl); Iris (Dv); Broom, Holy Thorn (F); Indian Paintbrush, Iris (Fes); Holm Oak, Lucombe Oak (GM)

CRISIS Waratah (Aus B); Cowkicks (Aus L); Aloe, Ephedra (DAl); Angelica (Dv); Speedwell (Hb); Pear (Ma)

CRITICISM Sphagnum Moss (Ask); Purple and Red Kangaroo Paw, Yellow Cowslip Orchid (Aus B); Brachycome, Yellow and Green Kangaroo Paw (Aus L); Beech, Chicory,

Impatiens (B); Aloe, Foothills Paloverde, Mala Mujer (DAl); Calendula, Snapdragon (Fes); Ulua (Haii); White Coral Tree (Him A); Date (Ma); Garden Mum (PF)

CYNICISM Ursinia, Wallflower Donkey Orchid (Aus L); Spotted Orchid (F); Baby Blue Eyes (Fes); Ukshi (Him I); Blackberry (Ma); Jelly Fish (Pac)

DAYDREAMING Red Lily, Sundew (Aus B); Welsh Poppy (Ba); Clematis (B, Fes); Sacred Datura (DAl); Rosemary (Dv); St John's Wort (Fes); Gul Mohar (Him I)

DELINQUENCY Red Helmet (Aus B); Saguaro (Fes); Macadamia, Stenogyne Calaminthoides (Haii)

DENIAL Cardon (DAl); Klein's Cholla Cactus (DAl); Sierra Rein Orchid (Peg); Dill (PF)

DEPRESSION Borage (AK, Dv); Red Beak Orchid (Aus L); Larch, Mustard, Pine (B); Mustard (B, Fes); Skullcap, Sugar Beet (Cal); Bisbee Beehive Cactus, Immortal, Rainbow Cactus (DAl); Zinnia (Dv); Black Cohosh, Olive, Scotch Broom, Yerba Santa (Fes); Moss Agate (Gem); Copper Beech, Sycamore (GM); Plemomele Fragrans (Haii); Blackberry, Daffodil, Primrose (Hb); Ashoka Tree (Him I); Orange (Ma); Grape Hyacinth, Periwinkle (Pac); Red Rose (PF); Cucumber (PVi)

DEPENDENCY Dog Rose, Red Grevillia (Aus B); Rose Damacea (Cal); Canyon Grape Vine (DAl); Black Cohosh, Bleeding Heart, Fairy Lantern, Milkweed (Fes)

DESPAIR Mint Bush, Waratah (Aus B); Cherry Plum, Gorse, Sweet Chestnut (B); Pine (B, Fes); Blackthorn (Ba); Indian Tobacco (DAl); Scotch Broom (Dv); Elm (Fes); Broom (Hb); Indian

Gooseberry, Soap Nut Tree (Him I); Orange (Ma)

DESPONDENCY Kapok Bush, Silver Princess (Aus B); Mauve Melaleuca (Aus L); Larch (B); Hornbeam (B, Fes); Flowering Currant (Ba); Scotch Broom (Fes); Cherry (Ma)

DETERMINATION (LACK OF) Peach Flowered Tea Tree (Aus B); Pink Impatiens (Aus L); Cardon, Ephedra (DAl); Penstemon (Fes)

DISHONESTY Fuchsia Grevillea, Red Feather Flower (Aus L); Devil's Claw, Syrian Rue (DAl); Basil, Deerbrush (Fes); Manna Ash (GM); Wiliwili (Haii); Honesty (Hb)

DISILLUSIONMENT Snake Bush, Wallflower Donkey Orchid (Aus L); Sacred Datura (DAl); Gentian, Star Tulip (Fes)

DISORIENTATION River Beauty (Ask); Bush Fuchsia (Aus B); Pencil Cholla Cactus, Queen of the Night, Staghorn Cholla Cactus (DAl); Stenogyne Calaminthoides (Haii); Corn, Indian Pink, Madia (Fes)

DOGMATIC Hibbertia (Aus B); White Coral Tree (Him A); Parvel, White Coral Tree (Him I)

DOMINATING Gymea Lily (Aus B); Vine (B); Soaptree Yucca (DAl); Willowherb (F); Tiger Lily (Fes); Hinahina-ku-kahakai (Haii); Nilgiri Longy Plant (Him I); Anemone, Sea Palm (Pac)

DREAMS – DISTURBED Grey Spider Flower (Aus B); Black-eyed Susan, Chaparral (Fes); Pa-nini-o-ka (Haii)

EGO (BALANCE) Sun Orchid (AK); Lace Flower, Round-leaved Sundew, Silka Spruce Pollen (Ask); Foothills Paloverde, Mountain Mahogany (DAl); Sunflower (Dv); Chrysanthemum,

Larkspur, Sunflower (Fes); Weeping WIllow, White Willow (GM); Thanksgiving Cactus, Water Poppy (Haii); White Narcissus (Hb); Flight (Him E); Yellow Silk Cotton Tree (Him I)

EMERGENCIES Fireweed, Labrador Tree, River Beauty, White Fireweed (Ask); Rock Rose (B); Red Clover (Dv); Pear (Ma)

EMOTIONAL BLOCKAGES Bluebell, Pink Mulla Mulla (Aus B); Compass Barrel Cactus (DAl); Baby Blue Eyes, Dandelion, Golden Ear Drops (Fes); Bay (GM); Amazon Swordplant (Haii)

EMOTIONAL CLEANSING/RELEASE Tree Like Heather (AK); Fireweed (Ask); Lavender, Onion (Dv); Chapparal, Deer Bush, Evening Primrose, Golden Ear Drops, Self-heal, Yerba Santa (Fes); Apple (GM); Marjoram (Hb); Moonsnail (Pac); Monkeyflower Bush, Swamp Onion (Peg)

EMOTIONAL DETACHMENT Pink Yarrow (AK); Sweetgale (Ask); Tall Yellow Top (Aus B); Mesquite (DAl); Bleeding Heart, Love Lies Bleeding, Tansy (Fes); Sweet Chestnut (GM); Cup of Gold (Haii); Green Rein Orchid (Peg)

ENDURANCE Willow (Ask); Banksia Robur, Macrocarpa (Aus B); Cardon, Soaptree Yucca (DAl); Penstemon (Fes); White Poplar (GM); Coconut (Ma)

ENERGY BOOST Amazon River Orchid, Victoria Regina Orchid (AK); Lady Slipper (Ask); Banksia Robur, Old Man Banksia (Aus B); Cherry, Sugar Beet (Cal); Fire Prickly Pear Cactus (DAl); Arnica, California Wild Rose, Cayenne (Fes); Bay, Buffalo Cactus, Hornbeam (GM); Pukiawe (Haii); Healing (Him E); Caster Oil Plant, Jack Fruit Tree (Him I); Orange (Ma); Red Spider Lily (Peg)

ENTHUSIASM Old Man Banksia (Aus B); Gorse (F); Bourgainvillea (Him A); Cherry, Corn (Ma)

ESCAPISM Bunchberry (Ask); Sundew (Aus B); Blue Topped Cow Weed (Aus L); Basil, Blackberry, California Poppy, Canyon Dudleya, Milkweed (Fes); Oriental Poppy (Hb); Gul Mohar (Him I); Coconut (Ma)

EXPRESSING – FEELINGS Poinsettia (AK); Dagger Hakea, Flannel Flower (Aus B); Fishhook Cactus, Ocotillo, Rainbow Cactus (DAl); Fuchsia, Onion, Scarlet Monkeyflower (Dv); Snapdragon (Dv, Hb); Golden Ear Drops, Indian Paintbrush, Pink Monkeyflower, Trumpet Vine (Fes); Birch, Holm Oak, Ivy, Larch, Mimosa (GM); Bluebell, Weigela (Pac); Blazing Star, Owls Clover (Peg)

EXPRESSING – IDEAS Bush Fuchsia, Turkey Bush (Aus B); Cosmos (Fes); Parrot (Him A); Tamarind Tree (Him I); Owls Clover, Trillium Red (Peg)

EXTROVERSION
  See **Introversion**

FAMILY PRESSURES/STRESS Boab (Aus B); Cat's Paw (Aus L); Canyon Grapevine, Mesquite, Organ Pipe Cactus (DAl); Nettles (Dv); Fairy Lantern, Red Clover, Sweet Pea, Tansy, Walnut (Fes); Chinese Violet, Plumbago, Poha (Haii); Tassel Flower (Him A, Him I); Mingimingi (NZ); Plumeria (Peg)

FATHERING Sunflower (AK); Mountain Mahogany (DAl); Baby Blue Eyes, Quince, Sage, Saguaro (Fes)

FEAR – GENERAL Dog Rose of the Wild Forces (Aus B); Dampiera (Aus L); Cherry Plum, Red Chestnut, Rock Rose (B); Scottish Primrose,

Thistle (F); Chamomile, Sweet Pea (Hb); Day-blooming Jessamine (Him A); Tomato (Ma)

FEAR – SPECIFIC Bog Rosemary, Tundra Rose (Ask); Dog Rose, Green Spider Orchid, Mulla Mulla (Aus B); Menzies Banksia (Aus L); Mimulus (B); Indian Root, Thurber's Gilia (DAl); St John's Wort (Dv); Black-eyed Susan, California Pitcher Plant, Fawn Lily, Pink Monkeyflower (Fes); Red Chestnut (GM); Avocado, Cotton, Ma'o (Haii); Blackberry, Cymbidium, Heather (Hb); Indian Almond (Him I); Choko, Loquat (NZ)

FEAR – UNKNOWN Red Clover, Wild Garlic (AK); Monk's Hood (Ask); Ribbon Pea (Aus L); Aspen, Mimulus (B); Garlic (Fes); Ivy, Leyland Cypress (GM); Cotton, Kukui (Haii); Flax (NZ); Snowdrop (Pac)

FLEXIBILITY Lamb's Quarters, Wild Rhubarb, Willow (Ask); Rock Water, Vine (B); Desert Willow, Foothills Paloverde (DAl); Quaking Grass, Rabbit Bush (Fes); Ash (GM); White Coral Tree (Him A); Fig (Ma)

FOCUS (MENTAL) Bunchberry, Golden Corydalis (Ask); Sundew (Aus B); Hops Bush, Pink Trumpet Flower, Yellow Boronia (Aus L); Fire Prickly Pear Cactus, Hedgehog Cactus (DAl); Madia, Peppermint, Shatsa Daisy (Fes); Hazel (GM); Neem, Tee Wood Tree (Him I)

FORGIVENESS Blue Elf Viola, Mountain Wormwood (Ask); Dagger Hakea, Mountain Devil (Aus B); Correa, Pixie Mope (Aus L); Pine (B); Immortal (DAl); Rowan (F); Elder, Hawthorn (GM); Hyssop (Hb); Tassel Flower, Tassel Flower (Him I); Raspberry (Ma); Salal (Pac); Clarkia, Prickly Poppy (Peg); Lilac (PF)

FREEDOM Cerato (AK); Mountain Wormwood (Ask); Rainbow Cactus, Tarbrush (DAl); Leyland Cypress (GM)

FRUSTRATION Blue Elf Viola (Ask); Banksia Robur, Wild Potato Bush (Aus B); Silver Princess Gum, Snake Bush, Ursinia (Aus L); Holly (B); Siberian Spruce (Ba); Blackberry, Indian Paintbrush, Iris, Wild Oat (Fes); Gorse (GM); Ulua (Haii); Cymbidium (Hb); Mussel (Pac); Verbena (PF)

GREED Goldenrod, Star Thistle, Trillium (Fes)

GRIEF Sturt Desert Pea (Aus B); Honeysuckle, Star of Bethlehem (B); Hackberry (DAl); Bleeding Heart (Dv, Fes); Borage, Golden Ear Drops (Fes); Hawthorn (Hb); Ashoka Tree, Radish (Him A); Indian Almond (Him I); Pear (Ma); Star Fish (Pac)

GROUP DYNAMICS Martagon Lily, Mullein (Dv)

GUILT Sturt Desert Rose (Aus B); Pine (B); Jumping Cholla Cactus (DAl); Golden Ear Drops, Mullein, Pink Monkeyflower (Fes); Sweet Chestnut (GM); Hyssop (Hb); Meenalih (Him A); Screw Pine (Him I); Strawberry (Ma); Polyanthus (NZ)

HAPPINESS Mountain Devil, Sunshine Wattle (Aus B); Star of Bethlehem (Aus L); Valerian (F); Manna Ash, Norway Maple (GM); Happiness (Him E); Cherry (Ma)

HATE Mountain Devil (Aus B); Black Kangaroo Paw, Cape Bluebell (Aus L); Holly (B); Black Cohosh, Oregon Grape, Snapdragon (Fes); Indian Mulberry (Him A)

HONESTY *See* **Dishonesty**

HOPE Cinnamon Rose, Japanese Rose (AK); Sunshine Wattle (Aus B); Star of Bethlehem (Aus L); Gorse, Sweet Chestnut (B); Beech (GM); Cherry (Ma)

HUMOUR (LACK OF) Little Flannel Flower (Aus B); Zinnia (Cal, Fes); Compass Barrel Cactus (DAl); Valerian (F); Leyland Cypress, Pittespora (GM); Fig (Ma)

HURT/PAIN Cotton Grass, Ladies' Tresses, River Beauty, White Fireweed (Ask); Sturt Desert Pea (Aus B); Illyarrie, Mauve Melaleuca, Menzies Banksia, Violet Butterfly (Aus L); Valerian (Cal); Aloe (DAl); Hawthorn May (Dv); California Wild Rose, Chamomile, Golden Ear Drops, Pink Monkeyflower, Yerba Santa (Fes); Beech, Mulberry (GM); Comfrey, Heartsease, Nettle (Hb); Tassel Flower (Him A); Weigela (Pac)

HYPERACTIVITY Black-eyed Susan, Jacaranda (Aus B); Morning Glory (Fes); Petunia (Hb); The Pongam, Yellow Canna (Him I)

HYPOCHONDRIA Peach Flowered Tea Tree (Aus B); Heather (B); Fuchsia, Purple Monkey-flower (Fes); Tiger's Jaw Cactus (PF)

IDENTITY CRISIS Columbine, Monk's Hood, Tamarack, Yellow Dryas (Ask); Sumach (Ba); Milkweed, Quaking Grass (Fes); Magnolia (GM); Strength (Him E)

IMMATURITY Bracken, Charlock (Ba); Faïry Lantern (Fes)

IMPATIENCE Aggression Orchid (AK); Black-eyed Susan (Aus B); Impatiens (B, Haii); Aloe (DAl); Calendula, Poison Oak (Fes)

IMPETUOUSNESS Kangaroo Paw (Aus B); Impatiens (B, Fes); Red Hot Cat Tail (Him I); Verbena (PF)

INADEQUACY Evening Star, Hackberry, Immortal, Queen of the Night (DAl); Buttercup, Evening Primrose, Goldenrod, Star Thistle (Fes)

INCEST (EFFECTS OF) Macrozamia (Aus L); Black Cohosh (Fes)

INDECISION Jacaranda, Paw Paw, Sundew (Aus B); Centuary, Scleranthus (B); Ratany, Soaptree Yucca (DAl); Cayenne (Dv); Cayenne, Mullein, Tansy (Fes); English Elm, Glastonbury Thorn, Pittespora (GM); Coffee (Haii); Cannon Ball Tree, Coconut Palm (Him I); Koromiko (NZ); Pipsissewa (Pac); White Petunia (PF)

INDEPENDENCE Angelsword, Southern Cross (Aus B); Box (Dv); Bleeding Heart, Fairy Lantern, Milkweed (Fes); Rose – wild (Hb)

INFERIORITY Buttercup (AK, Fes); Hibbertia (Aus B); Urchin Dryandra, Yellow Cone Flower (Aus L); Cardon (DAl); Rose Quartz (Gem); Spindle (GM); Vilayati Amli (Him A); Pineapple (Ma); Watermelon (NZ)

INHERITED BEHAVIOUR PATTERNS Fireweed (Ask); Boab (Aus B); Larch (B); Tarbrush (DAl); Black Cohosh (Fes); Macadamia, Ohai-ali'i (Haii); Nirjara (Him E); Agave Yaquinana (Peg)

INSECURITY Dog Rose, Tall Mulla Mulla (Aus B); Happy Wanderer (Aus L); Bouvardia, Cow Parsnip, Mala Mujer (DAl); Wild Garlic (Dv); Mallow (Dv, Fes); Rosemary, Star Thistle (Fes); Strength (Him E); Goldenrod (Him A); Viburnum (Pac)

INSENSITIVITY Flannel Flower, Kangaroo Paw, Red Helmet (Aus B); Orange Lesche-naultia, Red and Green Kangaroo Paw, Red Leschenaultia (Aus L); Calendula (Dv); Yellow Star Tulip (Fes); Awapuhi Melemele, Kamani

(Haii); Lady's Smock (Hb); Indian Coral, Sithihea (Him A)

INSPIRATION Blue Flag Iris (AK); Parakeelya (Aus L); Welsh Poppy (Ba); Iris (Dv); Iris (Fes); Rose White (Hb); Blackberry (Ma); Choke Cherry (Peg)

INTELLECT (IQ BOOSTER) Isopogon (Aus B); Lemon (Dv); Cosmos, Nasturtium, Peppermint (Fes)

INTIMACY Wisteria (Aus B); Fishhook Cactus, Klein's Pencil Cholla Cactus, Teddy Bear Cholla Cactus (DAl); Sticky Monkeyflower (Dv, Fes); Holy Thorn (F); Hibiscus, Pink Monkeyflower (Fes); Avocado (Haii)

INTOLERANCE Slender Rice Flower (Aus B); Yellow and Green Kangaroo Paw, Yellow Leschenaultia (Aus L); Green Rose (Aus L, Him I); Beech (B); Impatiens (B, Haii) Yellow Star Tulip (Fes); Date (Ma)

INTROVERSION Five Corners, Gymea Lily, Tall Mulla Mulla (Aus B); White Spider Orchid (Aus L); Mallow, Rosemary (Dv); Fawn Lily (Fes); Plane Tree (GM); Rhubarb (Hb); Green Rose, Water Lily (Him I)

INTUITION White Spruce (Ask); Bush Fuchsia (Aus B); Queen of the Night (DAl); Mimosa, Stags Horn Sumach (GM); Viburnum (Pac)

IRRATIONAL BEHAVIOUR Aspen (B); Scarlet Monkeyflower (Fes); Box (GM); Stenogyne Calaminthoides (Haii)

IRRESPONSIBLE BEHAVIOUR *See* **Responsibility**

IRRITABILITY Black-eyed Susan (Aus B); Leafless Orchid (Aus L); Beech, Impatiens (B); Poison Oak, Snapdragon (Fes); Mussel (Pac); Vanilla (PF)

ISOLATION Single Delight (Ask); Pink Mulla Mulla, Tall Mulla Mulla, Tall Yellow Top (Aus B); Green Rose, Veronica (Aus L); Water Violet (B); Mariposa Lily (DAl); Stonecrop (F); Love Lies Bleeding, Sweet Pea (Fes); Persian Iron Wood (GM); Flight (Him E); Heather (NZ); Cape Honeysuckle (Peg)

JEALOUSY Mountain Devil (Aus B); Red Feather Flower (Aus L); Holly (B, Fes); Desert Holly (DAl); Pretty Face, Trillium (Fes); Holm Oak (GM); Slow Match Tree (Him I); Grape (Ma)

JOY Borage, Chocolate Orchid (AK); Churning Bell, Tundra Rose (Ask); Apple Mint Bush, Little Flannel Flower (Aus B); Pink Everlasting Straw Flower, Red and Green Kangaroo Paw (Aus L); Aloe, Strawberry Cactus (DAl); Rhododendron (Dv); Gorse (F); Angel Trumpet, California Wild Rose (Fes); Catalpa, Gorse (GM); Ashoka Tree, Parval (Him A); Happiness (Him E); Apple, Orange, Spinach (Ma); Vanilla Leaf (Pac)

LAUGHTER (TONIC) Fun Orchid (AK); Zinnia (AK, Dv, Fes, PVi); Little Flannel Flower (Aus B); Strawberry Cactus (DAl); Verbascum (NZ)

LAZINESS Kapok Bush (Aus B); Red Feather Flower (Aus L); Peppermint (Dv); Veronica (NZ); Sycamore (Peg); Tiger's Jaw Cactus (PF)

LEARNING ABILITY Daisy (AK); Bush Fuchsia, Isopogon (Aus B); Chestnut Bud (B); California Wild Rose, Cosmos, Madia, Peppermint, Rabbit Bush (Fes); Hazel, Judas

Tree (GM); Poha, Ulei (Haii); Neem (Him I); Hangehange (NZ); Blue Camas (Pac); Silver Lace (PF)

LETHARGY (MENTAL) Red Beak Orchid (Aus L); Blackberry (Dv); Peppermint (Dv, Fes); Broom (F); Cosmos, Tansy (Fes); Sycamore (GM); Pua-kenikeni, Pua-Pilo, Water Poppy (Haii); Mast Tree (Him I); Corn (Ma); Tiger's Jaw Cactus (PF)

LONELINESS Violet (AK); Tall Yellow Top (Aus B); Parakeelya, Veronica (Aus L); Chaparral, Mesquite (DAl); Bleeding Heart, California Wild Rose, Nicotiana (Fes); Rose Quartz (Gem); Heartsease (Hb); Curry Leaf Tree, Soap Nut Tree (Him I); Grape (Ma)

LOVE (ABILITY TO) Heart Orchid, Love Orchid (AK); Tundra Rose (Ask); Black Kangaroo Paw, Mauve Melaleuca, Pink Everlasting Straw Flower (Aus L); Organ Pipe Cactus, Teddy Bear Cholla Cactus (DAl); Moonstone (Gem); Field Maple, Hawthorn (GM); Daffodil, Rosebud-red, Self-Heal (Hb); Malabar Nut Flower, Neem (Him A)

MALE/FEMALE BALANCE Arum Lily (AK); Green Fairy Orchid, Sitka Spruce Pollen (Ask); Niu (Haii); Rattlesnake Plantain Orchid, Red Ginger (Peg)
   See also **Sexuality**

MANIC DEPRESSION Peach Flowered Tea Tree (Aus B); Chamomile, Mustard (Fes); Copper Beech (GM); Stick Rorrish (Haii); Periwinkle (Pac)

MANIPULATIVE BEHAVIOUR Isopogon (Aus B); Fringed Lily Twiner, Pale Sundew (Aus L); Chicory (B, Fes); Devil's Claw, Klein's Pencil Cholla Cactus (DAl)

MATERNAL INSTINCTS – LACK OF Quince (Dv); Mariposa Lily (Fes); Moonstone (Gem); Niu, Noni (Haii)

MATERNAL INSTINCTS – UNFULFILLED Evening Primrose (Fes); Noni (Haii)
   See also **Mothering**

MEMORY (IMPROVING) Rosemary (AK); Isopogon (Aus B); Hairy Sedge (Ba); Comfrey, Fig Tree, Forget-me-not (Dv); Broom (F); Rabbit Bush, Rosemary (Fes); Yew (GM); Comfrey, Eyebright (Hb); Ulei (Haii); Teakwood Flower (Him A); Avocado (Ma); Periwinkle (Pac)

MEN – RELATING TO WOMEN Milky Nipple Cactus (DAl); Spider Lily (Haii); Rattlesnake Plantain Orchid (Peg)

MENTAL CHATTER Knotgrass, Wild Carrot (AK); Boronia (Aus B); White Chestnut (B, Fes); Star Primrose (DAl); Cosmos (Fes); Papaya (Haii); Salpglossis (Hb)

MENTAL HARMONY Jacob's Ladder, Willow (Ask); Nasturtium (Fes); Cherry Laurel (GM); Spider Lily (Haii); Curry Leaf, Red Hibiscus (Him A); Kohia (NZ); Iris (PF)

MENTAL ILLNESS W.A. Smoke Bush (Aus L); Indian Root, Sacred Datura (DAl); Yerba Santa (Fes); Stenogyne Calaminthoides, Stick Rorrish (Haii)

MOOD SWINGS Peach Flowered Tea Tree (Aus B); Scleranthus (B); Apricot (Cal); Buffalo Gourd (DAl); Chamomile (Dv); Bell Heather (F); Mustard (Fes); Silver Maple (GM); Cherry (Ma); Stock (PF)

MOTHERING Pumpkin (AK); Grove Sandwort, Northern Lady's Slipper, Spiraea (Ask); Bottlebrush (Aus B); Goddess Grasstree

(Aus L); Bog Asphodel (Ba); Desert Holly, Mala Mujer, Milky Nipple Cactus (DAl); Linden (Dv); Mariposa Lily (DAl, Fes); Iris, Milkweed, Pomegranate (Fes); Niu, Noni (Haii); Peach (Ma); Barnacle (Pac)

MOTIVATION Mountain Mahogany, Tarbrush (DAl); Mast Tree (Him I); Neoporteria Cactus (Peg)

NEGATIVITY (CLEARING) Forget-me-not (Hb); Purple and Red Kangaroo Paw (Aus L); Antiseptic Bush (Aus L); Crab Apple (B); Flowering Currant, Honesty (Ba); Crown of Thorns, Ephedra (DAl); Black Cohosh, Mountain Pennyroyal, Pink Yarrow, Yarrow (Fes); Holm Oak (GM); Day-Blooming Water Lily, Jade Vine, Spider Lily (Haii); Lungwort, Snapdragon (Hb); Christ's Thorn (Him A); Blackberry (Ma); London Pride (NZ); Sand Dollar (Pac); Okra (PVi)

NERVOUS BREAKDOWN Waratah (Aus B); Cherry Plum (B); Comfrey (Cal); Fairy Duster (DAl); Hau (Haii); Periwinkle (Pac)

NERVOUSNESS Waratah (Aus B); Chamomile (Cal, Fes); Fairy Duster (DAl); Dill, Garlic, Lady's Slipper, Lavender, Nicotiana (Fes); Horse Chestnut, Pear (GM); Hau (Haii); Banana (Ma); Marigold (NZ); Purple Nightshade (Peg)

NIGHT FEARS St John's Wort (Dv, Hb)

NIGHTMARES Rose of Sharon (AK); Green Spider Orchid (Aus B); Rock Rose (B); St John's Wort (Dv, Fes); Chaparral (Fes); Pa-nini-o-ka, Passion Flower (Haii); Swallow Wort (Him A)

NURTURING
  See **Mothering**

OBSESSION Boronia (Aus B); Rock Water (B);

Crab Apple (B, Fes); Jumping Cholla Cactus, Whitehorn (DAl); Filaree, Heather, Pink Monkeyflower, Purple Monkeyflower, Sticky Monkeyflower (Fes); Barnacle, Urchin (Pac)

OPPRESSION Tormentil (Hb); Jack Fruit Tree, Nilgiri Longy Plant, Yellow Champa (Him I)

OPTIMISM Sunshine Wattle (Aus B); Wild Violet (Aus L); Gorse (B, Fes); Buttercup (Ba); Strawberry Cactus (DAl); Scotch Broom (Dv); Spotted Orchid (F); Gentian, Penstemon (Fes); Blackberry, Cherry (Ma)

OVER-EXCITEMENT Lavender (Dv); Canyon Dudleya (Fes); Potato (Hb)

OVER-INTELLECTUAL BEHAVIOUR Crown of Thorns, Desert Holly (DAl); Nasturtium (Fes)

OVER-REACTING Vervain (B); Jumping Cholla Cactus, Ocotillo, Saguaro Cactus (DAl); Love Lies Bleeding (Fes); Parrot Tree (Him I)

OVER-SENSITIVITY Common White Spider, Hybrid Pink Fairy (Cowslip) Orchid, Pixie Mope (Aus L); Mimulus (B); Pink Yarrow, Zinnia (Dv); Daisy (F); Lady's Smock (Hb)

OVERWHELMED (FEELING) Dill (AK, Dv, Fes, Hb); Mint Bush, Paw Paw (Aus B); One-sided Bottlebrush, Pink Fairy Orchid (Aus L); Elm, Hornbeam (B); Buffalo Gourd, Jumping Cholla Cactus, Immortal, Woven Spine Pineapple Cactus (DAl); Daisy (F); Cosmos, Hornbeam, Larkspur, Red Clover, Scotch Broom (Fes); Nani-ahiahi (Haii); Spinach (Ma); Acorn, Rhododendron (NZ)

PANIC Red Clover (AK, Fes); Dog Rose of the Wild Forces, Yellow Leschenaultia (Aus L); Pencil Cholla Cactus (DAl); Buttercup (Hb); Sithihea (Him A); Vital Spark (Him E); Urchin (Pac)

PARANOIA Red Clover (AK); Hybrid Pink Fairy (Cowslip) Orchid (Aus L); Oregon Grape, Purple Monkeyflower (Fes); Stick Rorrish (Haii); St John's Wort (Hb); Spinach (Ma)

PATIENCE Brown Boronia, Yellow Leschenaultia (Aus L); Impatiens (B); Indian Tobacco (DAl); Pine (GM); Buttercup (Hb); Sithihea (Him A); Rain Tree (Him I); Lobelia (NZ); Pink Seaweed (Pac)

PERFECTIONISM Golden Waitsia, Yellow and Green Kangaroo Paw (Aus L); Fuchsia (Hb)

PERSEVERANCE Kapok Bush (Aus B); Woolly Banksia (Aus L); Kolokoltchik (Aus L); Gentian (B, Fes); Soaptree Yucca (DAl); Scotch Broom (Dv, Fes); Mountain Pride, Penstemon (Fes); Broom (Hb); Clematis (NZ); Washington Lily (Peg)

PESSIMISM
  See **Optimism**

POSSESSIVENESS Chicory (B); Lesser Stitchwort (Ba); Harebell (F); Bleeding Heart, Trillium (Fes)

POOR MOTHER/FATHER IMAGE Grove Sandwort (Ask); Sunflower (AK, Fes, Dv); Red Helmet (Aus B); Milky Nipple Cactus, Mountain Mahogany (DAl); Mariposa Lily (DAl, Fes); Baby Blue Eyes, Quince, Saguaro, Scarlet Monkeyflower (Fes); Rose Quartz (Gem); Sun Plant (Him I); Barnacle (Pac); Old Maid Pink/White (Peg)

PRE-CANCEROUS EMOTIONAL STATE Dagger Hakea, Southern Cross, Sturt Desert Rose (Aus B); Herkimer Diamond (Gem); Nani-ahiahi (Haii); Purple Crocus (Pac)

PREJUDICE Boab, Slender Rice Flower (Aus B);

Water Violet (B, Fes); Indian Mulberry, Malabar Nut Flower (Him A)

PRIDE Gymea Lily, Slender Rice Flower (Aus B); Vine (B); Poppy (Hb); Malabar Nut Flower (Him A); Banana (Ma)

PROCRASTINATION Jacaranda, Sundew (Aus B); Larch (B); Nasturtium (Ba); Pencil Cholla Cactus (DAl); Cayenne, Tansy (Fes); Blackberry (Fes, Ma); Corn (Ma)

PROTECTION FROM NEGATIVE EMOTIONS/THOUGHTS Fringed Violet (Aus B); Walnut (B); Pennyroyal (Cal, Dv); White Yarrow (Dv); Pink Yarrow (Dv, Fes); Mountain Pennyroyal, Oregon Grape (Fes); Yarrow (Fes, Hb); Kamani (Haii); White Rose (PF)

PROTECTION FROM OTHERS' NEGATIVITY Angel of Protection Orchid (AK); Shy Blue Orchid (Aus L); Walnut (B); Bistort (Ba); Fawn Lily (Fes); Banyan Tree (Him I); Tomato (Ma)

PROTECTION FROM STRESS Angel of Protection (AK); Yarrow (Ask); Pink Yarrow (Dv); Corn, Fawn Lily, Sweet Pea (Fes); Ti (Haii); Urban Stress Remedy (Him A); Banyan Tree (Him I)

PUBERTY Alpine Lily, Angelica, Calla Lily, Fairy Lantern, Morning Glory, Pretty Face (Fes)

RAPE (EFFECTS OF) Macrozamia (Aus L); Rippy Hillox (Him A); Mussel (Pac)

REBELLIOUSNESS Red Helmet (Aus B); Red Beak Orchid, Silver Princess Gum (Aus L); Saguaro (Fes)

REJECTION Illawarra Flame Tree (Aus B); Black Cohosh, Bleeding Heart, Evening Primrose, Holly, Oregon Grape, Pink Monkeyflower (Fes);

Ukshi (Him A); Tassel Flower (Him I); Euphorbia (NZ); Lemon Grass (PF)

RELATIONSHIP TO ONESELF Bird of Paradise (AK); White Desert Primrose (DAl)

RELATIONSHIP PROBLEMS Mountain Wormwood, Sweetgale (Ask); Bush Gardenia, Wedding Bush (Aus B); Purple Eremophila, Rabbit Orchid (Aus L); Hawthorn May (Dv); Scottish Primrose (F); Bleeding Hearts (Fes); Day-Blooming Water Lily, Jade Vine, Kukui, Night-Blooming Water Lily (Haii); Sweet Pea (Hb); Slow Match, Vilayati Amli (Him A)

RELATIONSHIPS – BREAK-UPS Bleeding Heart (AK); Twinflower (Ask); Snake Vine, Violet Butterfly (Aus L); Klein's Pencil Cholla Cactus (DAl); Bleeding Heart, Hawthorn May, Nettles (Dv); Rose Quartz (Gem); Amazon Sword Plant (Haii); Ixora, Pagoda Tree, Tassel Flower (Him I)

RELAXATION Zinnia (AK); Dampiera, Hop's Bush, Purple Flag Flower (Aus L); Vervain (B); Comfrey (Cal); Indian Root, Indian Tobacco (DAl); Dandelion (Dv, Fes); Dill, Lavender (Fes); Buttercup, Meadowsweet, Sage (Hb); Curry Leaf (Him A); Yellow Canna (Him I); Lettuce (Ma); Mussel (Pac)

REPRESSED EMOTIONS Bluebell (Aus B); Rainbow Cactus (DAl); Chaparral (DAl, Fes); Black-eyed Susan, Fuchsia, Golden Ear Drops (Fes); Awapuhi Melemele, Nani-ahiahi (Haii); Red Hibiscus (Him A); Jack Fruit Tree (Him I)

RESENTMENT Mountain Wormwood (Ask); Dagger Hakea (Aus B); Black Kangaroo Paw, Geraldton Wax (Aus L); Compass Barrel Cactus (DAl); Oregon Grape, Scarlet Monkeyflower (Fes); Drum Stick, Slow Match, Ukshi (Him A); Green Rose (Him I); Raspberry (Ma)

RESIGNATION Kapok Bush (Aus B); Star of Bethlehem (Aus L); Gorse (B); Tarbrush (DAl); Wild Rose (Fes); Plantain (Hb)

RESPONSIBILITY Colour Orchid (AK); Many-headed Dryandra (Aus B); Blue-Topped Cow Weed, Red Feather Flower, Wallflower Donkey Orchid (Aus L); Scleranthus (B); Ocotillo (DAl); Giant Redwood (GM); Strawberry (Ma)

RESTLESSNESS Red Grevillia (Aus B); W.A. Christmas Tree, Red Beak Orchid (Aus L); Agrimony, Scleranthus (B); Licorice (Cal); Zinnia (Dv); California Poppy, Morning Glory (Fes); Magnolia (GM); Swallow-wort (Him A); Rangoon Creeper (Him I)

RIGIDITY Bog Blueberry (Ask); Bauhinia, Hibbertia (Aus B); Beech, Rock Water, Water Violet (B); Prickly Pear Cactus (DAl); Spruce (Dv); Cherry Plum (GM); Ohai-ali'i (Haii); St John's Lily (Him A); Fig (Ma); Mussel, Twinflower (Pac)

SADNESS Desert Sturt Pea (Aus B); Mauve Melaleuca (Aus L); Cat's Paw (Aus L); Gentian (B); Mustard (B); Borage (Dv); Rhododendron (Dv, Ba); Double Snowdrop (Ba); Wolfberry (DAl); Colour Orchid (AK); Geranium (AK)

SARCASM Snapdragon (Fes); Uksi (Him I); Blackberry (Ma)

SCATTERED THINKING
  See **Focus (mental)**

SELF-CRITICAL BEHAVIOUR Bird of Paradise (AK); Alpine Azalea, Columbine, Lace Flower (Ask); Billy Goat Plum (Aus B); Pine (B); Foothills Paloverde, Indian Tobacco (DAl); Buttercup (Fes); Giant Redwood (GM); Uksi, Wood Apple Tree (Him I); Pineapple (Ma); Twinflower (Pac); Milkmaids (Peg)

SELF-DISCIPLINE Hibbertia (Aus B); Blue China Orchid (Aus L); Rock Water (B); Lawson Cypress (GM); Almond, Fig (Ma); Everlasting Pea (NZ); Surfgrass (Pac); Sycamore (Peg)

SELF-ESTEEM Buttercup (AK, Fes); Columbine, Tamarack (Ask); Five Corners (Aus B); Sturt Desert Rose (Aus B); Yellow Cone Flower (Aus L); Evening Star, Immortal (DAl); Echinacea, Sagebrush, Sunflower (Fes); Red Oak (GM); Daffodil, Star Jasmine, Thistle (Hb); Ukshi (Him A); Hidden Splendor, Strength (Him E); Rippy Hillox Plant (Him I); Viola-white (NZ); Vanilla Leaf (Pac); Sea Palm (Pac); Milkmaids (Peg)

SELFISHNESS Blue Leschenaultia, Fringed Lily Twiner (Aus L); Heather (B); Mala Mujer (DAl); Silverweed (F); Fawn Lily, Trillium (Fes); Tamarind Tree (Him I); Peach (Ma); Salvia (NZ)

SELF-PITY One-sided Bottlebrush (Aus L); Chicory (B)

SENSITIVITY TO EMOTIONALISM Angel of Protection Orchid (AK); Pink Yarrow (AK, Fes); Pennyroyal (Cal); Golden Yarrow (Fes); Banyan Tree (Him I)

SENSITIVITY TO THE ENVIRONMENT Radiation Essence (Aus B); Pink Fairy Orchid (Aus L); Yarrow Special Formula (Fes); IUG Kenya Energetic Protective Shield (Gem); Environmental Stress Remedy (Him A)

SENSITIVITY TO NEGATIVE THOUGHT-FORMS Angel of Protection Orchid (AK); Red Grevillia (Aus B); Pennyroyal (Cal); Chaparral, Golden Yarrow, Mountain Pennyroyal, Oregon Grape (Fes); Wild Fennel (NZ)

SEXUAL ABUSE Balsam Poplar (Ask); Flannel Flower (Aus B); Macrozamia (Aus L); Bisbee Beehive Cactus (DAl); Onion (Dv); Dogwood, Evening Primrose, Mariposa Lily, Pink Monkeyflower, Purple Monkeyflower (Fes); Prickly Poppy, Rippy Hillox (Him A); Orange (Ma); Nootka Rose (Pac)

SEXUAL HANG-UPS Wisteria (Aus B); Tufted Vetch (Ba); Basil, California Pitcher Plant, Evening primrose (Fes); Day-Blooming Water Lily (Haii); Water Lily (Him A); Down to Earth (Him E); Cannon Ball Tree (Him I); Mussel (Pac); Marigold (PF)

SEXUAL INSECURITY/INHIBITIONS Aggression Orchid, Basil, Fire Lily (AK); Balsam Poplar (Ask); Hibiscus, Martagon Lily, Sticky Monkeyflower (Dv); Calla Lily, Easter Lily, Rosemary, Sticky Monkeyflower (Fes); Bird Cherry (GM); Day-Blooming Water Lily, Pua Kenikeni (Haii); Karvi, Meenalih, Old Maid – white and pink (Him A); Purple Magnolia (Pac)

SEXUAL REVITALIZATION Canary Island Bellflower (AK); Queen of the Night (DAl); Hibiscus, Lady's Slipper (Fes); Day-Blooming Water Lily, Night-Blooming Water Lily (Haii); Night Jasmine, Water Lily (Him A); Ixora (Him A, Him I); Red Ginger, Shasta Lily (Peg)

SEXUALITY, ACCEPTANCE OF Arum Lily, Banana, Red Hibiscus (AK); Billy Goat Plum (Aus B); Basil, Pomegranate (Dv); Alpine Lily, Calla Lily, Manzanita (Fes); Bird Cherry (GM); Niu, Lehur (Haii); Courgette, Rose – red (Hb); Candystick (Pac); Lobivia Cactus, Mountain Pride (Peg)

SHARING Purple Nymph Waterlily, W.A. Christmas Tree (Aus L); Jojoba, Star Primrose (DAl)

SHATTERED FEELINGS Waratah (Aus B); Cowkicks, Violet Butterfly (Aus L); Echinacea, Sagebrush (Fes); Strength, Vital Spark (Him E); Rain Tree (Him I); Purple Crocus (Pac)

SHOCK River Beauty, White Fireweed (Ask); Emergency Essence (Aus B); Rescue Remedy, Star of Bethlehem (B); Arnica (Dv, Fes); Ulua (Haii); Red Clover (Hb); First Aid Remedy, Radish (Him A); Vital Spark (Him E); Pear (Ma)

SHYNESS Dog Rose (Aus B); Mimulus (B); Box, Buttercup (Dv); Mallow, Violet (Fes); Cherry Plum (GM); Red Tulip (Hb); Water Lily (Him I); Tomato (Ma)

SLEEP (DISTURBED) Boronia (Aus B); Chamomile (Cal, Fes); Yellow Ginger (Haii)

SPACED-OUT (FEELING) Clematis (B, Fes); Pink Fairy Duster (DAl); Rosemary (Fes)

STABILITY W. A. Smoke Bush (Aus L); Black Poplar, Horse Chestnut (GM); Coffee (Haii); Tamarind Tree (Him I); Narcissus, Pink Seaweed, Surfgrass (Pac); Salvia (PVi)

STRENGTH Red Grevillia (Aus B); Goddess Grass Tree, Happy Wanderer, Russian Forget-me-not (Aus L); Mimulus (B); Yew (Ba); Organ Pipe Cactus, Spineless Prickly Pear (DAl); Box (Dv); Elder, Cymbidium, Red Tulip (Hb); Strawberry, Tomato (Ma)

STRESS Labrador Tea (Ask); Crowea (Aus B); Purple Flag Flower, Yellow Flag Flower (Aus L); Peanut (Cal); Staghorn Cholla Cactus (DAl); Dill, Nettles, Valerian (Dv); Aloe Vera, Corn, Nicotiana, Self-heal, Sweet Pea (Fes); Alder (GM); Cotton, Hau (Haii); Dandelion (Hb); Goatsbeard, Surfgrass (Pac); Mock Orange, Sycamore (Peg); Sweet bell pepper (PVi)

SUBCONSCIOUS (CLEARING) Sage (AK); Forget-me-not (AK, Ask); Horsetail (Ask); Tarbrush (DAl); Chaparral, Mugwort (Fes); Yellow Ginger (Haii); Swallow Wort (Him A); Moonsnail, Poison Hemlock (Pac); Agave Yaquinana (Peg)

SUICIDAL THOUGHTS Waratah (Aus B); Cherry Plum (B); Urchin (Pac); Sunflower (PF)

SUPERIORITY Hibbertia (Aus B); Malabar Nut Flower (Him A)

TANTRUMS Scarlet Monkeyflower (Fes)

TEETH-GRINDING Black-eyed Susan (Aus B); Morning Glory (Cal, Fes)

TENDERNESS Venus Orchid (AK); Flannel Flower (Aus B); Noni (Haii); Date (Ma)

TERROR Green Spider Orchid, Grey Spider Flower (Aus B); Rock Rose (B); Rainbow Cactus, Teddy Bear Cholla Cactus (DAl); Tomato (Ma)

TOLERANCE *See* **Intolerance**

TRAPPED (FEELING) Red Grevillia, Sunshine Wattle (Aus B); Geraldton Wax, Russian Centaurea (Aus L); Honeysuckle, Larch (B); Nasturtium, Pine Cones (Ba); Cayenne (Dv); Stonecrop (F)

TRAUMA Northern Lady's Slipper, River Beauty (Ask); Fringed Violet (Aus B); Star of Bethlehem (B); Fireweed (Dv); Arnica (Dv, Fes); Dogwood, Echinacea, Golden Ear Drops (Fes); Beech, Larch, Monterey Pine (GM); Awapuhi Melemele, Kamani, Ulua (Haii); Ashoka Tree, Radish (Him A); Hibiscus, Rippy Hillox Plant (Him I); Jonquils (NZ); Hyacinth (Pac); White Hyacinth (PF)

TRUST Bog Rosemary, Prickly Wild Rose, White Violet (Ask); Flannel Flower (Aus B); Golden Glory Grevillea (Aus L); Centuary, Red Chestnut (B); Ephedra, Saguaro Cactus, Syrian Rose (DAl); Angelica, Buttercup, Mallow (Dv); Baby Blue Eyes, Oregon Grape (Fes); Hawthorn (GM); Bamboo Orchid (Haii); Marjoram, Ragwort, Rosemary, Snowdrop, White Narcissus (Hb); Slow Match (Him A); Spinach (Ma); Camellia (Pac)

TURMOIL Red Suva Frangipani (Aus B); Ephedra (DAl); Red Clover (Fes); Tormentil (Hb); Christ's Thorn (Him A)

UNDERSTANDING PROBLEMS One-sided Wintergreen (Ask); Pine (B); Bisbee Beehive Cactus (DAl); Love Lies Bleeding (Fes); Indian Coral, Malabar Nut Flower, Neem, White Coral Tree (Him A); Raspberry (Ma); Milkmaids, Pine Drops (Peg)

UNLOVED (FEELING) Mauve Melaleuca (Aus L); Holly (B, Fes); Crown of Thorns, Mariposa Lily, Mesquite (DAl); Sea Palm (Pac)

VICTIM MENTALITY Southern Cross (Aus B); Charlock, Urchin Dryandra (Aus L); Centuary (B); Canyon Dudleya, Larkspur, Love Lies Bleeding (Fes); Coral Bean, Immortal, Ocotillo, Star Primrose, Woven Spine Pineapple Cactus (DAl); Yellow Champa (Him I); Montbretia (NZ); Mussel (Pac); Dill (PVi)

VIOLENCE Mountain Devil (Aus B); Orange Spiked Pea Flower (Aus L); Black Cohosh, Dogwood, Scarlet Monkeyflower (Fes); Stick Rorrish (Haii); Red Silk Cotton Tree (Him I); Mussel (Pac)

VULNERABILITY Angel of Protection Orchid (AK); Buffalo Gourd, Pencil Cholla Cactus, Spineless Prickly Pear (DAl); White Yarrow (Dv); Golden Yarrow, Pink Monkeyflower, Sticky Monkeyflower (Fes); Viburnum (GM); Pansy, Windflower (Hb); Yellow Yarrow (PVi)

WILL-POWER Bunchberry (Ask); Blue China Orchid (Aus L); Aloe, Coral Bean, Desert Marigold, Pencil Cholla Cactus (DAl); Box, Cayenne (Dv); Blackberry, Cayenne, Mountain Pride, Tansy (Fes); Box (GM); Hinahina-ku-kahakai (Haii); Broom, Pansy, Sunflower (Hb) Manuka (NZ); Snowdrop, Surfgrass (Pac); Ettringite (Peg)

WOMEN – ACCEPTING FEMININITY Pomegranate (Fes); Quince (Dv); Hinahina-ku-kahakai, La'au'-aila, Lehua (Haii); Rattlesnake Plantain Orchid (Peg)

– RELATING TO MEN Baby Blue Eyes (Fes); Hinahina-ku-kahakai (Haii); Rattlesnake Plantain Orchid (Peg)

– STRENGTHENING FEMININITY Canary Island Bellflower, Pumpkin, Venus Orchid (AK); Pomegranate (Fes); Queen of the Night, Star Primrose (DAl); Zucchini (Dv); Alpine Lily, Mariposa Lily (Fes); La'au'-aila, Lehua (Haii); Lady's Mantle (Hb)

WORRY Crowea (Aus B); Brown Boronia, Golden Waitsia (Aus L); Agrimony, White Chestnut (B); Jumping Cholla Cactus, Melon Loco (DAl); Filaree, Garlic (Fes); St John's Wort (Hb); Narcissus, Pipsissewa, Urchin (Pac)

❄ SPIRITUAL ❄

ABANDONED (FEELING) Mesquite, Queen of the Night, Saguaro Cactus (DAl); Angelica (Fes)

ACCEPTANCE Eucalyptus (AK); Green Fairy Orchid, Icelandic Poppy (Ask); Five Corners, Red Suva Frangipani (Aus B); Pin Cushion Hakea (Aus L); Mallow (Dv); Shooting Star (Fes); Norway Maple (GM); Chamomile (Hb); Day-blooming Jessamine (Him A); Ixora – orange, white, pink (Him I); Windflower (Pac); Eclipse (PVi)

ALIGNMENT Chiming Bells, Paper Birch (Ask); Lotus (Dv, Fes); Apple, Harebell, Sea Pink (F); Pine (GM); Hawaiian Tree, Passion Flower (Haii); Malabar Nut Flower (Him I); Fuchsite (Peg); Viridiflora (PF)

ASTRAL TRAVEL Red Lily (Aus B); Kou (Haii); Mouse Ear Chickweed (Hb)

ATTUNEMENT (HIGHER REALMS) Angel Orchid, Angel of Protection Orchid, Channeling Orchid, Deva Orchid (AK); Arnica (Dv); Angelica, Forget-me-not (Fes); Judas Tree (GM); Nana-honua, Nani-ahiahi, Pa'u-o-hiiaka (Haii); Calypso Orchid, Hydrangea (Green), Holy Thorn, Indian Pipe, Spider Lily, Tagua (Peg)

AURA White Yarrow (AK); Crowea, Fringed Violet (Aus B); Pennyroyal (Cal); Aloe Vera (Cal, Fes); Arnica, Yarrow Special Formula (Fes); Auric Protector (Gem); Panini-awa'awa (Haii); St John's Wort, Yarrow (Hb); Aura Balancing and Strengthening Formula (Him A); Aura Cleansing (Him E); Curry Leaf Tree, Lotus, Portia Tree (Him I); Pear (Ma); Aloe Eru, Dutchman's Breeches, Okenite (Peg); Snowdrop, Vanadinite (Peg); Ligustrum (PF)

AWARENESS Rosemary (AK); Forget-me-not, Mullein (Dv)

BALANCE – MALE/FEMALE Arum Lily (AK); Green Fairy Orchid, Sitka Spruce Pollen (Ask); Niu (Haii); Red Ginger (Peg)

BALANCE – SEXUALITY/SPIRITUALITY Star Primrose (DAl); Red Ginger (Peg)

BEING HERE – RESISTANCE TO Fawn Lily, Milkweed, Manzanita, Shooting Star (Fes); Herkimer Diamond (Gem); Yellow Ginger (Haii); Oriental Poppy (Hb)

BELONGING Cow Parsnip (Ask); Tall Yellow Top (Aus B); Jojoba, Milky Nipple Cactus, Star Primrose (DAl); Baby Blue Eyes, Sweet Pea (Fes); Monterey Pine (GM); Maize (Hb); Arbutus (Pac); Chin Cactus (Peg)

BLOCKED SPIRITUALITY Indian Root (DAl); Cayenne, Lotus, Star Tulip (Fes); White Hibiscus (Him A); Lemon Balm (NZ)

BODY/SOUL BALANCE Apple Rose Hybrid (AK); Pineapple Weed (Ask); Great Sallow (GM); Red Hibiscus (Him I); Gruss an Aachen (PVi)

BOUNDARIES Corn (Fes, PVi); Rhubarb (Hb); Isan (Him E); Red Rata Vine (NZ); Nymphenburg (PVi)

CATALYST Cayenne, Tansy (Fes); Gratefulness (Him E); Peach (NZ); Camellia (Pac); Curry Leaf Tree, Hooded Ladies' Tresses (Peg)

CENTRING Red Clover (AK); Buffalo Gourd, Candy Barrel Cactus, Whitehorn (DAl); Daisy (F); Indian Pink, Lotus, Yerba Santa (Fes); Sweet Chestnut (GM); Alkanet, Gypsy Rose, Potato (Hb); Well-being (Him E); Ox-eye Daisy, Viburnum (Pac)

CHAKRA BALANCE Delph (AK); Early Purple Orchid (Ba); Lady's Slipper, Lotus (Fes); Herkimer Diamond (Gem); Lilac (GM); Lilac, Rhubarb (Hb); Chakra Tonic Formula (Him A); Drum Stick Tree (Him I); Blue Witch, Hydrangea, Indian Pipe, Red Spider Lily (Peg)

CHANGE (MAJOR) Mistletoe (AK); Bauhinia, Bottlebrush (Aus B); Leopardsbane, Spring Squill (Ba); Buffalo Gourd, Tarbrush (DAl); Elder, Lawson Cypress (GM); Wiliwili (Haii); Ixora – orange, white, pink (Him I); Brown Kelp, Poison Hemlock (Pac); Okenite, Tree Opuntia, Washington Lily (Peg)

CLEANSING Delph (AK); Fireweed (Ask); White Willow (GM); Lotus (Haii)

COMMITMENT Wedding Bush (Aus B); Prickly Pear Cactus, Teddy Bear Cholla Cactus (DAl)

COMPASSION Love Orchid (AK); Rough Bluebell (Aus B); Beech (B); Immortal, Mesquite (DAl); Poison Oak, Sunflower, Yellow Star Tulip (Fes); Lucombe Oak (GM); Parval (Him A); Christ's Thorn, Sithihea (Him I); Peach (Ma)

CONFIDENCE Paper Birch (Ask); Red Oak, Spindle (GM); Erigeron Daisy, Whau (NZ)

COURAGE Cattail Pollen, Yellow Dryas (Ask); Black-eyed Susan, Borage (Fes); White Poplar (GM); Wiliwili (Haii); Peace, Summer Squash (PVi)

DEATH AND DYING Victoria Regina Orchid (AK); Forget-me-not (AK, Fes); Bottlebrush, Bush Iris (Aus B); Hackberry, Sacred Datura (DAl); Snowdrop (F); Angels Trumpet, Chrysanthemum (Fes); Blackberry (Hb)

DENIAL Wolfberry (DAl); Deerbrush, Nicotiana (Fes); Dill (PF); Sierra Rein Orchid (Peg)

DESTINY Lady's Slipper, Shooting Star (Fes)

DIGNITY Rippy Hillox Plant (Him I); Bluebonnet (PF)

DIRECTION Silver Princess (Aus B); Pencil Cholla Cactus, Spanish Bayonet Yucca, White Desert Primrose (DAl); California Wild Rose, Chrysanthemum (Fes); Glastonbury Thorn, Lawson Cypress, Tamarisk (GM); Bamboo Orchid (Haii); Gypsy Rose, Speedwell (Hb); Bourgainvillea, Malabar Nut Flower (Him I); Peace Rose (NZ); Surfgrass (Pac); Ambassador (PVi)

EMPATHY Common White Spider Orchid (Aus L); Peach (Ma)

EMPOWERMENT – GENERAL Sitka Spruce Pollen (Ask); Desert Marigold, Klein's Pencil Cholla Cactus, Saguaro Cactus, Thurber's Gilia (DAl); Laurel, Thistle (F); Norway Maple, Plum (GM); Ettringite (Peg) – **AS A WOMAN (FEMININITY)** Southern Cross (Aus B); Mala Mujer, Melon Loco, Queen of the Night (DAl); Pomegranate (Dv); Calla Lily, Mountain Pride, Pomegranate (Fes); Hinahina-ku-kahakai (Haii); Ettringite (Peg) – **AS A MAN (MASCULINITY)** Southern Cross (Aus B); Mountain Mahogany (DAl); Agrimony, Calla Lilly, Larkspur, Mountain Pride, Nicotiana, Sunflower (Fes); Goddess (Him E); Ettringite (Peg)

EMPTINESS Mauve Melaleuca, Wallflower Donkey Orchid (Aus L); Spineless Prickly Pear (DAl); Sagebush (Fes); Osier (GM)

ENLIGHTENMENT 'Ili'ahi, Lotus (Haii); Indian Paintbrush (PF)

ETHERIC BODY Sweetgrass (Ask); Panini-awa'awa (Haii); Shasta Lily, Sourgrass (Peg)

FAITH Waratah (Aus B); Harebell (F); Angelica, Baby Blue Eyes, Borage, Gorse (Fes); Bamboo Orchid (Haii); Broom (Hb); Red-hot Cat Tail (Him A)

FOCUS Iceland Poppy (Ask); Lotus (Fes, Him I); Mamane (Haii); Bourgainvillea, Temple Tree (Him I)

GETTING OUT OF YOUR OWN WAY Canyon Dudleya, Fawn Lily, Sagebrush (Fes); Hoptree, Teddy Bear Cholla Cactus (DAl); Tree of Heaven (GM); Brown Kelp (Pac); Eclipse (PVi)

GROUNDED (FEELING) Northern Twayblade (Ask); Red Lily (Aus B); Thrift (Ba); Melon Loco, Milky Nipple Cactus (DAl); Bell Heather (F); Corn, Fawn Lily, Rosemary, Shooting Star, St John's Wort, Sweet Pea (Fes); Moss Agate (Gem); Black Poplar, Persian Iron Wood (GM); Buttercup, Maize, Plantain (Hb); Narcissus, Pink Seaweed, Windflower (Pac)

GROWTH Mullein (AK); Golden Corydalis, Spiraea (Ask); Arizona White Oak, Indian Tobacco, Teddy Bear Cholla Cactus (DAl); Scotch Broom (Fes); Gorse (GM); Mango (Haii); Bindweed (Hb); Dill (NZ)

GUIDANCE Rose of Sharon (AK); Hairy Butterworth, Monk's Hood, Shooting Star (Ask); Angelica, Mullein (Fes); Tulip Tree (Him I)

HUMANITARIAN FEELINGS Amazon River (AK); Yellow Cowslip Orchid (Aus B); Common White Spider Orchid (Aus L); Ocotillo (DAl); Naupaka-kahakai (Haii); Parval (Him A); Yellow Silk Cotton Tree (Him I); Kohekohe (NZ); Yellow Rose (PF)

HUMILITY Japanese Rose (AK); Gymea Lily (Aus B); Woolly Smokebush (Aus L); Golden Rod, Yellow Silk Cotton Tree (Him A); White Coral Tree (Him I); Banana (Ma)

INCARNATION Psyche/Soul Orchid (AK); Shooting Star (Fes); Herkimer Diamond (Gem)

INDEPENDENCE Evening Star (DAl); Tree Lichen (GM)

INNER CONFLICT Blue Elf Viola (Ask); Ratany (DAl); Fawn Lily (Fes); Pear (GM); Noho Malie (Haii); Gateway (Him E)

INNER HARMONY Aloe Vera, Sun Orchid (AK); Lotus (AK, Fes); Shooting Star, Twinflower (Ask); Immortal (DAl); California Poppy, Star Tulip (Fes); Ash (GM); Red Hibiscus (Him I)

INNER STRENGTH Agave, Arizona White Oak (DAl); Penstemon (Fes); Lapis Lazuli, Moss Agate (Gem); Ash (GM); Hidden Splendor, Well Being (Him E); Day-blooming Jessamine, Rain Tree (Him I); Sunstone (Peg); Christmas Cactus (PF); Nymphenburg (PVi)

INNOCENCE Forget-me-not (Ask); Devil's Claw (DAl); Deer Bush (Fes); Lily of the Valley, Moonsnail (Pac)

INSIGHT Hoop Petticoat Daffodil (AK); Azurite (Gem); Pine (GM); Tulip Tree (Him I); Eclipse (PVi)

INTEGRATION Passion Flower, Sage, Tibetan White Rose, Wild Rose Hybrid (AK); Golden Corydalis, Opium Poppy, Sweetgale, White Spruce (Ask); Queen of the Night (DAl); Basil, Lotus, Lady's Slipper, Shatsa Daisy (Fes); Gorse, Spindle (GM); Isan (Him E); Lady Eubanksia (PF); Laze Improved, White Lightnin' (PVi)

INTEGRITY Sturt Desert Rose (Aus B); Deer Bush, Echinacea (Fes); Tree of Heaven (GM); Sithihea (Him A)

INTUITION Lamb's Quarters, White Spruce (Ask); Queen of the Night (DAl); Eyebright (Dv); Forget-me-not (Fes); Horse Chestnut, Mimosa, Stags Horn Sumach (GM); Sunflower (Hb); Neem (Him A); Viburnum (Pac)

JOURNEY (SPIRITUAL) Chocolate Orchid (AK); Mint Bush (Aus B); Teddy Bear Cholla Cactus (DAl); Lotus (Fes, Him I); Lawson Cypress (GM); Cup of Gold, Lotus (Haii); Calypso Orchid, Star Thistle (Peg)

KARMIC PROBLEMS Boab (Aus B); Wood Anemone (Ba); Forget-me-not (Fes); Bamboo Orchid, Kukui (Haii); Rose Campion (PF)

LEARNING LIFE'S LESSONS Sage (Fes); Magnolia (GM); Coral Root – spotted (Peg)

LETTING GO Dampiera, Wallflower Donkey Orchid (Aus L); Agave, Indian Root, Rainbow Cactus, Strawberry Cactus (DAl); Bleeding Heart, Sage Brush (Fes); Crack Willow, Privet, Tree Lichen (GM); Marsh Woundwort, Ragwort (Hb); Leg Go (Him E); Salal, Sea Palm (Pac); Sycamore (Peg)

LISTENING (INNER VOICE) Higher Self Orchid, Mullein (AK); Twinflower (Ask); Candy Barrel Cactus (DAl); Calendula, Star Tulip (Fes); Orange Ruffles (PVi)

MATERIALISM Hedge hog Cactus (DAl); Silverweed (F); Chrysanthemum, Hound's Tongue, Trillium (Fes)

MEDITATION (AID) Horsetail, Paper Birch (Ask); Angelsword (Aus B); White Nymph Waterlily (Aus L); Blackberry (Dv); Angel's Trumpet, Fawn Lily, Star Tulip (Fes); Lotus (Fes, Him A, Him I); Stag's Horn Sumach, Tulip Tree (GM); 'Ili'ahi, Koa (Haii); Bourgainvillea (Haii, Him A); Chamomile, Lavender, Nasturtium, Salpglossis, Scarlet Pimpernel (Hb); Blue Dragon, Isan, Lotus (Him E); Temple Tree (Him I); Deer's Tongue (Peg)

MERIDIAN BALANCE Northern Lady's Slipper (Ask); Silver Maple (GM)

MOTIVATION Opium Poppy, Tundra Rose (Ask); Silver Princess (Aus B); Mountain Mahogany (DAl); California Wild Rose, Tansy (Fes); Mast Tree (Him I)

NATURE AWARENESS/ATTUNEMENT Alpine Azalea, Chiming Bells, Commandra, Green Bells of Ireland, Green Bog Orchid, Moschatel, Northern Twayblade, Spiraea (Ask); Deer Bush (B); Sweet Corn (Dv); Poison Oak, Yellow Star Tulip (Fes); Ash, Lilac, Rowan, Whitebeam, Yellow Buckeye (GM); Harebell (Hb); Gilia Scarlet (Peg)

NURTURING Grass of Parnassus, Spiraea (Ask); Hedgehog Cactus, Mariposa Lily (DAl); Mariposa Lily, Quince (Fes); Rose Quartz (Gem); Tulip Tree (GM)

ONENESS (UNIVERSAL) Green Fairy Orchid (Ask); Organ Pipe Cactus, Queen of the Night (DAl); Crack Willow (GM)

OPENING UP French Lavender, Passion Flower (AK); Icelandic Poppy (Ask); Pink

Mulla Mulla (Aus B); Dampiera (Aus L); Dandelion, Lotus, Passion flower (Dv); Lime, Scots Pine (F); Mugwort (Fes); Ilima (Haii); Jacob's Ladder (Hb); Soap Nut Tree (Him I)

PAST (LETTING GO) Bottlebrush (Aus B); Cape Bluebell (Aus L); Honeysuckle (B, Fes); Marsh Thistle (Ba); Indian Tobacco, Wolfberry (DAl); Rowan (F); Chrysanthemum, Forget-me-not (Fes); Mulberry (GM); Marsh Woundwort, Mugwort, Rose Bay Willow Herb (Hb); Prickly Poppy (Peg)

PAST LIFE (OVER-SPILL) Monk's Hood (Ba); Kukui, Noho Malie (Haii); Vinca Alba (Him I); Agave Yaquinana, Caterpillar Plant, Sunstone (Peg)

PAST LIFE PROBLEMS Past Life Orchid (AK); Black and White Spruce (Ask); Monk's Hood (Ba); Green Rose (Cal); Evening Primrose (Fes); Monterey Pine (GM); Naupaka-kahakai, Ohelo, Ulei (Haii); Gul Mohar, Red-hot Cat Tail (Him A); Vinca Alba (Him I); Agave Yaquiana, Everlasting, Prickly Poppy, Sunstone (Peg)

PEACE (INNER) Chiming Bells (Ask); Cow Parsnip (Ask); White Nymph Waterlily (Aus L); Agrimony (B); Scottish Primrose (F); Sage (Fes); Black Poplar, Holly, Italian Alder (GM); Koa (Haii); Lavender (Hb); Butterfly Lily, Gul Mohar, Indian Coral (Him A); Swallow Wort (Him I); Pear (Ma); Lasiandra (NZ); Sweet Bell Pepper (PVi)

PERCEPTION Cane Cholla Cactus, Indian Root, Sacred Datura (DAl); Sagebush, Shatsa Daisy (Fes); Kou (Haii); Brown Kelp (Pac); Choke Cherry (Peg)

PERSEVERANCE Teddy Bear Cholla Cactus (DAl); Mountain Pride (Fes); Washington Lily (Peg)

PERSPECTIVE Cane Cholla Cactus (DAl); Rabbitbrush (Fes); Kou (Haii); Green Rein Orchid (Peg)

POWER Sitka Spruce Pollen, Soapberry (Ask); Desert Marigold, Spineless Prickly Pear (DAl); Mountain Pride, Quince, Trillium (Fes); Plum (GM); Chives, Dill (PVi)

PREPARATION Mint Bush (Aus B); Marsh Woundwort (Hb)

PRETENDING Cane Cholla Cactus (DAl); Canyon Dudleya (Fes)

PROTECTION – GENERAL Angel of Protection Orchid, White Yarrow (AK); White Violet (Ask); Angelsword (Aus B); Sage (Cal); Angelica (Dv); Mountain Pennyroyal (Fes); Yarrow (Fes, Hb); Turquoise (Gem); Italian Alder (GM); Kamani (Haii); Monk's Hood, St John's Wort (Hb); Banyan Tree (Him I); Urchin (Pac) **– FROM PSYCHIC ATTACK** Yarrow (Ask); Fringed Violet, Grey Spider Flower (Aus B); Pennyroyal (Cal); Red Clover (Dv); Garlic, Purple Monkeyflower, St John's Wort (Fes); Yew (GM); Elder (Hb); IUG Kenya (IUG); Pa'u-o-hi-iaka, Ti (Haii); Tomato (Ma); Urchin (Pac); Vanilla (PF)

PSYCHO-SPIRITUAL BALANCE Victoria Regina Orchid, White Lily (AK); Green Rose (Cal); Creeping Thistle (Peg)

PURPOSE Ladies' Tresses, Paper Birch, Shooting Star (Ask); Silver Princess (Aus B); Hoptree, Soapberry Yucca, Spineless Prickly Pear (DAl); Apple, Bell Heather (F); Buttercup (Fes); Great Sallow (GM); Bourgainvillea, Plumeria (Haii); Geranium, Monk's Hood (Hb); Avocado (Ma); California Buckeye, Fuchsite, Pegasus Orchid Cactus, Sulcorebutia Cactus (Peg); Viridiflora (PF); Ambassador (PVi)

QUEST Red Oak (GM); Vinca Rosa (Him I)

QUIETNESS Twinflower (Ask); Strawberry Tree (GM)

REALITY Willow (Ask); Red Lily (Aus B); Angelica (Fes); Oak (GM)

REBUILDING LIFE Prickly Wild Rose (Ask); Cowkicks (Aus L); Echinacea (Fes); Coconut Palm, Rippy Hillox Plant (Him I)

RELATIONSHIPS Heart Orchid (AK); Papaya (Haii); Pagoda Tree (Him I); Pegasus Orchid Cactus (Peg)

RELEASING OLD PATTERNS Blueberry Pollen (Ask); Marsh Thistle (Ba); Foothills Paloverde, Immortal, Tar Bush, Whitehorn (DAl); Fairy Lantern (Fes); Azurite (Gem); Lime (GM); Rose Bay Willow Herb (Hb)

SELF-ACCEPTANCE Spring Gold (AK); Tamarack (Ask); Five Corners, Philotheca (Aus B); Aloe, Hedgehog Cactus, Ocotillo, Teddy Bear Cholla Cactus (DAl); Black-eyed Susan (Dv); Holy Thorn (F); Baby Blue Eyes, Buttercup, Purple Monkeyflower (Fes); White Willow (GM); Cornflower, Heather (Hb); Swallow Wort, Wood Apple Tree (Him I); Windflower (Pac); Milkmaids (Peg)

SELF-DOUBT Alpine Azalea (Ask); Happy Wanderer, Snake Vine (Aus L); Evening Star (DAl); Buttercup, Mullein (Dv); Bell Heather (F); Elder (GM); Rippy Hillox Plant (Him I)

SELF-FORGIVENESS Foothills Paloverde (DAl); Birch (GM); Screw Pine, Uksi (Him I); Prickly Poppy (Peg)

SELF-HEALING Co-ordination Orchid (AK); Self Heal (AK, Fes); Bog Rosemary (Ask); Aloe

(DAl); Gean Wood Cherry, Norway Maple (GM); Creeping Thistle (Peg)

SHADOW (DARK SIDE) Cinnamon Rose (AK); Sweet Chestnut (B, Fes, B); Moss (Ba); Cardon, Crown of Thorns, Mesquite (DAl); Black Co-hosh, Scarlet Monkeyflower (Fes); Ohelo (Haii); Heather (Hb); Indian Gooseberry (Him I)

STABILITY Lapis Lazuli, Moss Agate (Gem); Ash (GM); Gruss an Aachen, Royal Highness (PVi)

SOUL – AWAKENING Bush Iris (Aus B); Black-eyed Susan, Cayenne (Dv) – **DAMAGE** Slow Match Tree (Him I); Comfrey (PVi) – **LISTEN-ING TO** Jacob's Ladder (Ask); Angelsword (Aus B); Mesquite, White Desert Primrose (DAl); California Poppy (Dv); Mullein, Yellow Star Tulip (Fes); Lapis Lazuli (Gem); Great Scallop (GM); Nana-honua (Haii); Malabar Nut Flower, Tulip Tree (Him I)

SPIRITUAL BALANCE Lotus (Fes, AK); Chiming Bell (Ask); Pine (GM); Malabar Nut Flower (Him I)

SPIRITUAL GLAMOUR California Poppy, Canyon Dudleya (Fes); Thanksgiving Cactus (Haii); Ragoon Creeper, Red Silk Cotton Tree (Him A)

SUBTLE BODY BALANCE Delph (AK); Grass of Parnassus, Lady's Slipper, Sweetgrass (Ask); Sea Pink (F); Lotus (Fes); Herkimer Diamond, Turquoise (Gem); Privet (GM); Sun Plant (Him I); Wisteria (PF)

SUBCONSCIOUS/SUPERCONSCIOUS Rainbow Cactus (DAl); Lime (GM); Swallow Wort (Him I)

SURRENDER Arizona White Oak, Hoptree,

Prickly Pear Cactus (DAl); Snowdrop (F); Angel's Trumpet, Love Lies Bleeding (Fes); Naupaka Kahakai (Haii)

THERAPIST'S BALANCE Lady's Slipper, Northern Lady's Slipper (Ask); Leafless Orchid (Aus L); Eyebright (Dv); Calendula, Mallow (Fes); Strawberry Tree (GM); Healing (Him E); Leopard Lily (Peg)

TRANSCENDENCE Immortal, Rainbow Cactus, Wolfberry (DAl); Birch, Stonecrop (F); Love Lies Bleeding (Fes); Lotus (Him I); Grape (Ma)

TRANSFORMATION Mistletoe (AK); Chiming Bells, Fireweed, River Beauty (Ask); Bottlebrush (Aus B); Bisbee Beehive Cactus, Sacred Datura (DAl); Black-eyed Susan, Cayenne, Fireweed, Mallow (Dv); Love Lies Bleeding (Fes); Elder, Tamarisk (GM); Koa (Haii); Day-blooming Jessamine (Him A); Butterfly Lily, Sulcorebutia Cactus, Tree Opuntia (Peg)

TRANSITION Cow Parsnip (Ask); Bauhinia, Bottlebrush (Aus B); Rainbow Cactus, Ratany (DAl); Stonecrop (F); Angel's Trumpet, Filaree, Mugwort, Star Tulip (Fes); Gateway (Him E); Hairy Butterworth (Him I); Poison Hemlock (Pac); Gruss an Aachen (PVi)

TRANSPARENT SHIELD Coconut Palm, White Yarrow (AK); IUG Kenya (IUG); Vanadinite (Peg)

TRUTH Bladderwort, Cattail Pollen (Ask); Ratany, Syrian Rue (DAl); Plane Tree (GM); Ilima, Mamane (Haii)

UNCONDITIONAL LOVE Delph, Horn of Plenty Orchid, Sarah of Fleet (AK); Alpine Azalea, Harebell, Sphagnum Moss (Ask); Mountain Devil, Rough Bluebell (Aus B);

Snake Bush (Aus L); Cardon, Crown of Thorns, Desert Holly (DAl); Night Blooming Water Lily (Haii); Bourgainvillea (Him I); Grape (Ma); Washington Lily (Peg); India Hawthorn (PF)

UNDERSTANDING WHY Psyche/soul Orchid (AK); Sweet Chestnut (B); Sage (Dv); Birch (F); Rowan (GM); Scarlet Pimpernel (Hb); Coral root spotted (Peg)

UNIVERSAL BEING (CONNECTION) Channeling Orchid (AK); Bog Rosemary (Ask); Star Tulip (Fes); Ilima, Nana-honua, Passion Flower, Pa'u-o-hi-iaka (Haii); Tulip Tree (Him I); Yellow Silk Cotton Tree (Him I); Calypso Orchid, Christ Thorn (Peg)

UNIVERSAL TIMING Mountain Mahogany (DAl)

UNIVERSAL WILL Hoptree (DAl)

VISION Soapwort (Ba); Birch (F); Queen Anne's Lace (Fes); Hawks Weed, Nasturtium (Hb); Tulip Tree (Him I); Ox-eye Daisy (Pac)

VISUALIZATION Blackberry (Dv); Lotus (Fes); Hydrangea-green (Peg)

WISDOM Lotus (AK, Fes); Black Spruce, Silken Spruce Pollen, White Spruce (Ask); Scots Pine (F); California Poppy, Sage, Saguaro (Fes); Hazel, Tree of Heaven, Tree Lichen (GM); Sage (Hb); Indian Coral, Spotted Gliciridia (Him A); Puriri (NZ); California Baylaurel, Elephant's Head (Peg)

WORTHLESSNESS Yellow Mimosa (AK); Candy Barrel Cactus, Hedgehog Cactus, Immortal, White Desert Primrose (DAl); Rose Quartz (Gem); Elder (GM); Daffodil (Hb); Sun Plant (Him I)

SIX

SPECIFIC RECIPES FOR YOUR OWN USE

*If you do not feel sufficiently confident about choosing
flower essences to make your own personal prescription, here are some
recipes to help with common ailments for you to try.*

NOTE   All the recipes in this book are for your personal use. They are simplified versions of my professional recipes, which are also available directly from me (see Useful Addresses).

Some of the Pegasus remedies mentioned in these recipes are not included in the Encyclopaedia section of this book, but are available from Pegasus Products (*see* Useful Addresses).

❋ MAKING UP A REMEDY ❋

To make up your own remedies you will need several standard 20-ml tinted dropper bottles (available from most chemists), some spring water, a little brandy and some adhesive labels. It is a good idea to label each bottle with details like your name, the date you made the combination, a brief description of what this particular mix is for and the flower essences it contains.

- Rinse through a 20-ml stopper bottle with spring water.
- For each recipe, put 2 drops of each of the essences listed into the bottle.

- Add 1 teaspoon of brandy to the mix. This is used purely as a preservative. If you have a sensitivity to alcohol you may wish to use apple cider vinegar, vegetable glycerine or clear honey as a substitute for the brandy.
- Fill to the brim with spring water.

This is your course of treatment for the next two months. After a month it may be a good idea to stop taking the essence and review your condition. The emotional state, physical discomfort or other issue you were working on may have eased or even disappeared. If not, continue taking the combination until the course is completed. It is worth remembering that even when you have finished taking the remedy it will still be acting in your system for some time.

On regaining your balance there may be no need for further remedies for the time being. Alternatively you may become aware of another issue that is troubling you. In this case you will need to select appropriate remedies for your next prescription.

FIGHTING OFF DISEASE AND STRESS

STRESS BUSTER

- Black-eyed Susan (Aus B)
- Pink Fairy Orchid (Aus L)
- Peanut (Cal)
- Fairy Duster (DAl)
- White Carnation (PF)

An excellent de-stressor for when you are feeling over-stimulated and overwhelmed – burnt out, in short – by stressful situations and environments.

Brings calmness, filtering out the stress from all situations. Restores balance and resilience.

You can add 2 drops of Office Flower (Him A) to combat stressful office environments.

ENERGY BOOSTER

- Banksia Robur (Aus B)
- Leafless Orchid (Aus L)
- Cherry (Cal)
- Forsythia (Hb)
- Vanilla (PF)

A re-energizer and revitalizer for when you feel drained, tired or fatigued.

Restores deep-seated vitality and helps you to learn to work with consistency to avoid becoming depleted either physically, emotionally or mentally.

You can add 2 drops each of Bay (GM) and Vital

Spark (Him E) for extra potency.

ENVIRONMENTAL PROTECTOR

- Grass of Parnassus (Ask)
- Yarrow (Ask, Fes)
- Dill (Fes)
- Indian Pink (Fes)
- Viridiflora (PF)

For those feeling overwhelmed and sensitive to a city environment, whose nerves are frazzled by the fast and frantic pace of life. For those living and working in crowded and polluted surroundings. Vulnerability to electromagnetic radiation from computers, fluorescent lights, pollution and other noxious substances often manifests as allergic reactions.

This boosts and protects the energetic system against all kinds of environmental hazards. Eases stress and allows you to remain calm, centred and grounded.

Add 2 drops of Pink Fairy Orchid (Aus L) for extra potency.

PROTECTION FROM CHEMICAL POLLUTANTS

- Portage Glacier (Ask)*
- Sweet Grass (Ask)
- Fringed Violet (Aus B)
- Spruce (Cal)
- Lotus (Fes)
- Crossandra (PF)

This combination cleanses and detoxifies the system of environmental pollutants such as chemical residues and heavy metals, clearing vibrational debris and impurities from the body, mind and emotions. It also offers protection from pollution, rebuilds a suppressed immune system to alleviate allergic problems and guards against bacterial infections.

Add 2 drops each of Star Tulip (Fes) and Lily (PF) for extra potency.

*Portage Glacier Environmental Essence is available from Alaskan Flower Essences

IMMUNE BOOST

- K9 (AK)
- Macrocarpa (Aus B)
- Koenign van Daenmark (Cal)
- Echinacea (Haii)
- Celery (PVi)

Boosts immune resistance to all kinds of infections and speeds recovery. Restores balance to the immune system when it is over-stressed or over-worked; gives you greater mental control over your immune system. Builds resistance to auto-toxicity, enhances the body's natural defence network and invigorates the production of white blood cells – interferon – to fight viral or bacterial attack and infection which has over-powered the system.

Add 2 drops each of Rata Berries White (NZ) and Snapdragon (PF) for extra potency.

INFECTION FIGHTER

- Spinifex (Aus B)
- Pansy (Cal)
- Lungwort (Cal)
- Nasturtium (Dv)
- Drum Stick (Him A)

For helping to shake off viral infections such as colds and flu.

Eases the chills and aching associated with the pre-influenza state. Helps fight off infection by clearing viruses out of the system. Especially beneficial for respiratory and throat infections as well as fevers.

Add 2 drops each of Jasmine (Cal) and Tomato (PVi) for extra potency.

ANAESTHETIC CLEARING MIX

- Bottlebrush (Cal)
- Skullcap (Cal)
- Spruce (Cal)
- Morning Glory (Cal, Fes)
- Red Carnation (PF)
- White Hyacinth (PF)

Clears the effect of anaesthetic from the system. Acts as a tonic for a stressed nervous system and stimulates the cleansing of impurities and toxicity from the blood and lymphatic system. Releases the subtle anatomy from the shock and trauma of going through an operation. Enhances resistance to infection from bacteria and viruses, as immunity is weakened by an operation of any kind.

Add 2 drops each of Koenign van Daenmark (Cal) and Echinacea (PF) to boost immunity. To clear antibiotics from the system, use Coralroot Spotted (Peg).

HELP FOR SPECIFIC HEALTH PROBLEMS

ALLERGY ANTIDOTE

- K9 (AK)
- Green Rose (Cal)
- Eucalyptus (Fes)
- Wood Apple Tree (Him I)
- Lantana (PF)

For hayfever, asthma and other allergic problems.

Builds resistance to itching, watery eyes, runny nose and flu-type symptoms typical of an allergic reaction to grasses, pollens and so forth. Combats the breathing difficulties of asthma.

Add 2 drops each of Koenign van Daenmark (Cal) and Carrot (PF) for extra potency.

DIGESTIVE SOOTHER

- Paw Paw (Aus B)
- Sage (Cal)
- Chamomile (Dv, Fes)
- Curry Leaf (Him A)
- Jujube Tree (Him I)

For digestive upsets, nervous stomach, tension in the solar plexus, poor digestion, hyperacidity, ulcers and eating disorders.

Calms the stomach, aids digestion, promotes enzyme activity and assimilation of nutrients.

Add 2 drops each of California Pitcher Plant (Fes) and Moss Rose (PF) for extra potency.

FIRST AID

- **Fireweed (Ask)**
- **Waratah (Aus B)**
- **Cowkicks (Aus L)**
- **Arnica (Fes)**
- **Ashoka Flower and Tree (Him A)**
- **Jonquils (NZ)**
- **Grape Hyacinth (Pac)**

For shock, trauma and accidents.

Works on all levels – physical, mental and emotional – helping to rebuild them after shattering experiences. Clears grief, releases deeply held pain in the body after injury and trauma, restores the flow of energy and provides emotional stability in times of extreme stress.

CLARE'S FLORAL COMPLEXION CREAM

To an aqueous cream base, which is available from most chemists, add:

- **3 drops each of these essential aromatherapy oils:**
  Chamomile
  Jasmine
  Rose
- **Plus 2 drops of each of the following flower essences:**
  Billy Goat Plum (Aus B)
  Grapefruit (Cal)
  Luffa (Cal)
  Aloe Vera (Fes)
  Salvia (PF)

HEADACHE AND MIGRAINE

- **Menzies Banksia (Aus L)**
- **Clove (Cal)**
- **Feverfew (Cal)**
- **Green Rose (Cal)**
- **Narcissus (PF)**

For stress-related, tension-type headaches, migraines, and the neuralgia associated with menstruation.

Add 2 drops each of Black-eyed Susan (Aus B) and Crown of Thorns (Peg) for extra potency.

INSOMNIA

- **Macrocarpa (Aus B)**
- **Licorice (Cal)**
- **Valerian (Dv)**
- **St John's Wort (Fes)**
- **Swallow Wort (Him A)**

For insomnia and disturbed sleep.

An excellent tranquillizer bringing deep harmonizing sleep. Refreshes and recharges your whole being with vitality. Eases hyperactivity, excessive worry and fears in the subconscious, restlessness and nightmares.

JET LAG

- **Mulla Mulla (Aus B)**
- **Sundew (Aus B)**
- **Ylang Ylang (Cal)**
- **Thyme (GM)**
- **Speedwell (Hb)**

For preventing and easing jet lag, typified by fatigue and feelings of disorientation.

Protects you during air travel and realigns your system on all levels to reduce sensations of disorientation.

PRE-MENSTRUAL RELIEF

- **She Oak (Aus B)**
- **Evening Primrose (Cal)**
- **Mala Mijer (DAl)**
- **Pomegranate (Fes)**
- **Indian Almond (Him I)**
- **Japanese Magnolia (PF)**

For pre-menstrual symptoms caused by hormonal imbalance.

Eases over-emotional, agitated and irritable feelings, fluid retention and headaches. Aids absorption of iron, enhancing your strength and stamina during menstruation. Helps women to accept and accentuate their natural femininity.

Add 2 drops of Feverfew (Cal) for extra potency.

To tailor this mix for the menopause, add 2 drops each of Gooseberry (Cal) and Phytollica Diocia (Peg).

SUBTLE BODY PROTECTION

AURA PROTECTION AND REPAIR REMEDY

- **White Yarrow (AK)**
- **Fringed Violet (Aus B)**
- **Snowplant or Aloe Eru (Peg)**

A combination that repairs and mends holes in the aura, strengthening, enhancing and protecting the auric field.

Add 2 drops each of Wild Fennel (NZ) and Ligustrum (PF) for extra potency.

SUBTLE BODY HARMONIZER

- **Lotus (AK, Fes)**
- **Sweetgrass (Ask)**
- **Swamp Onion (Peg)**

A combination to clear blockages and discharge toxicity from the subtle bodies, bringing them all into correct alignment.

Add 2 drops of Live Forever (GM) for extra potency.

CHAKRA BALANCE

NOTE As a general rule of thumb, flowers that are the same colour as a certain chakra will benefit that particular energy centre (see Chapter 2 for a list of the chakras and their associated colours). The effects will also spill over into those areas of the body linked with that chakra.

- **Lady's Slipper (Ask)**
- **Sweetgale (Ask)**
- **Lotus (Him A)**
- **Drum Stick Tree (Him I)**
- **Viridiflora (PF)**

Helps to re-balance and restore smooth functioning to all the chakras.

Add 2 drops of Lilac (GM) and Hydrangea (Green) (Peg) for extra potency.

MERIDIAN RE-BALANCE

- **Sika Spruce Pollen (Ask)**
- **Silver Maple (GM)**
- **Tobacco (Cal)**

A potent remedy for clearing blockages in these energy channels, ensuring a smooth flow of qi and generally re-balancing the entire meridian system.

Add 2 drops each of Gladiola and Trumpet Vine-Nepal (Peg) for extra potency.

IMMUNOFLUIDIUM

- **Bottlebrush (Cal)**
- **Manzanita (Fes)**
- **Bells of Ireland (Peg)**

Strengthens, activates and binds the immunofluidium, improving the flow of nourishment to the cells. Aids in building immunity against bacterial infection by activating and stimulating the white blood corpuscles to detect and destroy viral and bacterial invaders.

Add 2 drops each of Paw Paw and Pokeweed (Peg) for extra potency.

ADDICTIONS

ANTI-ADDICTION REMEDY

- Blue China Orchid (Aus L)
- Morning Glory (AK, Cal, Fes)
- IUG Kenya (Gem)
- Nirjara (Him E)
- Rose Damaceria Bifera (Peg)

This is a basic mix for the addictive personality facing and dealing with the reasons behind addiction.

Releases patterns of abuse present in the general consciousness, strengthens the will to fight and break free of addictive habits, negates the need for stimulants. Detoxifies the system on all levels, especially focusing on the nervous system. Cleanses the aura and rehabilitates the whole energy system, leaving it refreshed and sparkling. Offers overall support in addiction therapy.

Add 2 drops each of Tundra Twayblade (Ask) and Spruce (Cal) for extra potency.

WITHDRAWAL REMEDY

The basic Anti-addiction Remedy (above) can be tailored towards specific addictions by adding 2 drops each of any or all of the following essences:

- Pennyroyal (AK, Cal, Fes)
- Sundew (Aus B)
- Skullcap (Cal)
- Californian Poppy (Fes)
- Sagebush (Fes)

This combination is for undoing the damage caused by heavy overuse of drugs. It repairs any deterioration in the nervous system, particularly that caused by morphine, counters 'spaced out' feelings, and encourages the letting go of habit patterns and lifestyles contributing to drug abuse, especially the tendency towards escapism. Mends holes in the aura resulting from drug abuse.

Add 2 drops of Red Lily (Aus B) for extra potency.

GIVE UP SMOKING

- Bo Tree (Cal)
- Tobacco (Cal)

Add 2 drops of each essence to the basic Anti-addiction Remedy.

Assists the will to give up smoking, providing emotional support. Re-oxygenates, repairs and improves the condition of the lungs after the long-term effects of smoke inhalation.

You may add Drum Stick (Him A) and Babies' Breath (PF) for any congestion and breathing difficulties.

KICKING CAFFEINE

- Skullcap (Cal)
- Coffee (Cal, Haii)

Add 2 drops of each essence to the basic Anti-addiction Remedy.

Clears the effects of caffeine from the nervous system, alleviating any deterioration due to long-term use of caffeine. Strengthens and detoxifies the overall energetic pattern of the liver. Revitalizes will-power when you are tempted to indulge.

ALCOHOL OVERUSE

- Avocado (Cal)
- Pennyroyal (Cal; Fes)
- Angelica (Cal, Fes)

Add 2 drops of each essence to the basic Anti-addiction Remedy.

NOTE Do not use extra alcohol or brandy as a base.

Helps to bring clearer insight into and understanding of the problems that lead to alcohol abuse. Cleanses the blood, protects the liver and kidneys and strengthens and repairs the etheric body, which can be damaged by alcohol's loosening effect on the

subtle bodies.
If you are only suffering from a typical hangover

after drinking too much at once, a good essence to take is Soberup (Him E).

❋ HAND PICKING YOUR OWN ESSENCES ❋

An ideal remedy can be created from the flowers growing in your own garden, suggests Ian White of Australian Bush Flower Essences.

Before picking and preparing the flowers it is important to feel still and calm, so if possible practise some form of meditation.

When searching for flowers in the garden choose those in full bloom with an intense, vibrant colour. Rinse a bowl with salt water, fill it with spring water and float the flowers in the bowl for 2–3 hours in the sunshine. After this time, or when the blooms have become limp, lift them from the liquid with a twig and return them to the soil.

This is your flower essence, made from your immediate environment and will help you to be more in tune with your surroundings.

- **To make the Mother Tincture – use ½ flower essence and ½ brandy.**
- **To make the Stock Essence – use ⅔ brandy and ⅓ spring water, then add 7 drops of Mother Tincture to every 25 ml.**
- **To make Dosage Bottles – use ¾ spring water and ¼ brandy, then add 7 drops of Stock Essence.**
- **Take 7 drops of this dosage essence morning and evening for two weeks.**

SEVEN

FLOWERS TO THE RESCUE

Case studies

❋ ENERGY MEDICINE ❋

Flower essences are unique in their ability to restore and enhance a sense of total well-being in mind, body and spirit.

Unlike most other remedies, flower essences act as catalysts to re-balance the body's vital energy. In doing so they provide the perfect antidote to stress-related upsets.

It is clear that stress in all its different guises disrupts and diminishes our natural life-force. Feeling tired and depleted, for example, is a sure sign that the body's energies have been thrown out of kilter. Upsets at this level inevitably precede other kinds of niggling minor ills and may eventually lead to more serious conditions.

We may take a holiday to escape the stresses of life when we start to feel run down. This temporarily recharges the batteries, but it will not get to the root of the problem. It is important that we redress the ingrained imbalance, which may originate and be linked to any shock or trauma that occurred many years ago.

Healers blessed with the ability to 'tap into' the body's energy may be able to bring all the systems back into balance. The problem with this is that we have to rely on someone else to rekindle our sense of well-being. The beauty of flower essences is that they have the power to evoke such changes. This means that you alone become responsible for inspiring your own happiness and good health.

To preserve an energetic equilibrium, we also have to become aware of those aspects of our personality and behaviour which are likely to upset the balance. Impatient people, for instance, who are easily irritated by the slowness or incompetence of others, merely agitate their own energy systems and always will – unless they find a way of tempering their impatience.

Many of these subtle remedies act on the mind, easing all kinds of emotional and mental turbulence. Feelings such as fear, guilt, anger, anxiety and irritability do not only detract from the pleasure of living. If left unchecked, they slowly and insidiously wear down the body's resistance to illness, leaving us vulnerable to all kinds of health problems. Negative, distracting emotions also cloud our vision making it difficult for us to see or understand our special role in life, so hindering any kind of spiritual development.

It should be stressed that flower essences are by no means cure-alls. They work best at nipping potential problems in the bud, so preventing illnesses from arising in the first place. However, these gentle remedies are also helpful at times when a more direct approach is required. Orthodox drugs, acting at the physical level, alleviate symptoms but do not give rise to a real sense of well-being.

Tranquillizers may ease discomfort by distancing us from reality and dulling our reaction to stress, but they do not provide us with the tools we need for coping with and overcoming it.

For complete healing it is necessary to instil feelings of harmony and balance in mind, body and spirit. This is where flower essences come to the rescue.

This scale of remedies (below) shows the difference between the various forms of medicine available to us.

The further up the scale you go, the more far-reaching are the benefits. Pharmaceutical drugs provoke profound physical changes, but they do not touch our emotional or spiritual well-being. In terms of our energy system, their effect can be likened to a sledgehammer, whose shattering impact can actually get in the way of complete healing.

In contrast, flower essences act at the higher emotional, mental and spiritual levels before filtering into the body. When taken in

SCALE OF REMEDIES

CLASSIFICATION	REMEDY/MEDICINE	MODE OF ACTION/SIDE-EFFECTS
Vibrational	Flower Essences	Acting at the subtle, emotional/psychological and spiritual energy levels, filtering down to the physical – no toxic side-effects.
Vibrational	Gems	Acting at the physical and subtle levels occasionally heightening symptoms – cleansing effect.
Like with like	Homoeopathy	Physical effect with reference to the emotional and psychological. Some side-effects and heightening of symptoms before they clear.
Natural	Aromatherapy (essential oils)	Natural chemicals with gentle influence on physical system with emotional/psychological benefits.
Natural	Herbal medicine	Natural chemicals with gentle physical effects.
Synthetic	Pharmaceutical drugs	Basic physical level with toxic physical and subtle side-effects.

conjunction with other forms of medicine, flower essences enhance their benefits and at the same time clear away any unwanted side-effects provoked by the more physical or 'denser' types of medicine. These gentle remedies can be used successfully alongside prescribed drugs to speed recovery from accidents or operations and help you overcome all kinds of disease. They will also bring benefit to those who are trying to wean themselves off anti-depressants, sleeping pills and other mood-elevating drugs.

❋ HOW DO FLOWER ESSENCES ❋ WORK THEIR WONDERS?

In many healing traditions, our natural disposition is believed to be one of perfect health and happiness. Unfortunately, all kinds of shock and stress conspire to shift us from this state of grace.

Given the right impetus, self-healing can be kicked into gear.

Flower essences act as catalysts in order to bring our energies back into balance so that we can begin to reach the potential for perfection which resides within our energetic blueprint. They have this capacity because they are able to vibrate at frequencies close to those of our own subtle energies. Vibrational flower essences are unique in their general effect of realigning and pulling the subtle anatomy back into order so the self-healing process can begin. They also act in a very specific way, by travelling to the area or areas most in need of attention.

The ideal combination of flower essences should be matched to your individual energetic blueprint. This sets up a sympathetic resonance, a dynamic conversation which constantly reminds the body of how it really should be. It's like sounding a chord that brings all the notes into perfect harmony.

THE ESSENCE PATHWAY

Flower essences appear to follow a particular pathway through the subtle anatomy. After a few drops are swallowed, the essence is taken up by the bloodstream before moving directly to the meridians, the energy channels which feed the life-force or qi into the body. The meridians form an energetic interface between the higher frequency subtle bodies and the physical body. From here the essences' life-force either enters the various chakras and subtle bodies or returns to the cells in the physical body.

Because of their ethereal nature, flower essences may at first be attracted to the subtle bodies. From here their beneficial vibrations may filter down into the physical body through the etheric body, chakras and the skin. However, a flower essence will also be instantly drawn to any place where vibrational imbalance exists. These areas act like a sponge, literally soaking up the essences' healing energy. Re-balancing occurs as toxicity, in the form of disharmonious frequencies, is flushed from the system. Flower remedies are particularly potent in inducing changes in the chakras and subtle bodies, although some also directly influence the physical body. The ultimate therapeutic action depends at which energetic level the being is out of balance.

These remedies also enhance the connection between spirit, mind and body. They facilitate the flow of information from the Higher Self or inner voice, which always knows what is best for us, so we become are far less likely to fall victim to emotional and physical problems in the first place. In other words, the remedies actually help to prevent the kind of problems that arise from ignoring what we instinctively know is right.

❋ READING THE SIGNS: THE BODY PHYSICAL ❋

For many people physical symptoms are the first sure sign that something is wrong. Seemingly minor problems such as headaches, stomach upsets or colds are the body's way of alerting you to the fact that you need to take steps to redress any imbalance. Such symptoms do not go away if they are ignored. They simply get worse and may spill into another system, giving rise to yet another source of physical discomfort.

To make it easier to recognize the source of your symptoms we must now look at the distinctive systems of the body. It is important to bear in mind, however, that all these systems are interconnected and that each exerts a profound influence over the others.

THE NERVOUS SYSTEM

The nervous system is rather like the body's telecommunication system because it is responsible for transmitting information around the body. It is composed of millions of tiny nerve cells called neurones which communicate with each other using weak electrical impulses. These cells are bundled together into fibres which spread, like branches, to form a vast and intricate network throughout the body.

The main branch runs from the brain, which masterminds the whole system, down through the spine. The brain assesses all the information coming into the body via the senses, then decides what action to take. For this reason the nervous system plays a vital role in enabling us to respond and adapt to ever-changing environmental conditions.

The nervous system is split into two parts, one we can control voluntarily (the voluntary system), and another which apparently functions below the level of consciousness (the autonomic system).

The Autonomic System

The autonomic system has received a great deal of attention in recent years because of its link with stress. It is divided into two branches, the 'activating' sympathetic part and the 'pacifying' parasympathetic part.

The sympathetic system comes into play when we need to handle emergencies or sudden changes. It gives rise to the so-called 'fight or flight' stress response characterized by a rush of energy , a racing heart and a feeling of alertness, changes caused by the secretion of the 'stress hormone', adrenaline. Once the stress has passed the parasympathetic system should take over to calm all the systems down, but thanks to the pressures of life today we often get stuck in sympathetic mode.

It now seems clear that our state of mind

can influence the autonomic nervous system and that we can 'talk ourselves into' becoming more relaxed.

Being the most reactive of all the systems, the nervous system is the first place were emotional upset takes its toll. From here it goes on to affect any system that is particularly weak and vulnerable.

SIGNS OF NERVOUS UPSET

- Increased heart rate; palpitations
- Rapid breathing
- Muscular tension
- Sweating, feeling flushed
- Disturbed digestion and a nervous 'knotted' stomach
- Irritability and edginess
- Restlessness
- Insomnia; lying awake worrying
- Aggressiveness
- Cravings for alcohol or nicotine
- Nervous habits such as nail-biting nails, foot-tapping or drumming repetitively with the fingers
- Loss of appetite or over-eating
- Inability to relax
- Feelings of being totally unable to cope – nervous breakdown.

CASE HISTORY: INSOMNIA

Rebecca, company director and self-confessed workaholic, was physically healthy but had suffered from insomnia for some time. She not only found it difficult to fall asleep, but also woke frequently during the night. By morning she was exhausted and felt she had not slept at all. She had also begun having slight pre-menstrual tension.

I PRESCRIBED

- Star of Bethlehem (B) for long, slow shock, since it transpired that her drive to achieve

stemmed from feeling unloved as a child. She had thus developed a strong desire to please and prove herself worthy of love

- Five Corners (Aus B), for her low self-esteem which had led to her desire to prove herself.
- Pomegranate (Fes), which helped her as a woman deprived of the nurturing needed for a positive self-image.
- A combination of Elm (B), Indian Pink (Fes), Chamomile and Valerian (Cal), to combat her feeling of being overwhelmed by the pressure of work and its debilitating effect on her nervous system, resulting in her sleeping problems.

Rebecca soon began to relax and found she could pace herself better at work. She reported feeling uplifted and more confident, and told me she had slipped into a regular sleeping pattern. The pre-menstrual tension also improved.

Now she began to wonder what her real purpose was in life.

I PRESCRIBED

- Silver Princess (Aus B) to help her realize her inner direction and purpose
- Zinnia (PVi) to keep her from taking life so seriously
- Pink Seaweed (Pac) to help her take stock before rushing into anything new
- Gruss an Aachen (PVi) and Ettringite (Pegasus Gem Essences) to integrate the change and help her to move in a new direction

CASE HISTORY: ANOREXIA NERVOSA

Although women are more susceptible to anorexia than men, at the age of 25 John had the classic symptoms of this illness.

He is a highly sensitive, gentle person whose problems began in childhood. John's mother was distant while his father's domineering, military style of discipline frightened him. John grew up feeling inadequate and reproached himself for not fulfilling his parents' expectations. He withdrew from life and his emotions, entering a fantasy world and following intellectual pursuits. The feelings of anxiety and inadequacy stayed with him, upsetting his nervous system and digestion, leading to severe weight loss over a period of time due to the need to control events by consciously starving himself.

I PRESCRIBED

- Chamomile (Cal) for calming and restoring the nervous system
- Indian Pink (Fes) and Star of Bethlehem and Pine (B) to clear the long, slow shock of his repressed childhood and the guilt and self-blame he took from his parents
- Scarlet Monkeyflower (Fes) to release his repressed anger and frustration with his parents
- Neem (Him A) to help him to feel safe with his emotions
- Paw Paw (Aus B) and Turquoise and Gold (Gem) for anorexia and to facilitate absorption of vital nutrients

While taking the remedies John lost the anorexic mind-set and began to put on weight and felt happier and more able to be himself. He also began standing up to his father in a quiet but positive way.

THE IMMUNE SYSTEM

Like an army, the immune system defends the body from invaders such as viruses, bacteria and other potentially harmful organisms.

White cells, or leukocytes, act as soldiers and move freely around the body via the bloodstream to target the site of infection. The first battalion to arrive on the scene when something like a stomach bug enters the system is made up of granular leukocytes. These cells are armed with chemical weapons which immobilize and often destroy bacteria.

The rest of the army is broken down into two divisions of lymphocytes which are produced in the lymph glands and spleen. The T-lymphocytes are like the body's intelligence service, for they are concerned with recognizing foreign invaders. As well as viruses they regard implanted tissue as alien and prompt its rejection. The thymus gland, which orchestrates the functioning of the immune system, endows the T-cells with their discerning qualities.

If the T-cells verify an invasion, the immune system is switched to 'red alert'. Some of the T-cells possess deadly weapons which they then put to use.

Blymphocytes are also brought into play. These cells make antibodies which act as straitjackets, immobilizing the invader until it can be attacked.

The B-cells have memories and can remember what type of antibody to make if it meets the same virus again. This means the invader can be dealt with more efficiently next time, and that any resulting symptoms will be mild. In the case of allergy, the B-cells start making a specific sort of antibody called IgE. During the scuffle between antibody and invader, inflammatory chemicals such as histamine are released which cause the typical allergic symptoms such as a runny nose, watery eyes, etc.

The way the immune system functions is complex and remains to be fully understood. However, we know that if over-worked or sabotaged it may fail to know the difference between an enemy and something innocuous – or even between an enemy and the body's own tissues. In auto-immune diseases such as rheumatoid arthritis and ME, it appears to turn on its own cells.

Shock, long-standing stress, a poor diet and/or environmental pollutants appear to act as immuno-suppressants. Some researchers have found that certain negative emotions such as grief and feelings of despair are particularly effective at disarming the immune system. In contrast, unconditional love seems to strengthen its reserves.

SIGNS OF POOR IMMUNITY

- Frequent colds, sore throats, swollen glands
- Recurrent bacterial and/or viral infections
- Allergies
- Aching joints and muscles
- Depression, irritability, anxiety, emotional upset
- Lank, greasy hair
- Dull, blotchy skin
- Watery eyes
- Itchy, streaming nose
- Bleeding gums
- A reduction in the amount of time it takes cuts and grazes to heal
- Low or fluctuating energy levels – making it necessary to rely on stimulants such as coffee
- Dull headaches
- General lack of vitality

CASE HISTORY: FLU

Charlotte (a busy literary agent) had been laid low for a week with Asian flu, with the usual symptoms of fever, aching joints and a sore throat. Then the virus moved to her chest, giving rise to congestion and a debilitating cough. She was keen to avoid taking antibiotics, especially since the person who had passed the virus on to her had had the flu for eight weeks despite taking two courses of antibiotics.

I PRESCRIBED
- Pansy (Cal) for clearing viruses
- K9 (AK), a natural antibiotic
- Koenign van Daenmark (Cal) to boost the immune system
- Eucalyptus (Fes) for the chesty cough

Charlotte's recovery was speedy. Within a matter of days the flu symptoms and chestiness had cleared; she felt her healthy self again.

Another good remedy is Coralroot Spotted (Peg), which helps to clear the effects of antibiotics from the system.

CASE HISTORY: HERPES VIRUS

Aged 32, Helen had first caught herpes from her boyfriend; after they'd broken up it continued to flare up for about five days in every month, making her feel depressed, unclean and unable to contemplate a long-term relationship.

She had a history of susceptibility to viral infections, having contracted scarlet fever and whooping cough when she was three, then glandular fever in her late teens.

I PRESCRIBED
- Pansy (Cal) and Spinifex (Aus B) for fighting the herpes virus
- Chamomile (Fes) and Hau (Haii) for repairing and restoring the nervous system
- Koenign van Daenmark (Cal) and K9 (AK) for boosting her immunity
- Illyarrie (Aus L) to help her to realize she had the strength to cope
- Billy Goat Plum (Aus B) for her feelings of revulsion associated with having herpes

After taking the course of treatment Helen noticed that the recurrences were becoming less frequent; then they ceased completely and have not come back for over two years.

CASE HISTORY: ME

Angela was 40 and had for the last three years been suffering from ME, which was getting progressively worse. She was exhausted and ached all over. She was confined to bed most of the time as she was unable to walk or stand for more than a few moments.

Talking with her, I learned that as a child she had been pushed academically and told she was not clever enough to make the grade. She'd started taking drugs to evade reality, and had continued to use them heavily until her late thirties when she'd realized she needed professional help. However, the drugs had already taken a severe toll on her immune system and she had developed ME when at her lowest ebb, with no job, relationship or other form of support. She had been in and out of many relationships, all of them either unproductive or destructive.

I PRESCRIBED

- Star of Bethlehem (B) for the long, slow shock of childhood and drug abuse
- Morning Glory (AK, Cal) to clear the toxic effects of drugs
- Pansy (Cal) as an antiviral and immune-booster
- Comfrey (Cal, Fes) to strengthen the nervous and muscular system
- Dandelion (Fes) to ease psychological tension stored in muscles
- Dill (Fes) to lift depression and to help her develop a healthier perspective on her emotional problems

Angela reported that she was finding it easier to relax and felt less stressed. The burning aching in her body, especially in her legs, had eased and she was able to do simple (though previously impossible) daily tasks without getting exhausted.

Now was the time for a follow-on prescription.

I PRESCRIBED

- Koenign van Daenmark (Cal) to boost the immune system
- Gold (Gem) to encourage assimilation of vital nutrients
- Tomato (PVi) to help her throw off the disease
- Zinnia (PVi) to lift her outlook on life and inspire humour
- First Aid Remedy (Him A) as an all-round booster

Slowly but surely Angela grew stronger, reporting increased energy levels and an ability to be mentally detached from her problems. She has also overcome her dependency on addictive, destructive relationships. She continues to feel better each day.

CASE HISTORY: ECZEMA

Charlie, aged 3, had developed very bad eczema (linked to an allergy to dairy products). In addition, his birth had been traumatic and he appeared to be shy, fearful and apprehensive.

I PRESCRIBED

- Arnica (Fes) for traumatic birth
- Mimulus (B) for shyness and timidity
- Sweet Chestnut (B) for anxiety
- Aspen (B) for apprehension
- Aloe Vera and Luffa (Fes, Cal) for his skin condition
- Koenign van Daenmark (Cal) to boost the immune system

A month later the eczema began to clear and Charlie appeared to be more confident and less fearful. Before the end of the second course his eczema had completely disappeared; there has been no recurrence.

THE LYMPHATIC SYSTEM

The lymphatic system is closely linked to the immune system because it plays a vital role in whisking away dead bacteria, disabled viruses and other debris from the tissues.

Lymph itself is a colourless, faintly opalescent fluid which bathes the body's cells, furnishing them with nutrients and cleansing them of wastes and other impurities. In this respect it is rather like blood. Lymph, however, is not pumped around the body by the heart. It flows freely, relying on full, rhythmic breathing along with the contraction and relaxation of major muscles in the body for its circulation.

The network of lymphatic vessels are intimately connected with the main circulatory system. Blood seeps from its own vessels into those of the lymphatic system where it is cleansed and reconditioned before returning again to the veins and arteries.

Each organ has its own lymph supply, and the system itself has its own organs. The spleen, thymus, tonsils, adenoids, appendix and Peyer's patch are all part of this complex purification system. So too are bundles of sinus tissue called lymph nodes. The main ones are found under the arms, in the neck, behind the knees and in the groin. They can be felt as small lumps beneath the skin. Inside these nodes, lymphocyte cells are busy detoxifying wastes by engulfing or destroying them.

During an infection, the lymph nodes often swell and feel tender as battle gets underway within.

Eating food laden with fats, sugars, salt, additives and preservatives, as well as drinking alcohol and coffee, tends to 'pollute' the lymphatic system. The lymph fluid draws liquids from the tissues to dilute these toxins, which is what makes you look puffy and feel waterlogged when there is a problem with your lymphatic system.

SIGNS OF LYMPHATIC DISORDER

- **Puffiness**
- **Bags under the eyes**
- **Skin blemishes**
- **Cellulite**
- **Congestion**
- **Swollen, tender lymph glands**

CASE HISTORY: SWOLLEN GLANDS

Sarah, a 27-year-old public relations officer, was distressed by the presence of painful boils under her armpits. She had been prescribed a course of antibiotics which had not helped.

Her lymphatic system was sluggish, she tended to gain weight easily, felt nauseous after eating and suffered from poor circulation.

I PRESCRIBED

- Chamomile (Cal, Fes) and Hau (Haii) for emotional stress and nervous conditions affecting the stomach
- K9 (AK) and Koenign van Daenmark and Pansy (Cal) for boosting the immune system
- Moss Agate (Gem), Yellow Ginger (Haii) and Luffa (Cal) for clearing toxins from the blood and her whole system, reducing lymphatic swelling and clearing the skin

During the first week Sarah came out in rash, which soon disappeared to be followed by a sore throat, which in turn cleared quickly along with the boils themselves. She felt wonderful.

Not long afterwards she went out drinking to celebrate her birthday. That night her whole arm swelled up and the lumps reappeared.

Sarah doubled her dosage and by morning both the swelling and the boils had gone.

THE RESPIRATORY SYSTEM

Oxygen is the vital spark that kindles the physical energy necessary for powering life processes. Many ancient traditions teach that air, not food, is responsible for vitality, for it facilitates the flow of life-force.

Breathing brings oxygen from the air into the lungs. Here the gas dissolves in the blood and is taken up by the complex iron-rich molecule, haemoglobin, present in the red cells or corpuscles.

In this form oxygen is distributed to every cell in the body. The by-product of cell respiration, carbon dioxide, then combines with water in the red cells and is carried back to the lungs before being exhaled out into the atmosphere.

Full rhythmical breathing is best for the mind and body as it assures a continuous flow of oxygen to the cells and the swift removal of carbon dioxide. At rest, a typical man breathes around 8 litres of air a minute – a woman somewhat less. If deprived of oxygen for as little as three minutes, brain cells die and the heart struggles to keep beating.

Although breathing happens automatically, normal breathing patterns are easily disrupted. Sudden temperature changes such as stepping outdoors on a frosty day or into a very hot sauna make us gasp and temporarily hold our breath. Everyday stresses also play havoc with breathing patterns, although we tend not to notice. When anxious, fearful, angry or frustrated our breathing becomes rapid and shallow, a phenomenon known as hyperventilation.

Hyperventilation makes the heart pound, the head spin and the legs turn to jelly. Shallow breathing reduces the body's oxygen supply, leading to feelings of tiredness, lethargy and faintness as well as difficulty concentrating and frequent yawning.

Heavy air pollution also undermines our oxygen supply. Car exhaust fumes are rich in carbon monoxide, which competes with oxygen for haemoglobin in the blood. Other noxious chemicals include nitrogen oxides and hydrocarbons, which irritate the lungs and nasal passages – triggering asthma attacks, exacerbating chest troubles and increasing our vulnerability to chest infections and allergic rhinitis.

SIGNS OF RESPIRATORY PROBLEMS
- **Shortness of breath**
- **Coughing**
- **Wheezing**
- **Frequent colds**
- **Hayfever and asthma**
- **Bronchitis**
- **Weakness and dizziness**
- **Anxiety**
- **Feelings of panic**

CASE HISTORY: HAYFEVER

Michael, a businessman in his late forties in a stress-charged profession, had been suffering from hayfever since he was 12 years old. Each year during the second week of June symptoms of itchy eyes, sneezing and a streaming nose would begin and continue until the end of July, signifying a typical allergy to grass pollens.

His normal treatment was to take anti-histamines, although he had also unsuccessfully tried the inoculation method for several years.

I PRESCRIBED

- Pink Fairy Orchid (Aus L) for feeling frenzied and overwhelmed by stress and the environment
- Eucalyptus and Green Rose (Cal) for allergic reactions and hayfever
- Koenign van Daenmark (Cal) to boost immunity

Michael began taking the combination a few months before the start of the hayfever season. That year he was symptom-free. He has repeated this treatment for three years, and to date his hayfever has not recurred.

CASE HISTORY: SINUSITIS

Rosemary's sinus problems began at the age of 24, following an infection she appeared to pick up in a public swimming pool. As a child she had frequent chest infections; she had contracted tuberculosis when she was 20 and it left her with a weakness in the chest area. She had great difficulty shaking off winter colds and was very sensitive to cold winds and dust.

I PRESCRIBED

- Moss Agate (Gem) and Jasmine (Cal) to clear the nasal passages and sinuses
- Drum Stick (Him A) for lung and bronchial conditions
- Eucalyptus (Cal, Fes) to help breathing
- Echinacea (Haii) to boost the immune system
- Tomato (PVi) to ease the hold this condition had on her system

Her sinus condition has cleared and she is now able to breathe more easily. She reports feeling better than she has done in over 20 years.

THE CIRCULATORY SYSTEM

The circulatory system is closely linked to the respiratory system, as one of its main functions is to transport oxygen-laden blood from the lungs to the tissues and return it again, this time carrying carbon dioxide.

The heart is responsible for pumping an incredible five litres of blood around the body every minute. It starts beating when we are still in the womb, just a few weeks old, and continues to pulsate independently under the orchestration of its own inbuilt pacemaker for the rest of our lives.

The heart was once believed to be the seat of emotion – not surprisingly, perhaps, for feelings like anxiety, fear, anger, excitement and passion are felt here. Grief in particular seems to tear at the heart, hence the saying 'broken-hearted'.

This vital pump forces blood along highly elastic vessels which spread through the body becoming increasingly fine as they reach the extremities. Tiny blood capillaries feeding the skin surface may be just one cell thick. Blood itself contains a variety of cells including the haemoglobin-rich red blood corpuscles and the white lymphocytes.

Along with oxygen, other nutrients absorbed from the digestive tract, hormones secreted by the glandular system and other chemicals are all circulated around the body in the blood.

As blood comes into close contact with every part of the body, its composition is a particularly good reflection of what is happening at the cellular level.

A tendency towards good or bad circulation tends to be inherited, but it can also be influenced by lifestyle. Tension held in the muscles interferes with the swift flow of blood to certain parts of the body. Such deprived regions tend to feel cold. It is interesting to note that people who have experienced a great deal of trauma in childhood often tend to have poor circulation.

SIGNS OF CIRCULATORY UPSET

- **Sluggish circulation**
- **Cold hands and feet**
- **Chilblains in winter**
- **Irregular heart beat**
- **Palpitations**
- **Dizziness and feeling faint**
- **Blurred vision**
- **Nosebleeds**
- **Constant fatigue**

CASE HISTORY: CIRCULATORY PROBLEMS

Anne, who runs a small family business, was 52 when she was diagnosed as suffering from nervous angina. She had flu-like symptoms all the time and experienced pins and needles as well as pains down her left side. Every 10 days she would get nighttime palpitations lasting for 10 minutes. Anne woke frequently during the night in a sweat, her pulse racing.

She was also suffering from water retention which caused her legs to swell, as well as cold hands and feet due to poor circulation.

She had been taking several angina tablets a day to open the arteries, as well as tranquillizers to soothe her nerves.

I PRESCRIBED

- Rose Quartz and Ruby (Gem) for childhood sadness, as her parents had argued all the time and she had always been trying to keep the peace. Her very repressive father made her angry, but she would not express this feeling

- Bleeding Heart (Peg) for regulating blood-pressure and circulation
- Yellow Ginger (Haii), Avocado (Cal) and Redwood (Peg) for cleansing the blood and strengthening the vessels
- Saguaro (Cal, Fes) to cleanse the lymphatic system and so ease fluid retention

After the first course of treatment Anne's circulation had improved, she had not felt the need to take a tranquillizer for a month and her angina pains had lifted. Five days after finishing the essences she experienced some discomfort and was given a repeat prescription. She has now come off the tranquillizers completely and is now down to taking just one angina tablet a day.

THE DIGESTIVE SYSTEM

The digestive system is responsible for extracting and absorbing essential nutrients from the foods we eat, as well as for disposing of wastes that would otherwise congest and clog up the system.

Digestion begins in the mouth, where food is pulverized by chewing and mixed with saliva which contains mild starch-digesting enzymes. It then passes to the stomach where digestion begins in earnest. Here food is mixed with a potent gastric juice rich in hydrochloric acid which creates an environment suitable for protein-digesting enzymes to carry out their task.

All kinds of emotional upset, from fear and frustration to anger and anxiety, upset the flow of gastric juice. While an over-secretion of acid gives rise to heartburn, under-secretion means food lingers in the stomach causing indigestion and feelings of heaviness.

On leaving the stomach, food passes into the small intestine, a long and convoluted tunnel where starches are broken down into sugars and digestion is completed.

According to the traditions of Chinese medicine, emotions are processed in the digestive tract as well as foods. If sensations such as anger or fear are not properly dealt with, tension accumulates in this area giving rise to symptoms such as stomach knots and colicky pains.

Everything we absorb into the bloodstream through the intestinal walls is passed on to the liver, a remarkable organ which emulsifies fats and changes sugar into glycogen so it can be stored away until it is needed. The liver also detoxifies any undesirable chemicals such as alcohol and the food additives taken in with the vital nutrients. The liver functions best when we eat simply prepared, natural foods and keep regular eating and sleeping patterns; when over-burdened with rich, fatty foods and impurities we feel nauseous and headachy, as if slightly hungover. From an emotional viewpoint, the liver is affected by angry outbursts more than anything else.

Foods that have not been broken down for nutrients then enter the large intestine or colon, where any water is reabsorbed and wastes are gathered for elimination. Eating plenty of fibre-rich vegetables and foods helps to speed digestion and prevent wastes from stagnating in the bowel.

Elimination is also carried out by two other organs in the body: the kidneys and the skin. The kidneys, like the liver, filter the blood to remove unwanted salts and noxious wastes. These are expelled in a diluted form as urine. The kidneys also play a vital role in maintaining the balance of body fluids by eliminating excess water and conserving it when in short supply.

Sweat glands in the skin secrete water that contains dissolved mineral salts and small quantities of other wastes through microscopic pores at the surface, helping to keep the body free of impurities. Wearing natural fibres such as cotton and wool allows the skin to breathe and perspire more freely than synthetics do.

SIGNS OF DIGESTIVE UPSET

- **Indigestion/heartburn**
- **Bloating and wind**
- **Knots in the stomach**
- **Colicky cramps**
- **Diarrhoea**
- **Constipation**
- **Nutritional deficiencies**
- **Fluid retention**
- **Cystitis**
- **Blemished skin**

CASE HISTORY: WIND AND BLOATING

Susan was experiencing abdominal discomfort due to bloating, wind and constipation which had become worse during her divorce from a husband who was both difficult and vindictive. During this period of intense emotional stress she had also started to react to city pollution, suffering hayfever-type symptoms.

Her childhood was traumatic. Susan had been brought up during the Second World War years by very strict parents who would not tolerate any show of emotion. She had suffered from constipation as a child and was allergic to dairy produce.

I PRESCRIBED

- For the past:

    Star of Bethlehem (B) for long, slow shock
    Sweet Chestnut (B) for suppressed anxiety and not being able to express emotion
    Mimulus (B) for timidity and fearfulness

Agrimony (B) for the British tendency to be stiff-upper-lipped as a protective mechanism

Vervain (B) for trying too hard to please and over-exerting herself

- For the present:

Chamomile (Cal, Fes) for stress that leads to a nervous stomach

Cedar (Cal) to cleanse the digestive system and ease wind, bloating and constipation

Eucalyptus (Cal, Fes) to ease breathing and clear pollutants from the lungs

Susan feels she has been able to clear the emotional upset of her childhood and present life. The wind and bloating have subsided, the constipation has cleared and her allergic reactions are less pronounced.

CASE HISTORY: GASTRIC ULCER

After three unsuccessful operations to treat an ulcer condition, Karen came to me for help. The ulcer flared up roughly every three months, causing her to wake in the night with severe pain under her ribcage. At these times she would feel cold, shivery and headachy, as if in a state of shock.

She was found to be allergic to milk and dairy products generally.

Karen had also suffered long, slow shock as a child because her mother had never been there to nurture her and she was left to look after her younger brother most of the time. She had also been traumatized when her first child was stillborn. She had turned her fear and panic inward on herself.

I PRESCRIBED

- Star of Bethlehem (B) for shock
- Rock Rose (B) for fear and panic
- Sweet Chestnut (B) for deep anguish and anxiety
- Green Rose (Cal) for suppressed shock which had turned inwards
- Crowea (Aus B) for continuous worry linked to stomach ulcers
- Cedar (Cal) to soothe the stomach and colon
- Pennyroyal (Cal, Fes) to protect her from negativity

Karen's ulcer seems to have been calmed, for she has not experienced any repeat attacks and is now sleeping peacefully through the night.

THE ENDOCRINE AND REPRODUCTIVE SYSTEMS

The endocrine system describes the body's so-called 'ductless glands', namely the pineal, pituitary, thyroid, parathyroid, adrenal, pancreas and thymus glands. They all secrete hormones – chemical 'messengers' which play a vital role in controlling and co-ordinating important processes such as metabolism and growth. Our behaviour and emotions are influenced to a degree by the hormones circulating in our bloodstream. Each gland and its hormones has a specific job to do. While some enable us to cope with changes in our environment, others orchestrate the rhythms that regulate our sleep and fertility patterns.

The pituitary is the gland which ensures that all the other glands work together in harmony. In spite of its epithet 'master gland', it in turn falls under the influence of the hypothalamus, a region of the brain that detects and responds to emotional upset.

Stressful events such as relationship problems and conflicts at work can throw the entire endocrine system into turmoil. Is it any wonder that stress has such a disruptive effect on so many bodily processes?

Hormones produced by the pituitary gland also control the activities of the reproductive organs in both men and women. Although not officially part of the endocrine system, they too produce hormones. Along with the other glands they are also responsive to emotional upset. Reproductive problems such as irregular periods are often one of the first signs that the whole endocrine system is under stress.

Sex drive is thought to be regulated by the hormone testosterone, which is produced in males by the testes and in females in smaller quantities by the adrenal glands. Male fertility is fairly consistent, which may explain why men tend to be less susceptible to emotional highs and lows. Female fertility, in contrast, is a cyclical affair marked by distinct fluctuations in the two predominantly feminine hormones, oestrogen and progesterone. Hormonal changes may precipitate or enhance all kinds of feelings from irritability and anger to sadness and security, which is the reason why all women suffer from premenstrual mood changes. It is only when stress is added that these emotions can spiral out of control.

A woman's ability to conceive or sustain a pregnancy can also be affected by stress-induced emotions. In instances where there is no biological reason for infertility, negative attitudes and beliefs may underlie problems with conception. A woman who has, for instance, grown up believing that being a parent is incredibly difficult – a view probably passed on to her by her own parents – may subconsciously fear starting a family.

Pregnancy itself is a particularly emotional time, due to the hormonal upheavals that take place and because it raises all kinds of anxieties such as 'Will I love my baby?', 'Am I ready to be a mother?' Emotional turbulence during this time may play a part in exacerbating symptoms such as morning sickness and feelings of exhaustion.

As the birth approaches it is natural to feel increasingly apprehensive and scared by the pain of labour, feelings that are sensed by baby. Excessive fear at this time may encourage the baby to remain in a breech position. Interestingly, in India flowers are thought to bring about mental and emotional balance during birth. During the early stages of labour an Indian mother will bathe in water steeped with flowers.

Flower essences help to replace negative feelings such as fear and anxiety with a sense of excitement and anticipation.

SIGNS OF UPSET

- Lack of sex drive or desire
- Pre-menstrual tension
- Absence of periods
- Irregular periods
- Period pains
- Infertility
- Mood swings in pregnancy
- Morning sickness
- Postnatal depression
- Menopausal problems
- Impotency in men

CASE HISTORY: THE PROBLEMS OF PREGNANCY

Mary had been married for eight years and although she was three months pregnant she had in the past experienced problems both conceiving and carrying a baby to full term. She had miscarried four years previously, had to have polyps removed from her uterus, then suffered another miscarriage two years later, in both instances at nine and a half weeks.

She was very anxious about losing her baby, and

her highly stressed job only made matters worse.

I PRESCRIBED

- Star of Bethlehem (B) for past long, slow shock resulting from her parents' divorce when she was 14. It was very traumatic and set up a stress pattern which continued to affect her life
- Hornbeam (B) for strength to cope
- Chamomile (Cal, Dv, Fes) to soothe the nerves and clear stress
- Pomegranate (Fes) and Watermelon (Cal) to stabilize the baby and the whole reproductive area
- Crystal Rescue (Gem) to boost self-healing and buffer both mother and baby from any future stress or shock

This combination was taken as a four-month course of treatment.

At seven months Mary reported having had a trouble-free pregnancy and asked for more remedies for the last two months and for the birth itself.

I PRESCRIBED

- A repeat of the Pomegranate (Fes) and Watermelon (Cal)
- Cauliflower (PVi) to help the baby through the birth process
- Vanadinite (Peg) to act as a protective shield for mother and baby

The birth was trouble-free; both mother and baby are thriving.

CASE HISTORY: MENOPAUSE

At 50, Jane began going through the menopause, suffering hot flushes and panic attacks. She had always suffered from pre-menstrual tension and depression around the time of her period. She was also finding her work as a counsellor highly stressful, as she tended to take her clients' emotional problems to heart.

I PRESCRIBED

- Pomegranate (Fes), Gooseberry and Phytollaca Dioica (Peg) for the reproductive area and hormonal balance
- Candysticks (Pac) for releasing pelvic tension and to boost energy levels
- Correa (Aus L) for learning to accept her limitations in helping others
- Pink Fairy Orchid (Aus L) to filter out the emotional stress of those around her

Jane felt all her menopausal symptoms ease, especially the hot flushes, and she had ceased having panic attacks. She now feels more like her normal self again.

CASE HISTORY: PRE-MENSTRUAL TENSION

For some time Sophie had been experiencing severe pre-menstrual tension. She generally felt exhausted and overwhelmed by stress due primarily to her two young children: one was not sleeping through the night and the other was having mild learning difficulties.

I PRESCRIBED

- Star of Bethlehem (B) for past long, slow shock caused by the fact that her mother had not been very nurturing
- Vervain (B) for over-exertion brought on by trying too hard to please and achieve
- Chamomile (Fes) for sleep loss due to the effects of stress on her nervous system
- Pomegranate (Fes) for re-balancing the reproductive area
- She Oak (Aus B) for pre-menstrual hormonal imbalance and water retention
- Noni (Haii) for awakening the maternal

instincts of nurturing, caring and love so she could find it easier to cope with being a mother

- Illyarrie (Aus L) for strength to overcome difficulties without feeling overwhelmed
- Leafless Orchid (Aus L) to find energy from within to keep working without becoming physically depleted
- Russian Kolokoltchik (Aus L) to help conquer adverse conditions
- First Aid Remedy (Him A) as an overall booster

The month after Sophie started taking the prescription she did not have any pre-menstrual tension; the following month she experienced mild symptoms; since then she has been symptom-free and has felt much more balanced, with the energy to cope with a young family.

THE SKELETAL AND MUSCULAR SYSTEMS

The bones, joints, muscles and ligaments provide the body with structure, strength and suppleness. They work together, enabling us to move with ease and comfort.

The spine is the linchpin of the skeletal system. It is made up of 24 drum-shaped vertebra separated by discs of fibrous tissue which act as shock-absorbers. As babies our spines are relatively straight. Curves slowly develop as we spend more and more time upright.

Its S-shape endows the spine with remarkable resilience to physical impact. Sadly this does not prevent us getting backache brought on by poor posture and emotional tension. Those who suffer from bad backs often tend to bear the troubles of the world on their shoulders and feel overwhelmed by responsi-

bilities. As the archetypal providers and supporters, married men with families are the classic example.

Joints form the connections between two or more adjacent parts of the skeleton. They are held together by ligaments, tough elastic fibres which allow the joints to bend to allow movement and flexibility. Inflammation of the joints, as in the case of arthritis, is traditionally thought to be caused by wear and tear or disease. However, all kinds of inflammatory chemicals, such as those produced during an allergic reaction, contribute to certain forms of arthritis.

Muscles move the joints and bones. There are 620 we can move of our own accord, plus many more involuntary ones in the heart, blood vessels, intestines and so on that we cannot control.

Emotional tension is readily transmitted to the muscles. From early in life we often develop a habit of tensing certain muscles. Most people tend to raise their shoulders and tense the neck muscles when they feel threatened. We all develop our own ways of responding to stress. Repressed emotions, whether painful or pleasurable, are also stored in the muscles as tension, giving rise to a sort of 'muscular armour'. Such ingrained tensions not only limit our freedom of movement, they also stifle energy – which may explain why our natural vitality dwindles as we age.

SIGNS OF UPSET

- Muscular aches
- Tension in the neck and shoulders
- Back aches and pains
- Slipped discs
- Stiff, sore joints
- Arthritis
- Rheumatism
- Poor posture

CASE HISTORY: HIP REPLACEMENT

Juliet was 48 when she discovered she needed to have a hip replacement. As the day for the operation approached she became increasingly fearful and was unable to eat.

I PRESCRIBED

- Indian Pink (Fes), Hau (Haii) and Chamomile (Cal) for stress affecting the nervous system and stomach
- Star of Bethlehem (B) for shock brought on by any operation
- Gold (Gem) for healing the skeletal system
- Russian Kolokoltchik (Aus L) for courage and strength

The operation was very successful and Juliet's recovery amazed her doctor. After just four weeks she reported no pain, bruising or swelling and could walk without crutches. She continued with the remedies to consolidate the treatment, adding Crystal Rescue (Gem) for self-healing, Ohai-ali'i (Haii) to help knit and strengthen the bones and Comfrey to help repair and rebuild muscle tissue. A month later she completely regained her mobility and could even run upstairs.

CASE HISTORY: ARTHRITIS

Margaret developed extremely painful arthritis in her hands and knees. She was taking the usual combination of anti-inflammatory agents, painkillers and paracetamol. At the same time she was exhausted and was not absorbing nutrients properly from her food.

I PRESCRIBED

- Moss Agate (Gem) for the inflammation
- Azurite (Gem) for arthritis
- Gold (Gem) to aid the assimilation of nutrients
- Koenign van Daenmark (Cal) for auto-immune problems
- Morning Glory (Cal, Fes) to clear the toxic effects of the medication she had been taking

Margaret charted her condition from December to mid-May. For the first 20 days the pain continued, but the next day it started to ease. Five days later it had disappeared and has not recurred since.

She now has more energy than before and, now able to kneel and squat without discomfort, she has resumed her passion for gardening.

❋ THE MIND – THOUGHTS AND EMOTIONS ❋

Nobody understands exactly how the mind functions. Our thoughts, feelings and emotions ultimately depend on our outlook on life. This in turn is linked to our personality and shaped by upbringing and personal experiences.

For simplicity's sake the mind is regarded as the seat of consciousness, intelligence, thought, reasoning, memory, imagination, creativity, emotions and instinctive drives.

These functions take place within the brain, the most complex and highly developed structure that exists.

The brain is composed of millions and millions of interconnecting nerve cells which pass snippets of information, in the form of chemical messages, from one to another.

Certain regions of the brain are associated with different functions. The most ancient reptilian region comprising the spinal cord, brain stem and mid-brain controls our most basic survival and reproductive instincts.

The next layer is the paleomammalian brain, also known as the limbic system. This is the control centre for emotions and states of mind such as fear, panic, pleasure and bliss. It is here that responses such as affection, sexual behaviour, altruistic impulses and even love originate. Bodily functions such as thirst, hunger, temperature and sexual drive are also regulated by this region.

The cerebral cortex is biologically the most recent region of the brain. It seems to have evolved once humans had overcome the basic function of survival and found time to sit around thinking, learning new skills, creating things and so forth. The cortex is where perception, memory, judgement and the intellect, something loosely defined as cognition, occurs.

The 'thinking' brain is responsible for mental activity. It is divided into two parts or hemispheres, the left and right, which deal with information in rather different ways. In modern Western society greater emphasis is placed on the logical, rational and analytical thinking which occurs in the left hemisphere. Recently we have begun to realize the importance of the right brain, which is concerned with creativity, inspiration and imagination. 'Whole brain thinking' is not only more effective, it also makes life seem richer.

Although the brain has a seemingly infinite capacity to store knowledge, in our information-orientated age there is a danger of mental over-stimulation. By trying to make sense of it all, our minds become filled with swirling thoughts and an internal chatter which we cannot switch off.

When mentally exhausted we cannot think clearly or concentrate properly, we become forgetful and find it hard to make decisions. When the mind is in turmoil, thinking is distorted and so too is the way we act or behave.

The famous psychoanalyst R. D. Lang pointed out that mental turmoil may also arise when something we are told or seems to be fact is at odds with what we instinctively know or sense. Suspicions of being deceived and lied to can, he claimed, torment us to the point of insanity.

Similarly, powerful emotions like anger, fear and rage undermine our ability to think in a clear and rational manner. Emotions are part of our ancient inheritance and we probably share them in common with our distant ancestors. The psychologist Carl Jung referred to the 'collective unconscious' as being the hopes, fears and anxieties which all human beings hold in common.

It is natural and healthy for us to experience the whole gamut of emotions. However, certain ones such as anger and fear are seen as socially unacceptable, perhaps because they remind us of our primitive origins or just because they make us feel uncomfortable. We suppress them, learning from childhood that it is 'wrong' to lose our temper or break down in tears. Both Sigmund Freud and Carl Jung believed that repressed emotions do not go away; they stay in our psyche and crop up in our dreams. Without an outlet they become bottled up inside until the pressure becomes so intense that we may literally blow a fuse.

Negative emotions will not do us much harm if they are fleeting. However, if they become part of our behavioural response they slowly and insidiously wreak havoc on the system.

We inherit many behavioural patterns from our parents. As young children we copy the way they react to situations and handle their emotions. We also acquire perceptions about ourselves, others and the world in general from them. Their attitudes and opinions undoubtedly influence the way we think of and view life. It is believed that all experiences, even those we cannot consciously remember from childhood, are stored in the subconscious mind. From here they exert an influence on our behaviour and on the way we react to other people and situations in our lives.

This influence may be appropriate when we are growing up for it gives us a sense of structure and security. In later life, however, these inherited views and attitudes may no longer be helpful – can even be limiting – and their value to us has to be reassessed.

Thousands of years ago wise men realized we can only see things for what they really are when are minds are clear, still and free from cluttering thoughts. They developed meditative techniques for calming the mind and subduing the disruptive effects of our emotions. They also taught that, to be free of negative emotions, we have to find ways of turning seemingly negative situations into ones that can have a positive outcome. After all, what we think of as reality is really all in the mind.

SIGNS OF MENTAL AND EMOTIONAL UPSET

- Confusion
- Inability to think clearly
- Persistent unwanted thoughts
- Forgetfulness
- Inability to make decisions
- Poor concentration
- Feelings of being overwhelmed by emotions of all kinds
- Emotional outbursts
- Mood swings
- Feelings of being on an emotional roller-coaster, out of control

CASE HISTORY: STRESS

Elizabeth, a self-styled company director, had built her own business into a growing concern. Despite being extremely successful in her career, she always found herself in relationships with men in which she felt abused. These played havoc with her self-esteem and were a continual source of worry. She felt confused, overwhelmed and unable to sleep properly. Her tumultuous emotional life was beginning to affect her work. She could not concentrate or make decisions and was in danger of ruining her business.

I PRESCRIBED
- Paw Paw (Aus B), for feeling overwhelmed and burdened by decisions
- Scleranthus (B) to encourage decisiveness and belief in her own intuition
- Stress/Tension (Him A) for general tension and nervous stress
- Scarlet Monkeyflower (Fes), Montbretia (NZ) and Ettringite (Peg Gem) for her difficulties with relationships
- Lehua (Haii) for bringing self-esteem by increasing sensuality and joy in femininity
- Russian Kolokoltchik (Aus L) to help her conquer adverse conditions

Elizabeth recovered her strength and sense of being centred. She spent some time on her own and began to feel more positive about herself, realizing that she did not need the sort of destructive relationships in which she was always trying hard to please someone else, but never succeeding. Later she was drawn to a man who was gentle, kind yet strong in his own way, who treated her with the respect she desired and deserved. Her business and her new relationship continue to flourish.

SPIRITUAL HARMONY

Most people feel there must be more to us than merely mind and body. The dictionary defines spirit is the vital force, soul, the immortal part of us. It is not something that can be measured or analysed by science. None the less, this elusive part of us has a profound influence on our behaviour, beliefs and the kind of relationships we form. The spirit is the real person and is unique to each one of us, whereas the soul is viewed as that essential spark of creation that is part of the universal soul from which we all originate. This is what gives us being and existence, connects us to all living things.

Spiritual harmony is best described as an awareness of, a knowing of who you are, why you are here and what your particular purpose is in life. This brings a tremendous feeling of well-being, an abundance of vital energy and a real sense of security and belonging or being 'at home' in the world. Spiritual harmony manifests when your personality or ego is in touch with and works together with the deeper aspect of yourself, your soul.

At the same time you are still aware of a kind of spirituality that is indefinable. This is the highest form of existence which usually lies just on the edge of your consciousness. The spirit and soul seem to give us a great deal of freedom, but luckily if we stray too far from our true path, warning signals are sent out – which we ignore to our cost.

It is interesting that we begin life full of energy and sparkle. As children we often have a clear picture of what we wish to do with our lives, too. We may speculate that during those early years the ego/personality is more in touch with or in tune with the inner spirit/soul. As adults many of us end up in relationships, jobs or environments which leave us feeling empty, unfulfilled and craving something to make our lives more meaningful. From the spiritual point of view, we are lost.

Over 50 years ago Dr Edward Bach understood that physical disease is the direct outcome of emotional upset, which arises from a conflict between the soul/spirit and the mind/ego. He wrote:

Man has a soul which is his real self – it ever guides, protects and encourages us, leading us always for our utmost advantage. The soul knows what environment and what circumstances will best enable us to develop virtues which we lack and wipe out all that is wrong in us. So long as our souls and personalities are in harmony, all is joy and peace, happiness and health. When our personalities are led astray from the path laid down by the soul, either by our own worldly desires or by the persuasion of others, a conflict arises. This conflict brings disease...which will never be eradicated except by spiritual and mental effort.

So we might view disease, whether physical, mental, emotional or spiritual, as the way our soul tries to attract our attention and make us realize that we are straying too far from our path, giving us the opportunity to take steps to regain our sense of inner harmony.

In difficult times, most people find themselves wondering why life seems so hard and full of suffering. One explanation is that we are here to learn certain lessons and can only do so by experience. Certain religions hold that the soul may incarnate over and over again into a succession of physical bodies to master lessons that can only be learned from a material existence. These lessons include how to give love without expecting anything in return and how to be compassionate.

The concept of reincarnation holds that life throws in our path a series of challenges that have to be met. As each situation arises we have to decide how we are going to deal with it. The choices we make constantly shape the rest of our lives. We create our own destiny. No two souls have ever walked an identical path; each chooses his or her own.

The notion of karma is part and parcel of a belief in reincarnation. What it basically suggests is that 'you reap what you sow'. In other words, what you have done and thought in the past are affecting you now. Similarly what you are doing and thinking now affects your future. We are creating our own good or bad karma all the time.

If you are going through a time of pain and suffering, you may be paying off some past transgressions. If you are one of those lucky people who seems to be in the right place at the right time, you may be reaping the benefit of past good deeds. It's a sort of universal justice system.

If someone wrongs you it is best to forgive him or her, knowing that in due course justice will be done, if not in this lifetime then in the next. Any feelings of resentment, hatred, ill-will or contempt will tie you to the person for whom you feel such antipathy. Eventually you will have to undo those karmic ties.

Philosophers and sages contemplating the meaning of humanity throughout the ages have come to the conclusion that our reason for being is to achieve purity of spirit and matter. It was once said by Rama Teph, a 2nd-dynasty Nubian Pharoah, that man's special purpose is to have his head in heaven but his feet firmly planted in the earth. To be a complete human being we must be both spirit and matter, beautifully combined together, each of us blending these two aspects in a unique way.

Sometimes we try so hard to find spiritual harmony that we literally get in our own way. The same problem occurs if we take this quest too seriously, overcomplicating the whole process and missing the simplicity of it all. Life is best viewed as an adventure which enables the spirit to meet challenges, to rise above limitations, to grow in wisdom and vision. We don't need to take this spiritual quest too seriously – discovering our true nature can be fun. Life and this journey would be soulless without the essential element of humour. The art lies in taking life seriously in a non-serious way.

The beauty of succeeding is that it brings inner strength, a belief in your ability to achieve whatever you choose to do, a sense of purpose and a feeling of being in harmony with other people, with animals and the nature kingdom.

SIGNS OF DISHARMONY

- Feeling ill at ease with yourself and life
- Lack of fulfilment
- Feeling empty, insecure, alone
- Feeling that your life is not as you would like it to be
- Feeling out of control; needing to manipulate life and control others
- Lack of flexibility and adaptability with the environment
- No sense of direction or purpose
- Feeling spiritually impoverished
- Feeling disconnected from nature

CASE HISTORY: SHOCK

David was a wealthy businessman who suddenly lost all his money in a stock-market crash. He was shattered and traumatized. His life was falling apart, as money had given him his sense of security; he no longer saw any reason for living. His relationship with his wife began crumbling; he seemed paralysed, aimless, exhausted and at times suicidal. He turned to alcohol for comfort.

I PRESCRIBED

- Emergency Essence (Aus B) for shock
- Fringed Violet and Waratah (Aus B) for his black despair and suicidal feelings
- Okenite (Peg Gem) to help him cope with and integrate the changes in his life
- Gruss an Aachen (PVi) for intense challenge and fears associated with this evolutionary process, to calm, stabilize and offer him support to move forward
- Shooting Star (Ask) to understand his purpose in life
- Fuchsite (Peg Gem) to have a clearer image of himself and his role in the future

David stopped using alcohol as an emotional crutch. He became positive and dynamic, which made him feel empowered. He realized that money did not bring him happiness and that his purpose in life was to initiate more ethical projects linked to saving the environment via the world he knew best, that of business and high finance. He was then head-hunted for a highly paid position to establish such ventures, enabling him to use money in a way that helped others. By his example he has instigated a change in consciousness and a realization in those he now works with that business can be both ethical and commercially viable.

EIGHT

EXTRA ADVICE FOR PRACTITIONERS

*Practitioners of both complementary
and orthodox medicine will find flower essences invaluable tools for
helping others to help themselves. Like many natural remedies and therapies
they are excellent for easing the ill-effects of stress. Yet flower essences go
further, highlighting the underlying patterns leading to emotional distress
and its physical repercussions. They do so by cultivating self-awareness,
helping others to see and understand the reasons why they are
not feeling as well as they could be.*

From the patient's or client's point of view it can be extremely beneficial to have someone with greater experience to help them become aware of their negative behavioural patterns and emotional responses, then guide them towards the most appropriate remedies.

As Dr Edward Bach pointed out over half a century ago:

The physician of the future will have two great aims...firstly to assist the patient to a knowledge of himself and to point out to him the fundamental mistakes he may be making, the deficiencies of his character which he should remedy and the defects in his nature which must be eradicated and replaced by the corresponding virtues.

Secondly to administer remedies to help his physical body gain strength and to assist the mind to become calm, widen its outlook and strive towards perfection, thus bringing peace and harmony to the whole personality. Such remedies exist in nature...

These remedies are, of course, the flower essences for which he is famed.

Anyone prescribing these remedies needs to act as a finely tuned instrument, as a receptor, resonator and reflector for the patient. Clearly each practitioner will wish to evolve his or her own appropriate way of treating patients, and this will vary according to the actual needs of people coming for help. It is essential to be flexible, adaptable and creative in your approach to diagnosing and prescribing the flower essences. However, the following method can be used as a practical guide for those wishing to work with these remedies.

BUILDING UP A FLOWER ESSENCE REPERTOIRE

Ideally you should aim to have about one hundred remedies at your fingertips. In order to choose the most useful ones it is important to familiarize yourself with the major flower essence families listed in the Encyclopaedia section of this book. Slowly read through them all, placing a tick beside those that reflect the sort of problems you most frequently come across.

If you specialize in treating certain kinds of symptoms, such as women's problems, it will be useful to look at the Ailment Chart (Chapter 6); this will tell you at a glance which are the most appropriate remedies for each type of condition.

Even when you have composed your repertoire it is important to keep abreast of new additions to the flower essence families.

GIVING A DIAGNOSTIC SESSION

During the 10 years that I have been working with flower essences in a professional capacity, I have found that straight discussion with the patient combined with a good working knowledge of the remedies does not always provide a clear enough picture of the more deep-seated problems involved. I have found that using a pendulum as a diagnostic tool helps me to be accurate in the selection of essences. The pendulum prevents the practi-

tioner's opinions and ideas from impinging on the selection of essences, making the whole procedure far more objective.

Almost without exception everyone can become proficient at using a pendulum with a little practice.

Before you begin a diagnosis, arrange the Stock bottles of flower essence in neat, orderly rows before you so they are easily accessible. Then ask the patient to place one finger on each test bottle in turn. Gently lay one hand over the patient's to create a link with him or her. Holding the pendulum in the other hand, you will find that it begins to move one way or the other, giving a distinct 'yes' or 'no' the instant you make contact with the patient.

Pick out each of the chosen remedies from the batch of Stock bottles and put them to one side. These are the essences the patient has selected for him- or herself with assistance from you, acting as a mirror for or extension of the patient.

It is quite acceptable to have diagnosed up to 15 different essences. The real art then lies in making sense of what they can tell you about your patient.

I have found that each remedy is either for the patient's past, present or future condition.

- **The past – childhood and other early traumas.**
- **The present – immediate emerging emotions as well as the patient's psychological and physical state at the moment of treatment.**
- **The future – protection from and prevention of certain mental and emotional states which have their roots in the past and present, and which could easily manifest as major blockages later on.**

To find out which how many drops of each essence are needed, use the pendulum again. Count slowly from one to three; the pendulum will indicate a 'yes' when the correct number is reached. The number of drops required will also tell you to which life phase that particular essence applies:

- Essences for the past – 3 drops of each.
- Essences for the present – 2 drops of each.
- Essences for the future – 1 drop of each.

With experience you will begin to see that one remedy naturally follows on from and connects with the others. In this way you will begin to build up a picture of your patient, using the past as a starting point, progressing to current problems and ending with future issues. It is in relating and making the connection between each particular remedy that your insight and intuition will come into play.

Emily was suffering from recurrent migraines and nervous stomach upsets. At the time she was working as a computer analyst in London and felt highly stressed.

During a diagnostic session the following essences were chosen for her:
- **Past –**
  Star of Bethlehem (B) for long, slow shock. Emily suggested that this related to childhood. She was always trying very hard to prove herself in order to please her authoritarian father, but never felt up to the mark
  Vervain (B) for overriding the stress pattern set up in childhood. She had become forceful, highly strung and prone to exhausting herself through over-effort
- **Present –**
  Indian Pink (Fes) for stress from the environment
  Chamomile (Cal, Fes) for the effect of stress on the nervous system and stomach
  Amethyst (Gem) for stress resulting in migraine-type headaches
  Illawarra Flame Tree (Aus B) to cultivate self-approval, confidence and inner strength

Environmental Stress Remedy (Him A) to protect against radiation given out by her computer and contributing to her headaches
- **Future –**
  Chicory (B) for countering feelings of self-pity which could impair her improvement

Occasionally the pendulum will keep swinging, telling you that 4 drops of a particular essence are needed. This suggests stress stemming from a past life, a possible trauma that is spilling over into this lifetime and creating a blockage. This will need to be addressed before complete healing can take place.

Past-life traumas are often responsible for irrational fears that do not stem from childhood. A fear of water, for instance, could indicate that the person died by drowning in a previous existence.

The essence in the 4-drop position could also pertain to the birth experience. If it was traumatic there may be a reluctance to be here, which may manifest itself as daydreaming, escaping to a fantasy world. Someone who was born with the umbilical cord wrapped around his neck may have a problem swallowing, or may dislike having anything close-fitting around his neck (such as a tie or polo-neck shirt).

WHAT TO SAY AND WHAT NOT TO SAY

The whole reason for prescribing flower essences is to help patients become aware of their own stress patterns, enabling them to take back responsibility for their health and happiness. Handing back power to the individual is in fact the first stage of the self-healing process. It is therefore extremely important for you to inform and involve the patient throughout the entire procedure.

You will need to give a brief description of what the essence is for, such as shock in the past. If the patient is relaxed and feels able to trust you, he or she will hopefully fill in the missing information by telling you the nature of the past trauma.

The Encyclopaedia or Ailment Chart in this book can be used to discuss the descriptions of each essence with patients.

It is not a good idea to discuss issues such as reincarnation and past lives with patients during an initial consultation. If they already hold other beliefs they may feel uncomfortable with such concepts or react against them. Respect their views and you may find, in time, that they become more open-minded to these possibilities.

It is essential, however, that you give patients a brief description of the body's energy systems – the aura, chakras and subtle bodies, so they are able to understand how shock and stress affect the system (see Chapter 2).

❈ COMBINING FLOWER ESSENCES ❈ WITH OTHER THERAPIES

Flower essences can be used in conjunction with both complementary and orthodox medicines because they are totally safe and free from any side-effects. They are a perfect complement to all kinds of natural healing therapies, particularly aromatherapy and acupressure, enhancing their effectiveness in relieving symptoms and speeding the rate of recovery.

FLOWER ESSENCES AND AROMATHERAPY

Flower essences and essential oils work particularly well together. As both belong to the plant world, they have a special affinity for one another. While essential oils are only extracted from aromatic plants, flower essences can be made from those with little or no perfume, which greatly enhances the range of flora you can work with.

Even when essential oils and flower essences do come from the same plant you will notice that their properties may be different – although there may be overlaps. This is because their vibrational qualities are not identical. Generally speaking, the vibration of flower essences is higher and more ethereal than that of essential oils. While essential oils tend to work primarily at a physical level, they can also have some psychological benefits. Flower essences, in contrast, concentrate their influence mainly on our thoughts and emotions, benefits which filter into the physical body. This means that a practitioner using essential oils can draw on a flower essence to provide a particular vibration that cannot be found in any of the essential oils. The converse is just as true. Used in combination the benefits of each become more profound and far-reaching.

When selecting flower essences to complement essential oils, always opt for those whose qualities are most relevant for that particular person. Whether they come from the same or completely different flowers or plants is irrelevant. Add a drop or two of the chosen flower essence to a massage oil. This will bring to the blend a vibrational quality that complements that of the essential oil, making the treatment more complete.

FLORAL ACUPRESSURE

This is a budding form of therapy which is proving to be highly beneficial. Many find that improvements for all kinds of conditions occur faster and are more dramatic when appropriate flower essences are applied to certain acupuncture points on the skin.

Drs Vasudeva and Kadambii Barnao (Australian Living Flower Essences) and Drs Atul and Pupa Shah (Himalayan Aditi Flower Essences) have done pioneering work in this field. Their research is geared towards discovering which particular essences work best on key acupressure points. From their findings Drs Vasudeva and Kadambii Barnao have drawn up 'Floral Acu-maps' which can be obtained directly from the suppliers (see Useful Addresses).

I find that flower essences are particularly effective when used in combination with Shen Tao, thought by some to be the Mother of Acupuncture. This is a special kind of acupressure which differs from the traditional approach in that it accesses the extraordinary as well as the main meridians. The extraordinary meridians are seen as the reservoir, whereas the main meridians are seen as the rivers. They have a powerful influence on the whole subtle anatomy so the benefits they bring are emotional, mental and spiritual as well as physical. However, Shen Tao shares many key points with ordinary acupressure.

Useful Acupressure Points

The 'Hegu' or 'Hoku' acupoint is arguably the best pain-relieving point on the body. It is found on the back of the hand in the web between thumb and forefinger.

Good essences to use here are those that are also have pain-relieving or relaxing qualities (see Ailment Chart, Chapter 5).

For headaches and other pains, Living Essences of Australia recommends either Dampiera (a mental and muscle relaxant) for dissolving rigidity in mind and body, or Menzies Banksia to help you to go with the pain rather than resist and so intensify it.

In Shen Tao acupressure this point, known as 'Joining Valley', is also used for treating colds, constipation, laryngitis (sore throats) migraines and arthritis.

The 'Shenmen' acupoint on the ear is excellent for relieving stress and promoting relaxation. It can be found just inside the rim at the tip of the ear.

Four Living Essences of Australia essences you can use here are:

- **Pink Fairy Orchid** – good for stress from environmental factors such as noise.
- **Hybrid Pink Fairy (Cowslip) Orchid** – helps ease stress caused by over-sensitivity to other people. Especially useful for easing pre-menstrual emotional and mental tension.
- **Yellow Flag Flower** – for when stress has taken all the sparkle out of life, making people dull and grim.
- **Purple Flag Flower (Bush Iris)** – releases stress which has been building up in the body. Acts as a valve for dispelling pressure.

In Shen Tao the 'Daling' point works wonders for calming the emotions. It can be found on the underside of your wrist, lying in the centre of the wrist crease. Use essences here that are appropriate for your particular emotional disturbance (see Ailment Chart).

For clearing the mind and lifting the spirit, one of the best points to work on is the 'Baihui' acupoint. Take a line from the top of each ear lobe and continue to the crown of the head. The Baihui point lies where these two lines meet.

Excellent essences to use here are Lotus (Him A) or Leafless Orchid (Aus L) to re-balance energy after excessive emotional or physical drain. Place a drop of either essence here every 15 minutes for an hour or so and you will find yourself revitalized.

In Shen Tao, working with the 'Shining Sea' point not only clears the mind but also helps to treat fluid retention, irregular periods and joint problems. It is found on the inner ankle directly behind the ankle bone.

FLOWER ESSENCES AND ORTHODOX MEDICINE

Many general practitioners realize that stress may be responsible for their patients' health problems, but feel powerless to help. While tranquillizers and other such drugs may help someone over a particularly bad patch, they do not provide the tools needed for dealing with stress. They tend to dull perception and subdue the stress response.

Tranquillizers also have less desirable side-effects and tend to be addictive; coming off them suddenly can give rise to frightening withdrawal symptoms. Flower essences can safely be given to patients to help them cope with their particular source of stress. Many open-minded general practitioners are now adding flower essences such as Star of Bethlehem (B) for general shock to their prescription list.

As a flower essence practitioner you may frequently see patients who want to wean themselves off tranquillizers, anti-depressants and any other mood-altering drugs but are worried about withdrawal symptoms. Flower essences can help to free them from their dependency, ease any side-effects and clear the system of any imbalance that has been caused by long-term use of medicinal drugs.

❋ HELPING YOURSELF ❋

As a practitioner it is easy to be affected by the problems of others. If steps are not taken to protect your own emotional well-being, you could start to feel energetically drained. With this in mind I have composed a special 'practitioner mix' for boosting energy levels and safeguarding against exhaustion.

- Delph (AK)
- Fringed Violet (Aus B)
- Leafless Orchid (Aus L)
- Lotus (Haii)
- Rose Gallica Officialis (Peg – not listed in the Encyclopaedia but available from Pegasus Products)

Use 2 drops of each essence.

❋ PROVING THE ESSENCES WORK ❋

Some people argue that flower essences act as placebos, in other words that they make us feel better simply because we believe they are doing us good.

This does not explain, however, the numerous incidences in which flower essences have brought benefits to animals, babies and young children, who obviously do not know that what they are being given is 'supposed to' bring relief.

To test the placebo argument scientifically, Michael Weisglas PhD conducted a double-blind test on the Bach Flower Remedies in 1979. Neither he nor his subjects (who were suffering from depression) knew beforehand who had received and taken the remedies and who took the placebos. Results showed that those who were given the remedy mix reported experiencing a feeling of well-being, growth and self-understanding and acceptance, a better sense of humour and increased creativity, while those who took the placebo reported no significant change.

Dr Weisglas concluded that the effect of the remedies does not depend on the belief or faith of the user.

For at least five years I have conducted my own investigations into many flower essences. I have recently tested all the Bach remedies, the Orchids of the Amazon and most of the Californian remedies, as well as many others. During my teaching courses I typically give one particular anonymous remedy to 10 people and ask each one to describe its properties. Without fail their descriptions of the essence, its qualities and place of action are accurate.

At their clinic in Delhi, Drs Atul and Pupa Shah (Aditi Himalayan essences) combine flower essences with other natural therapies such as homoeopathy, acupuncture, aromatherapy and crystal therapy. They claim great success in treating all kinds of problems including mental retardation, the problems of childhood, tumours, infertility and pregnancy problems, arthritis and any condition related to stress and tension such as irritable bowel syndrome, insomnia and hypertension. They have also found that flower essences work extremely well in conquering addictions. To prevent their own expectations from getting in the way of their assessments, the Shahs often ask other doctors to assess the improvements in their patients' conditions.

A new area of research involves observing the changes in the body's energy field after a patient has taken different essences. I asked Harry Oldfield to use his electro-scanning machine (which in effect photographs the aura) in an attempt to see what happened when certain flowers and their essences were introduced into my energy field. Looking at Figures 1 and 2 (*see plate section*) it seems clear that flower essences indeed have a measurable effect. This surely paves the way for further research into this field of investigation.

NINE

CONCLUSION

Medicine of the future

It is time to realize that we must take responsibility for our own well-being. This is perhaps the hardest lesson to learn. How much easier it is to place the blame for our unhappiness and failing health onto something extraneous to ourselves.

In reality, how we feel is a reflection of the way we live our lives, how we think and act, and how we respond to other people and events.

Anyone who is constantly anxious, irritable, frustrated or depressed should heed these signs and look inwards to discover the real source of his or her discomfort.

Flower essences enhance self-knowledge and understanding, helping us to take back responsibility for our own health, happiness and fulfilment. This is tremendously empowering. Knowing you are able to take care of yourself brings great rewards. As your confidence and inner strength flourish you will feel more in control of life and of your own destiny. Deep down you will experience a sense of safety and security that does not hinge upon anyone or anything else.

In the search for inner harmony we become aware that our own welfare is inextricably linked and interconnected to the well-being of everything else that exists in nature. Essentially what this means is that if we fail to respect and care for our home, the planet, and all living creatures, we in turn will suffer the consequences. We clearly can no longer afford to see ourselves as separate from everything around us.

As a race we seem to have forgotten this sense of duty and are threatening the very existence of life on earth. The World Conservation Centre in Cambridge, England, tells us that of the 270,000 species of flora inhabiting the earth, 41,000 are under threat. In Britain alone 27,000 flowering plants are struggling for survival, accounting for a staggering 10 per cent of the entire global population.

Survivors of certain indigenous peoples like the Native Americans and Australian

Aborigines, who have a long tradition of living in harmony with the natural environment, regard the earth as a gift from the creator to be tended, nurtured and protected for future generations. Indeed, Native American peoples always think ahead for 'seven generations' to come before taking any action that may affect the course of nature. The wise men or spiritual leaders of such peoples are so alarmed at the way we are treating our home that they are finally breaking their silence and are now prepared to share their wisdom and knowledge with us.

The most dramatic instance of this occurred back in 1988, when Alan Ereira was in Colombia researching a documentary and chanced upon the Lost City of Taironas, as well as the descendants of those who had once inhabited this remarkable place – the Kogi. Breaking their 400 years of self-imposed isolation, the Kogi priests or Mamas asked him to film a message to give to the world, an urgent warning about the destruction of the planet: *'You are killing the earth and we must teach you how to stop.'*

The Kogi live in the Sierra Nevada de Santa Marta, hidden away at the remote northern tip of Colombia. They call their home 'the heart of the world'. The Sierra could easily be described as a Garden of Eden. It is like the planet in miniature, boasting the whole spectrum of landscapes and climates. Its lush Caribbean coastline gives way to tropical rainforests, mountainous peaks and even desert in some areas. Every animal and every plant has its ecological niche in this equatorial zone.

Long ago the Sierra was inhabited by the Taironas – Indians who dressed in gold and lived in magnificent cities amid fields and orchards. They were all but annihilated by the Spanish conquistadors in the sixteenth century. Some survivors managed to flee up into the mountains where they settled and remained hidden from the world. The Kogi are directly descended from these people and are living proof that a harmonious existence with nature is neither fanciful, unrealistic or something that belongs to a bygone age. They are intelligent, sensitive people who dress in white; they walk barefoot to keep in touch with the earth. They see those of us in Western society as primitive and uncouth, calling us the ignorant 'Younger Brother'.

According to the Kogi story of creation, in the beginning was the mother. She is spirit, she is water, the life-force that makes things alive – she is Aluna. The mother conceives all possibilities, everything that can be.

Aluna gave birth to nine daughters or worlds, of which only one was capable of fertile growth, the earth. She then created humans to look after this world. But then 'Younger Brother' was created in the heart of the world. He was too dangerous to live among the Kogi, so he was given knowledge of machinery and sent far away across the sea.

The Kogi believe that if Younger Brother returns to the heart of the world, then the whole world will die.

During the last 20 years the Kogi have witnessed what they regard as the return of Younger Brother. They have watched settlers move into the Sierra, forcing them to move higher and higher up into the mountains. They see the havoc these intruders are wreaking on the land by ripping down trees and digging up the earth, and this simply reconfirms their own beliefs.

As the elder brothers they see themselves as the caretakers or gardeners of the earth who are responsible for looking after nature. The philosophy of harmony underpins everything that they do. The Kogi Mamas, the priests, the enlightened ones, mentally work with Aluna to keep everything in balance, viewing themselves as guardians of the planet with a duty to keep humanity's spirituality alive. They believe that if we fail to be in harmony with ourselves we jeopardize not only our own health but also the harmony of the world. When this happens the life energy will become dangerous and uncontrolled. 'You will see new diseases appearing for which you have no medicine,' the Kogi tell us. They do not know about AIDS or BSE or the other diseases affecting people, animals and plants, but they know that new diseases have arisen because they are in touch with the deeper instincts of the world.

We do not have to have to look far afield to realize the truth in what the Kogi are saying. Throughout the world the indigenous countryside is slowly and insidiously changing. Fields and hedgerows, woodlands and forests are constantly being demolished to make way for new houses, roads and other 'developments'. We have allowed such changes to take place because of our desire for an increasingly materialistic society. We are now paying the price for our greed, as stress and pollution take their toll on our health.

We may feel that we are powerless to avert such global tragedy. However, just as we are capable of taking charge of our own well-being, so too can we take back responsibility for looking after the planet. Time and again it has been shown that when one person changes his or her perceptions and starts to see new solutions to personal and world problems, there is a knock-on effect, instigating a shift in the collective consciousness of the rest of humanity.

The Kogi do not see the death of the planet as an inevitability. They believe there are other options open to us.

The rediscovery of flower remedies has come at a time when it is most needed, as the future of the planet hangs precariously in the balance. Only by experiencing how they can help us to alter our perceptions and take back our own power will we really appreciate the value and importance of the world around us.

At the same time, flower essences appear to be offering us a way of finding inner balance by enhancing our well-being at a time when many other systems are failing us. In this respect they may truly be the medicine of the future.

USEFUL ADDRESSES

Clare G. Harvey
Middle Piccadilly Natural
Healing Centre
Holwell
Nr Sherborne
Dorset
DT9 5LW
Tel: (01963) 23468/23774
or
The Hale Clinic
7 Park Crescent
London W1N 3HE
Tel: (0171) 637–3377
*Clare can supply flower remedies
and is available for consultation.
Teaches two-year professional
course*

SUPPLIERS OF FLOWER ESSENCES

Australia/New Zealand
Bush Flower Essences
8a Oaks Avenue
Dee Why
NSW 2099
Australia
Tel: (02) 972 1033

Living Essences of Australia
Box 355
Scarborough
Perth
W. Australia 6019
Tel: (09) 244 2073

**New Perception Flower
Essences**
PO Box 160–127
Titirangi
Auckland 7
NZ
Tel: (09) 817 7775

Europe
Bach Flower Remedies
The Hale Clinic
7 Park Crescent
London W1N 3HE
Tel: (0171) 637–3377
*Bach Flower Remedies are also
available from Boots the Chemists
and most healthfood stores and
chemists in the UK*

Bailey Essences
7/8 Nelson Road
Ilkley
West Yorks
LS29 8HH
England
Tel: (01943) 602177

Findhorn Flower Essences
'Mercury'
Findhorn Bay
Findhorn, Forres
Morayshire
IV36 0TY
Scotland
Tel: (01309) 690129

**Flower and Gem Remedy
Association**
Suite 1
Castle Farm
Clifton Road
Deddington
Oxon, OX15 0TP
England
Tel: (01869) 337349
Major UK supplier

Green Man Tree Essences
2 Kerswell Cottages
Exminster
Exeter
Devon
EX6 8AY
England
Tel: (01392) 832005

Harebell Remedies
Monybluie
Corsock
Castle Douglas
Kirkcudbrightshire
DG7 3DY
Scotland

Healing Herbs – The Flower Remedy Programme
PO Box 65
Hereford
HR2 0UW
England
Tel: (01873) 890218
Healing Herbs remedies are also available from The Hale Centre and most healthfood stores and chemists in the UK

IUG (Ivan U. Ghyssaert) Kenya
Gem Realisations SA
Mont-de-Plain
C. P. 67
CH–1605 Chexbres
Switzerland
Tel: (02) 19 46 23 90

Korte Phi Essenzen Orkid
Alpenstrasse 25
D–78262 Gailingen
Germany
Tel: (49) 77 74 7004

Laboratoire Deva Elixirs Floreaux
BP 3-38880 Autrans
France
Tel: (33) 76 95 3587

India
Himalayan Aditi Flower Essences
Complementary Medicine
Research Centre
15 (E)
Jaybahrat Society
3rd Road
Khar (W)
Bombay 400 052
Tel: (91 22) 648 6819

Himalayan Flower Enhancers
Bundaleer
Lot 100 Dromedary Trail
Tilba Tilba
NSW 2546
Australia

Himalayan Tree Essences
Available from the Flower and Gem Remedy Association (*see above*)

USA/Canada
Alaskan Flower Essence Project
PO Box 1329
Homer, AL 99603
USA
Tel: (907) 235–2188

Aloha Flower Essences
PO Box 2319
Kealakekua, HI 96750
USA
Tel: (808) 328–2529

FES and California Research Essences
Available from the Flower and Gem Remedy Association (*see above*)

Desert Alchemy
PO Box 44189
Tucson, AZ 85733
USA
Tel: (602) 325–1545

Flower Essence Services
PO Box 1769
Nevada City, CA 95959
Tel: (916) 265–9163
Producers and distributor of FES Quintessentials line of North American flower essences. North American distributor for Healing Herbs English Flower Essences

Master's Flower Essences/Yoga Flower Remedies
14618 Tyler Foote Road
Nevada City, CA 95959
USA
Tel: (916) 292–3345
Please send $3 for catalogue and ordering

Pacific Essences
PO Box 8317
Victoria, BC V8W 3R9
CANADA
Tel: (604) 384–5560

Pegasus Products
PO Box 228
Boulder, CO 80306
USA
Tel: (303) 667–3019/
1 (800) 527 6104
Pegasus Gem Remedies mentioned in this book are also available from this address

Perelandra Inc.
Box 3603
Warrenton, VA 22186
USA
Tel: (703) 937–2153

Petite Fleur Essences Inc.
8524 Whispering Creek Trail
Fort Worth, TX 76134
USA
Tel: (817) 293–5410

PROFESSIONAL COURSES IN FLOWER AND GEM REMEDIES

Australia/New Zealand
Bush Flower Essences
8a Oaks Avenue
Dee Why
NSW 2099
Australia
Tel: (02) 972 1033

Living Essences of Australia
Box 355
Scarborough
Perth
W. Australia 6019
Tel: (09) 244 2073

Europe
Healing Herbs – The Flower Remedy Programme
PO Box 65
Hereford
HR2 0UW
England
Tel: (01873) 890218

The International Federation for Vibrational Medicine
Suite 1
Castle Farm
Clifton Road
Deddington
Oxon

OX15 0TP
England
Tel: (01869) 337349
Can also supply details of qualified IFVM Practitioners in Flowers and Gems
Courses are held at:
Middle Piccadilly Natural
Healing Centre
Holwell
Nr Sherborne
Dorset
DT9 5LW
Tel: (01963) 23468/23774

USA/Canada
Alaskan Flower Essence Project
PO Box 1329
Homer, AL 99603
USA
Tel: (907) 235–2188

Flower Essence Society
PO Box 459
Nevada City, CA 95959
Tel: (916) 265–9163
Educational and research organization

Master's Flower Essences/Yoga Flower Remedies
14618 Tyler Foote Road
Nevada City, CA 95959
USA
Tel: (916) 292–3345
Correspondence postal course

Perelandra Inc.
Box 3603
Warrenton, VA 22186
USA
Tel: (703) 937–2153
For two-year professional course in flowers and gem remedies

INTRODUCTORY COURSES

UK
Marion Bielby
17 Bristol Road
Auguston
Ilkeston
Derbyshire
DE7 5HZ
Tel: (01159) 323373

Anne Mari Clarke
61 Granville Road
Limpsfield
Oxted
Surrey
RH8 0BY
Tel: (01883) 715977

Margaret Gallier
19 Maxwell Drive
Hazelmere
Bucks
HP15 7BX
Tel: (01494) 715745

Christine Parr
30 Glencoe Road
Bushey
Herts
WD2 3DS
Tel: (0181) 930–5851

Sue Sem
31 Burr Close
London E1
Tel: (0171) 481–4393

Gail Shaw
93 Station Road
Hayling Island
Hants
PO11 QEE
Tel: (01705) 462250

QI GONG SCHOOL OF CHINESE HERITAGE

Flat 3
15 Dawson Place
London W2 4TM
England
Tel: (0171) 229–7187

KIRLIAN AND AURA PHOTOGRAPHY

IFVM
Harry Oldfield
The School of Electro-Crystal
Therapy
17 Long Drive
South Ruislip
Middlesex
HA4 0HL
England
Tel: (0181) 841–1716

Erik Pelham
Kirlian photographer and
Devic analyst
Cooks Farm
Tothill
Alford
Lincs
LN13 0NJ
Tel: (01507) 450382

PHOTOGRAPHY

The authors would like to
thank the following for their
wonderful photographs:

'Helmut Maier'
Archives of Flower Slides
Kornbergst 7
D–73092 Heiningen
Germany
*For photographs of the Edward
Bach Flowers and others*

Regina Hornberger
Im Rotbad 8
D–72076 Tübingen
Germany
Tel: (0049) 7071 62619

Carol Bruce
Mill End Cottage
211 Slade Road
Stroud
Gloucs
GL5 1RT
England
Tel: (01453) 758046

PROFESSIONAL ORGANIZATIONS

**The British Complementary
Medicine Association (BCMA)**
The Administrator
St Charles Hospital
Exmoor St
London W10 6DZ
England
Tel: (0181) 964 1206
*The organization for complemen-
tary medicine in the UK*

**The International Federation
for Vibrational Medicine
(IFVM)**
Suite 1
Castle Farm
Clifton Rd
Deddington
Oxon
OX15 0TP
England
Tel: (01869) 337349
*Membership insurance allows
practitioners to practise flower
and gem essence therapy within
the constitution of the IFVM.
Affiliated membership insurance
allows practice and healing to
the BCMA (see above) code of
conduct. THe IFVM is a member
of the BCMA*

FURTHER READING

Edward Bach, *Heal Thyself* (C. W. Daniel Co. Ltd, 1931; reprint 1990)

Julian Barnard, *A Guide to the Bach Flower Remedies* (C. W. Daniel Co. Ltd, 1979; 1994)

Julian and Martine Barnard, *The Healing Herbs of Edward Bach* (Ashgrove Press, 1988)

David Bohm, *Wholeness and Implicate Order* (Routledge and Kegan Paul, 1980)

Barbara Ann Brennan, *Hands of Light* (Bantam New Age Books, 1988)

Jillie Collings, *The Ordinary Person's Guide to Extraordinary Health* (Aurum Press, 1993)

John and Farida Davidson, *Harmony of Science and Nature* (Wholistic Research Company, 1986–8)

Patricia Davis, *Subtle Aromatherapy* (C. W. Daniel Co. Ltd, 1991)

Richard Gerber, M. D., *Vibrational Medicine* (Bear and Co, 1988)

Kate Greenaway, *Language of Flowers* (F. Warne, 1977)

Eliana Harvey and Mary Jane Oatley, *Acupressure – Shen Tao* (Hodder and Stoughton, 1994)

Stephen W. Hawkings, *A Brief History of Time* (Paul Banton Press, 1988; 1993)

Liz Hodgkinson, *Reincarnation – The Evidence* (Piatkus, 1989)

Steve Johnson, *Flower Essences of Alaska* (Alaskan Flower Essence Project, 1992)

Anodea Judith, *Wheels of Light* (Llewellyn, 1987)

Patricia Kaminski and Richard Katz, *Flower Essence Repertory* (The Flower Essence Society, 1994)

Cynthia Athina Kemp, *Cactus and Company – Patterns and Qualities of Desert Alchemy Flower Essences* (Desert Alchemy, 1993)

Andreas Korte, *Orchids, Gemstones and Their Healing Energies* (Bauer Berlag, 1993)

Jacob Liberman, *Light Medicine of the Flower* (Bear & Co, 1991)

Sue Minter, *The Healing Garden* (Headline, 1993)

Dr Hiroshi Motoyama, *Theories of the Chakras' Bridge to Higher Consciousness* (The Theosophical Publishing House, 1981)

Harry Oldfield and Roger Coghill, *The Dark Side of the Brain* (Element Books, 1988)

Sabina Pettitt, *Energy Medicine – Pacific Flower and Sea Essences* (Pacific Essences, 1993)

A Practitioner's Research Guide to Hawaiian Tropical Flower Essences (Aloha Essences, 1993)

Daniele Ryman, *The Aromatherapy Handbook* (Century, 1984)

Drs Rupa and Atul Shar, *Aditi Himalaya Essences* (Aditi, 1993)

Rudolf Steiner, *Cosmic Memory: Atlantis and Lemuria* (Harper & Row, 1981)

Gregory Vlamis, *Flowers to the Rescue* (Thorsons, 1986; 1994)

Nora Weeks, *The Medical Discoveries of Edward Bach Physician* (C. W. Daniel Co. Ltd, 1940; 1983)

Ian White, *Bush Flower Essences* (Bantam Books, 19xx)

Ruth White, *Working with your Chakras* (Piatkus, 1993)

Christine Wildwood, *Flower Remedies for Women* (Thorsons, 1994)

Machelle Small Wright, *Flower Essences* (Perelandra, 1988)

Nature vol. 333, no 30 (June, 1988)

Nature vol. 334, no 28 (July, 1988)

Newsweek March 28, 1994

INDEX